THE AMERICAN PSYCHIATRIC ASSOCIATION PRACTICE GUIDELINE FOR THE Pharmacological Treatment of Patients With Alcohol Use Disorder

Guideline Writing Group

Victor I. Reus, M.D., *Chair*
Laura J. Fochtmann, M.D., M.B.I., *Vice-Chair, Methodologist*
Oscar Bukstein, M.D., M.P.H.
A. Evan Eyler, M.D., M.P.H.
Donald M. Hilty, M.D.
Marcela Horvitz-Lennon, M.D., M.P.H.
Jane Mahoney, Ph.D., R.N., PMHCNS-BC
Jagoda Pasic, M.D., Ph.D.
Michael Weaver, M.D.
Cheryl D. Wills, M.D.
Jack McIntyre, M.D., *Consultant*

Systematic Review Group

Laura J. Fochtmann, M.D., M.B.I., *Methodologist*
Joel Yager, M.D.
Seung-Hee Hong

Steering Committee on Practice Guidelines

Michael J. Vergare, M.D., *Chair*
Daniel J. Anzia, M.D., *Vice-Chair*
Thomas J. Craig, M.D.
Deborah Cowley, M.D.
Laura J. Fochtmann, M.D., M.B.I., *Consultant, Methodologist*
David A. Kahn, M.D.
John M. Oldham, M.D.
Carlos N. Pato, M.D., Ph.D.
Joel Yager, M.D., *Consultant*

APA Assembly Liaisons

John P. D. Shemo, M.D., *Chair of Area Liaisons*
John M. de Figueiredo, M.D.
Marvin Koss, M.D.
Annette L. Hanson, M.D.
Bhasker Dave, M.D.
Robert M. McCarron, D.O.
Jason W. Hunziker, M.D.

APA wishes to acknowledge the contributions of APA staff (Jennifer Medicus, Seung-Hee Hong, Samantha Shugarman, Michelle Dirst, Kristin Kroeger Ptakowski). APA and the Guideline Writing Group especially thank Laura J. Fochtmann, M.D., M.B.I.; Jeremy Kidd, M.D.; Seung-Hee Hong; and Jennifer Medicus for their outstanding work and effort in developing this guideline. APA also thanks the APA Steering Committee on Practice Guidelines (Michael Vergare, M.D., Chair), liaisons from the APA Assembly for their input and assistance, and APA Councils and others for providing feedback during the comment period.

Contents

Acronyms/Abbreviations

AA Alcoholics Anonymous

ACCME Accreditation Council for Continuing Medical Education

AHRQ Agency for Healthcare Research and Quality

ALT Alanine aminotransferase

APA American Psychiatric Association

ASAM American Society of Addiction Medicine

AST Aspartate aminotransferase

AUD Alcohol use disorder

AUDIT Alcohol Use Disorders Identification Test

AUDIT-C Alcohol Use Disorders Identification Test–Concise

CAGE Cut down, Annoyed, Guilty, Eye-opener

CBI Combined behavioral intervention

CBT Cognitive-behavioral therapy

CDT Carbohydrate-deficient transferrin

CI Confidence interval

COMBINE Combined Pharmacotherapies and Behavioral Interventions for Alcohol Dependence

CRAFFT Car, Relax, Alone, Forget, Friends, Trouble

CrCl Creatinine clearance

DSM-III-R *Diagnostic and Statistical Manual of Mental Disorders*, 3rd Edition, Revised

DSM-IV *Diagnostic and Statistical Manual of Mental Disorders*, 4th Edition

DSM-IV-TR *Diagnostic and Statistical Manual of Mental Disorders*, 4th Edition, Text Revision

DSM-5 *Diagnostic and Statistical Manual of Mental Disorders*, 5th Edition

eGF Estimated glomerular filtration rate

FDA U.S. Food and Drug Administration

GGT Gamma-glutamyl transferase

GRADE Grading of Recommendations Assessment, Development and Evaluation

GWG Guideline Writing Group

HIV Human immunodeficiency virus

ICD-10 *International Classification of Diseases*, 10th Revision

IM Intramuscular

IRR Incidence rate ratio

MBSCT Modified behavioral self-control therapy

MCV Mean corpuscular volume

MDD Major depressive disorder

MET Motivational enhancement therapy

MI Motivational interviewing

MM Medical management

NIAAA National Institute on Alcohol Abuse and Alcoholism

NIMH National Institute of Mental Health

NNT Number needed to treat

NQF National Quality Forum

OPRM1 Genotype Opioid receptor μ 1 genotype

OR Odds ratio

OTC Over-The-Counter

PCM Primary Care Management

PEth Phosphatidylethanol

Project MATCH Matching Alcoholism Treatments to Client Heterogeneity

PTSD Posttraumatic stress disorder

QTc Corrected QT interval

RCT Randomized controlled trial

RD Risk difference

SNP Single nucleotide polymorphism

SRG Systematic Review Group

TSF Twelve-step facilitation

USPSTF U.S. Preventive Services Task Force

WMD Weighted mean difference

Introduction

Overview of the Development Process

Since the publication of the Institute of Medicine (now known as National Academy of Medicine) report, *Clinical Practice Guidelines We Can Trust* (Institute of Medicine, Committee on Quality of Health Care in America 2001), there has been an increasing focus on using clearly defined, transparent processes for rating the quality of evidence and the strength of the overall body of evidence in systematic reviews of the scientific literature. This guideline was developed using a process intended to be consistent with the recommendations of the Institute of Medicine (Institute of Medicine, Committee on Quality of Health Care in America 2001), the *Principles for the Development of Specialty Society Clinical Guidelines* of the Council of Medical Specialty Societies (2012), and the requirements of the Agency for Healthcare Research and Quality (AHRQ) for inclusion of a guideline in the National Guidelines Clearinghouse. Parameters used for the guideline's systematic review are included with the full text of the guideline; the development process is fully described in the following document available at the American Psychiatric Association (APA) Web site: http://www.psychiatry.org/File%20Library/Psychiatrists/Practice/Clinical%20Practice%20Guidelines/Guideline-Development-Process.pdf.

Rating the Strength of Research Evidence and Recommendations

Development of guideline statements entails weighing the potential benefits and harms of the statement and then identifying the level of confidence in that determination. This concept of balancing benefits and harms to determine guideline recommendations and strength of recommendations is a hallmark of GRADE (Grading of Recommendations Assessment, Development and Evaluation), which is used by multiple professional organizations around the world to develop practice guideline recommendations (Guyatt et al. 2013). With the GRADE approach, recommendations are rated by assessing the confidence that the benefits of the statement outweigh the harms and burdens of the statement, determining the confidence in estimates of effect as reflected by the quality of evidence, estimating patient values and preferences (including whether they are similar across the patient population), and identifying whether resource expenditures are worth the expected net benefit of following the recommendation (Andrews et al. 2013).

In weighing the balance of benefits and harms for each statement in this guideline, our level of confidence is informed by available evidence, which includes evidence from clinical trials as well as expert opinion and patient values and preferences. Evidence for the benefit of a particular intervention within a specific clinical context is identified through systematic review and is then balanced against the evidence for harms. In this regard, harms are broadly defined and may include serious adverse events, less serious adverse events that affect tolerability, minor adverse events, negative effects of the intervention on quality of life, barriers and inconveniences associated with treatment, direct and indirect costs of the intervention (including opportunity costs), and other negative aspects of the treatment that may influence decision making by the patient, the clinician, or both.

Many topics covered in this guideline have relied on forms of evidence such as consensus opinions of experienced clinicians or indirect findings from observational studies rather than research from randomized trials. It is well recognized that there are guideline topics and clinical circumstances for which high-quality evidence from clinical trials is not possible or is unethical to obtain (Council of Medical Specialty Societies 2012). For example, many questions need to be asked as part of an assessment, and inquiring about a particular symptom or element of the history cannot be separated out for study as a discrete intervention. It would also be impossible to separate changes in outcomes due to assessment from changes in outcomes due to ensuing treatment. Research on psychiatric assessments and some psychiatric interventions can also be complicated by multiple confounding factors such as the interaction between the clinician and the patient or the patient's unique circumstances and experiences. The GRADE working group and guidelines developed by other professional organizations have noted that a strong recommendation or "good practice statement" may be appropriate even in the absence of research evidence when sensible alternatives do not exist (Andrews et al. 2013; Brito et al. 2013; Djulbegovic et al. 2009; Hazlehurst et al. 2013). For each guideline statement, we have described the type and strength of the available evidence as well as the factors, including patient preferences, that were used in determining the balance of benefits and harms.

The authors of the guideline determined each final rating, as described in the section "Guideline Development Process," and is endorsed by the APA Board of Trustees. A *recommendation* (denoted by the numeral 1 after the guideline statement) indicates confidence that the benefits of the intervention clearly outweigh harms. A *suggestion* (denoted by the numeral 2 after the guideline statement) indicates greater uncertainty. Although the benefits of the statement are still viewed as outweighing the harms, the balance of benefits and harms is more difficult to judge, or either the benefits or the harms may be less clear. With a suggestion, patient values and preferences may be more variable, and this can influence the clinical decision that is ultimately made. Each guideline statement also has an associated rating for the *strength of supporting research evidence*. Three ratings are used: *high*, *moderate*, and *low* (denoted by the letters A, B, and C, respectively) and reflect the level of confidence that the evidence for a guideline statement reflects a true effect based on consistency of findings across studies, directness of the effect on a specific health outcome, precision of the estimate of effect, and risk of bias in available studies (Agency for Healthcare Research and Quality 2014; Balshem et al. 2011; Guyatt et al. 2006).

Proper Use of Guidelines

The APA Practice Guidelines are assessments of current scientific and clinical information provided as an educational service. The guidelines 1) should not be considered as a statement of the standard of care or inclusive of all proper treatments or methods of care; 2) are not continually updated and may not reflect the most recent evidence, as new evidence may emerge between the time information is developed and when the guidelines are published or read; 3) address only the question(s) or issue(s) specifically identified; 4) do not mandate any particular course of medical care; 5) are not intended to substitute for the independent professional judgment of the treating provider; and 6) do not account for individual variation among patients. As such, it is not possible to draw conclusions about the effects of omitting a particular recommendation, either in general or for a specific patient. Furthermore, adherence to these guidelines will not ensure a successful outcome for every individual, nor should these guidelines be interpreted as including all proper methods of evaluation and care or excluding other acceptable methods of evaluation and care aimed at the same results. The ultimate recommendation regarding a particular assessment, clinical procedure, or treatment plan must be made by the clinician in light of the psychiatric evaluation, other clinical data, and the diagnostic and treatment options available. Such recommendations should be made in collaboration with the patient, whenever possible, and incorporate the patient's personal and sociocultural preferences and values in order to enhance the therapeutic alliance, adherence to treatment, and treatment outcomes. For all of these reasons, the APA cautions against the use of guidelines in litigation. Use of these guidelines is voluntary. APA provides the guidelines on an "as is" basis and makes no warranty, expressed or implied, regarding them. APA assumes no responsibility for any injury or damage to persons or property arising out of or related to any use of the guidelines or for any errors or omissions.

Rationale

The goal of this guideline is to improve the quality of care and treatment outcomes for patients with alcohol use disorder (AUD), as defined by DSM-5 (American Psychiatric Association 2013). The guideline focuses specifically on evidence-based pharmacological treatments for AUD but also includes statements related to assessment and treatment planning that are an integral part of using pharmacotherapy to treat AUD. AUD pharmacotherapy is a topic of increasing interest given the burden of AUD in the population and the availability of several U.S. Food and Drug Administration (FDA)–approved medications for this disorder. For these reasons, the AHRQ undertook a systematic review of AUD pharmacotherapy in outpatients (Jonas et al. 2014), which serves as the foundation of the systematic review for this practice guideline. The guideline does not apply to the use of these same medications for indications other than AUD. It also does not address the management of individuals who are intoxicated with alcohol, who require pharmacotherapy for the acute treatment of alcohol withdrawal, or who are experiencing other acute medical problems related to alcohol use. Evidence-based psychotherapeutic treatments for AUD, including cognitive-behavioral therapy (CBT), twelve-step facilitation (TSF), and motivational enhancement therapy (MET) (Anton et al. 2006; Martin and Rehm 2012; Project MATCH Research Group 1998b), also play a major role in the treatment of AUD, but specific recommendations related to these modalities are outside the scope of this guideline.

Worldwide, the estimated 12-month adult prevalence of AUD is 8.5%, with an estimated lifetime prevalence of 20% (Slade et al. 2016a). In the United States, AUD has estimated values for 12-month and lifetime prevalence of 13.9% and 29.1%, respectively, with approximately half of individuals with lifetime AUD having a severe disorder (Grant et al. 2015). Rates of AUD in U.S. adults vary by race/ethnicity (Delker et al. 2016; Grant et al. 2015), with 12-month prevalence rates being highest among American Indians and Alaska Natives (19.2%) as compared with whites (14.0%), Hispanics (13.6%), African Americans (14.4%), and Asian Americans and Pacific Islanders (10.6%). Onset of AUD is most commonly between ages 18 and 29, and men are more likely to be diagnosed with the disorder as compared to women (12-month prevalence in the United States 17.6% vs. 10.4%; Grant et al. 2015). However, in recent decades, differences between men and women in patterns of alcohol use have become less pronounced (Slade et al. 2016b; White et al. 2015), and overall rates of AUD appear to be increasing (Grant et al. 2015).

AUD places a significant strain on both the personal and public health of the U.S. population. According to a 2006 Centers for Disease Control and Prevention–sponsored study (Bouchery et al. 2011), AUD and its sequelae cost the United States $223.5 billion annually and account for significant excess mortality (Kendler et al. 2016). Globally, AUD is associated with a substantial burden of disease in terms of years of life lost to premature mortality, disability-adjusted life years, and years lived with disability (Whiteford et al. 2013). Additionally, problematic alcohol use has been linked to motor vehicle accidents (Kelly et al. 2004); poor academic performance (Williams et al. 2003; Wolaver 2002); increased risk of suicide (American Psychiatric Association 2016; Darvishi et al. 2015); increased criminal activity, including intimate partner violence perpetration (Okuda et al. 2015); increased risk for death by overdose (Jones et al. 2014); and increased transmission risks for human immunodeficiency virus (HIV) and other sexually transmitted infections (Monroe et al. 2016; Rashad and Kaestner 2004; Williams et al. 2016). Additionally, many symptoms of AUD relate to the inability to regulate alcohol use, and relapse of AUD is common (Dawson et al. 2007; Moos and Moos 2006; Tuithof et al. 2014). Associated impairments in insight often lead to delays in accessing care (Chapman et al. 2015). Access to care can also be challenging because AUD often co-occurs with other psychiatric disorders (Grant et al. 2015), and each disorder will need to be treated. Furthermore, the co-occurrence of AUD and other psychiatric disorders reduces treatment outcomes for both types of disorders (Drake et al. 2001) and can be an unrecognized source of treatment resistance.

Despite its high prevalence and numerous negative consequences, AUD remains undertreated. Effective and evidence-based interventions are available, and treatment is associated with reductions in the risk of relapse (Dawson et al. 2006) and AUD-associated mortality (Timko et al. 2006). Nevertheless, fewer than 1 in 10 individuals in the United States with a 12-month diagnosis of AUD receive any treatment (Grant et al. 2015; Substance Abuse and Mental Health Services Administration 2014). Receipt of evidence-based care is even less common. For example, one study found that of the 11 million people in the United States with AUD, only 674,000 received psychopharmacological treatment (Mark et al. 2009). Furthermore, treatment availability and the type of treatment provided can vary based on geography and, in the United States, insurance coverage (Hagedorn et al. 2016; Mark et al. 2015), including formulary restrictions (Harris et al. 2013). In a systematic literature review focused on this disparity, Hagedorn et al. (2016) identified contributing factors at the level of patients (e.g., lack of awareness of treatment options) and clinicians (e.g., perceived low demand and low confidence in the efficacy of pharmacotherapy). Other clinician barriers to prescribing medications for AUD include an inability to provide suitable psychosocial co-interventions and lack of familiarity with medications (Harris et al. 2013; O'Malley and O'Connor 2011). These and other gaps in the care of individuals with AUD suggest that greater efforts are needed to develop and test quality measures related to AUD treatment (Patel et al. 2015; Pincus et al. 2016; Seibert et al. 2015; Thomas et al. 2013; Watkins et al. 2011). Accordingly, this practice guideline provides evidence-based statements aimed at increasing knowledge and the appropriate use of medications for AUD. The overall goal of this guideline is to enhance the treatment of AUD for millions of affected individuals, thereby reducing the significant psychosocial and public health consequences of this important psychiatric condition.

Guideline Statement Summary

Assessment and Determination of Treatment Goals

1. APA *recommends* (**1C**) that the initial psychiatric evaluation of a patient with suspected alcohol use disorder include assessment of current and past use of tobacco and alcohol as well as any misuse of other substances, including prescribed or over-the-counter medications or supplements.
2. APA *recommends* (**1C**) that the initial psychiatric evaluation of a patient with suspected alcohol use disorder include a quantitative behavioral measure to detect the presence of alcohol misuse and assess its severity.
3. APA *suggests* (**2C**) that physiological biomarkers be used to identify persistently elevated levels of alcohol consumption as part of the initial evaluation of patients with alcohol use disorder or in the treatment of individuals who have an indication for ongoing monitoring of their alcohol use.
4. APA *recommends* (**1C**) that patients be assessed for co-occurring conditions (including substance use disorders, other psychiatric disorders, and other medical disorders) that may influence the selection of pharmacotherapy for alcohol use disorder.
5. APA *suggests* (**2C**) that the initial goals of treatment of alcohol use disorder (e.g., abstinence from alcohol use, reduction or moderation of alcohol use, other elements of harm reduction) be agreed on between the patient and clinician and that this agreement be documented in the medical record.
6. APA *suggests* (**2C**) that the initial goals of treatment of alcohol use disorder include discussion of the patient's legal obligations (e.g., abstinence from alcohol use, monitoring of abstinence) and that this discussion be documented in the medical record.
7. APA *suggests* (**2C**) that the initial goals of treatment of alcohol use disorder include discussion of risks to self (e.g., physical health, occupational functioning, legal involvement) and others (e.g., impaired driving) from continued use of alcohol and that this discussion be documented in the medical record.
8. APA *recommends* (**1C**) that patients with alcohol use disorder have a documented comprehensive and person-centered treatment plan that includes evidence-based nonpharmacological and pharmacological treatments.

Selection of a Pharmacotherapy

9. APA *recommends* (**1B**) that naltrexone or acamprosate be offered to patients with moderate to severe alcohol use disorder who

   - have a goal of reducing alcohol consumption or achieving abstinence,
   - prefer pharmacotherapy or have not responded to nonpharmacological treatments alone, and
   - have no contraindications to the use of these medications.

10. APA *suggests* (**2C**) that disulfiram be offered to patients with moderate to severe alcohol use disorder who

    - have a goal of achieving abstinence,
    - prefer disulfiram or are intolerant to or have not responded to naltrexone and acamprosate,
    - are capable of understanding the risks of alcohol consumption while taking disulfiram, and
    - have no contraindications to the use of this medication.

11. APA *suggests* (2C) that topiramate or gabapentin be offered to patients with moderate to severe alcohol use disorder who

- have a goal of reducing alcohol consumption or achieving abstinence,
- prefer topiramate or gabapentin or are intolerant to or have not responded to naltrexone and acamprosate, and
- have no contraindications to the use of these medications.

Recommendations Against Use of Specific Medications

12. APA *recommends* (1B) that antidepressant medications not be used for treatment of alcohol use disorder unless there is evidence of a co-occurring disorder for which an antidepressant is an indicated treatment.
13. APA *recommends* (1C) that in individuals with alcohol use disorder, benzodiazepines not be used unless treating acute alcohol withdrawal or unless a co-occurring disorder exists for which a benzodiazepine is an indicated treatment.
14. APA *recommends* (1C) that for pregnant or breastfeeding women with alcohol use disorder, pharmacological treatments not be used unless treating acute alcohol withdrawal with benzodiazepines or unless a co-occurring disorder exists that warrants pharmacological treatment.
15. APA *recommends* (1C) that acamprosate not be used by patients who have severe renal impairment.
16. APA *recommends* (1C) that for individuals with mild to moderate renal impairment, acamprosate not be used as a first-line treatment and, if used, the dose of acamprosate be reduced compared with recommended doses in individuals with normal renal function.
17. APA *recommends* (1C) that naltrexone not be used by patients who have acute hepatitis or hepatic failure.
18. APA *recommends* (1C) that naltrexone not be used as a treatment for alcohol use disorder by individuals who use opioids or who have an anticipated need for opioids.

Treatment of Alcohol Use Disorder and Co-occurring Opioid Use Disorder

19. APA *recommends* (1C) that in patients with alcohol use disorder and co-occurring opioid use disorder, naltrexone be prescribed to individuals who

- wish to abstain from opioid use and either abstain from or reduce alcohol use and
- are able to abstain from opioid use for a clinically appropriate time prior to naltrexone initiation.

Guideline Statements and Implementation

Assessment and Determination of Treatment Goals

STATEMENT 1: Assessment of Substance Use

APA *recommends* **(1C)** that the initial psychiatric evaluation of a patient with suspected alcohol use disorder include assessment of current and past use of tobacco and alcohol as well as any misuse of other substances, including prescribed or over-the-counter medications or supplements.

Implementation

For any patient who is undergoing an initial psychiatric evaluation, it is important to assess the patient's use of tobacco, alcohol, and other substances, as well as any misuse of prescribed or over-the-counter (OTC) medications or supplements (see Guideline II, "Substance Use Assessment," in the APA *Practice Guidelines for the Psychiatric Evaluation of Adults*; American Psychiatric Association 2016). In individuals with AUD, both the 12-month and lifetime odds ratios (ORs) of nicotine use and other substance use disorders are increased (Grant et al. 2015), which supports the need to inquire about past as well as current use. In addition, knowledge of past and current use can inform treatment planning. Information can be obtained through face-to-face interviews, standardized assessment tools, laboratory testing, and input from collateral sources such as family members, other health professionals, medical records, history of electronic prescriptions, or prescription drug monitoring program data.

In face-to-face interviews with the patient, a nonjudgmental and open-ended approach to questions is typically most informative. The interviewer can begin by seeking the patient's permission to ask about or discuss alcohol and other substance use before actually doing so, respecting and documenting the wishes of patients who do not choose to discuss this information, and speaking openly with the patient about the confidentiality of the information and any limits on confidentiality that may exist. Questioning and terminology should be adapted to the individual patient on the basis of such factors as age and culture. The specific substances that are asked about will vary with the clinical context and may include, but are not limited to, alcohol; caffeine; cannabis; hallucinogens; inhalants; opioids; sedatives, hypnotics, and anxiolytics; stimulants, including amphetamine-type substances, cocaine, and other stimulants; tobacco; and other substances. Questions about misuse of prescribed or OTC medications or supplements can often be introduced while the clinician is taking a history of the patient's prescribed medications. Depending on the substance(s) being used, additional follow-up questions will generally be needed to delineate the route, quantity, frequency, pattern, typical setting, and circumstances of use as well as self-perceived benefits and psychiatric and other consequences of use. In terms of alcohol use, it can be helpful to identify the type of alcohol used (e.g., beer, wine, distilled spirits).

For a variety of reasons (e.g., stigma, memory impairment, potential for negative consequences), individuals may underreport the type or extent of alcohol or other substance use. In addition to information about use that can be gained from collateral sources or laboratory studies, aspects of the patient's history may signal a need to probe further in identifying problematic alcohol or other substance use. For example, additional questioning may be needed to explore issues such as family discord; academic or occupational problems; difficulties with mood, sleep, or sexual functioning; or specific physical symptoms (e.g., gastrointestinal distress) or symptom patterns (e.g., anxiety or headaches after every weekend). Observations made during the interview can provide additional clues to possible use (e.g., an odor of cigarettes or alcohol on the patient's breath, physical signs of injection drug use, slurred speech, tremulousness or other evidence of alcohol or substance intoxication or withdrawal).

Information from self-report rating scales can complement information from the face-to-face interview (Guideline II, American Psychiatric Association 2016). The DSM-5 Self-Rated Level 1 Cross-Cutting Symptom Measure (available online at http://www.psychiatry.org/practice/dsm/dsm5/online-assessment-measures) permits initial screening; patients can be asked for additional details on substance use items through administration of the DSM-5 Level 2—Substance Use measure (American Psychiatric Association 2013).

Balancing of Potential Benefits and Harms in Rating the Strength of the Guideline Statement

Benefits

Assessment of the current and past use of alcohol is beneficial in verifying that AUD is present and in identifying its severity and longitudinal course. Knowledge of the patient's current pattern of alcohol use provides important baseline data for assessing the effects of subsequent interventions. Individuals with AUD often use tobacco and other substances. Identifying these conditions, if present, is important in developing a treatment plan that can reduce associated symptoms, morbidity, and mortality. Information about past use is also beneficial in identifying potential health risks from prior use and monitoring for relapse of other substance use disorders.

Harms

Some individuals may become anxious or annoyed if asked multiple questions, including questions about use of substances, during the evaluation. This could interfere with the therapeutic relationship between the patient and the clinician. Another potential consequence is that time used to focus on assessment of tobacco, alcohol, and other substance use could reduce time available to address other issues of importance to the patient or of relevance to diagnosis and treatment planning.

Patient Preferences

Although there is no specific evidence on patient preferences related to assessment in individuals with AUD, clinical experience suggests that the majority of patients are cooperative with and accepting of these types of questions as part of an initial assessment.

Balancing of Benefits and Harms

The potential benefits of this recommendation were viewed as far outweighing the potential harms. (See Appendix B, Statement 1 for additional discussion of the research evidence.) This recommendation is also consistent with Guideline II, "Substance Use Assessment," as part of the APA *Practice Guidelines for the Psychiatric Evaluation of Adults* (American Psychiatric Association 2016). The level of research evidence is rated as low because there is minimal research on the benefits and harms of assessing tobacco, alcohol, and other substance use as part of the psychiatric evaluation. However, screening for use of tobacco, alcohol, and other substances has been studied in other settings, such as primary care. In addition, expert opinion suggests that conducting such assessments as part of the initial psychiatric evaluation improves the identification and diagnosis of substance use disorders (for additional details, see American Psychiatric Association 2016).

Differences of Opinion Among Writing Group Members

There were no differences of opinion. The writing group voted unanimously in favor of this recommendation.

Quality Measurement Considerations

As described in the APA *Practice Guidelines for the Psychiatric Evaluation of Adults* (American Psychiatric Association 2016), individuals who were identified by peers as experts in psychiatric evaluation assessed patients for use of alcohol or other substances at consistently high rates, whereas assessment of past and current tobacco use were also high but showed opportunity for improvement. The typical practices of other psychiatrists and mental health professionals are unknown, but rates of tobacco use screening have been declining among psychiatrists practicing in ambulatory settings (Rogers and Sherman 2014). Data from ambulatory settings (Glass et al. 2016) suggest that many individuals receive screening for alcohol use, but approximately one-third of individuals do not. Rates of screening for use of other substances, including misuse of prescribed or OTC medications, are likely to be less than rates of screening for either tobacco or alcohol use.

Several existing measures are of relevance to this recommendation. National Quality Forum (NQF) Measure 110, "Bipolar Disorder and Major Depression: Appraisal for Alcohol or Chemical Substance Use," assesses the percentage of patients with depression or bipolar disorder, with evidence of an initial assessment that includes an appraisal for alcohol or substance use (www.qualityforum.org/QPS/0110). In terms of tobacco use, the NQF-endorsed Measure 0028, "Preventive Care & Screening: Tobacco Use: Screening & Cessation Intervention," assesses the percentage of adult patients who are screened every 2 years for tobacco use and who receive cessation counseling intervention if identified as a tobacco user (www.qualityforum.org/QPS/0028). Several other NQF-endorsed treatment performance measures are related to screening for tobacco use in inpatient settings. In addition, an expert panel convened by the RAND Corporation has suggested that detailed specification development and pilot testing would be appropriate for a potential AUD-related quality measure on screening for substance use, including tobacco use, in individuals with an Alcohol Use Disorders Identification Test–Concise (AUDIT-C) score of greater than or equal to 5 (Hepner et al. 2017). The American Society of Addiction Medicine also has proposed a measure on screening for tobacco use disorder (American Society of Addiction Medicine 2014). Before adopting any measures, it is important to determine whether the measure has been validated in the population and setting of interest. Thus, it is recommended at this time that only measures specified or endorsed for outpatients be used in that treatment setting.

The most effective manner to assess and report on measures related to substance use is unclear. Several options for reporting are in practice, and have been proposed.

As described in the APA *Practice Guidelines for the Psychiatric Evaluation of Adults* (American Psychiatric Association 2016), a comprehensive measure could be derived that assesses the percentage of patients seen in an initial evaluation who are screened for the use of tobacco, alcohol, or other substances as well as for the misuse of prescribed or OTC medications.

Because existing measures already include a tobacco use screening measure, it may be preferable to focus new measure development on assessment of current and past alcohol use. Such a measure could be paired with a distinct measure on assessment of substance use. Alternatively, a measure on the assessment of alcohol use could be paired with a measure that determines whether treatment for AUD was initiated.

In practices that use an electronic health record, a measure on the assessment of past and current alcohol use could be implemented by measuring for the presence or absence of text in corresponding fields labeled "past alcohol use" and "current alcohol use." This approach would aim to ensure that assessment has occurred and is documented in a patient's record but would allow for maximum flexibility in how clinicians document findings of their assessments without endorsing use of a specific scale or method of assessment. Regardless of the approach that is chosen, quality improvement activities derived from this recommendation, including performance measures, should not oversimplify the process of assessing alcohol use, as alcohol use is commonly underreported by patients and often requires use of clinical interviewing skills to elicit accurate information. Exceptions to the denominator of the measure should be specified and might include individuals who are unable to participate in the evaluation because of their current mental status. Other exceptions might also be appropriate.

STATEMENT 2: Use of Quantitative Behavioral Measures

APA *recommends* **(1C)** that the initial psychiatric evaluation of a patient with suspected alcohol use disorder include a quantitative behavioral measure to detect the presence of alcohol misuse and assess its severity.

Implementation

Quantitative behavioral measures should be used during the initial psychiatric evaluation of a patient with AUD to detect the presence of alcohol misuse and determine its severity. The intent of using a quantitative behavioral measure is not to establish diagnosis but rather to complement other aspects of the screening and assessment process. Depending on the measure, it can also serve as a baseline measure to judge the effects of treatment. Co-occurring psychiatric conditions or cognitive impairment may limit some patients' ability to complete self-report instruments. In these circumstances, it may be necessary to place greater reliance on collateral sources of information such as family members or staff members of sober living homes or community residence programs, if applicable.

A number of validated scales and screening tools have been developed (Jonas et al. 2012a, 2012b). Although recommending a particular scale is outside the scope of this practice guideline, considerations in choosing a scale include the age of the patient, clinical setting, time available for administration, and therapeutic objective (i.e., screening vs. diagnosis vs. ongoing monitoring). For example, the CAGE questionnaire (Ewing 1984) has been studied as a screening tool for AUD and asks whether the individual felt a need to cut down on drinking, was annoyed by criticism of drinking, felt guilty about drinking, or had a morning eye-opener. CAGE does not provide enough information to suggest a diagnosis of AUD or to be used in monitoring alcohol use in patients with known AUD (do Amaral and Malbergier 2008). In addition, it is less sensitive in screening for mild to moderate AUD than are some other measures. The CRAFFT screening tool is intended to be developmentally appropriate for adolescents and includes questions about being in a car driven by someone who was using alcohol or drugs, use of alcohol or drugs to relax or when alone, forgetting what was done while using alcohol or drugs, being told by family or friends to cut down on use, and getting into trouble while using alcohol or drugs (Knight et al. 1999). On the other hand, the AUDIT (Saunders et al. 1993) and its shortened form, the AUDIT-C (Bush et al. 1998), are more appropriate for use with adult patients, including pregnant women (Burns et al. 2010). With both the AUDIT and the AUDIT-C, interpretation of the resulting score differs by sex and by age, with women and individuals age 65 and older having lower score thresholds than men or adults under age 65. The National Institute on Alcohol Abuse and Alcoholism (NIAAA) one-question screen, which is useful in identifying problematic drinking in primary care settings (Smith et al. 2009), asks, "How many times in the past year have you had X or more drinks in a day?", where X is 5 for men and 4 for women, with a response greater than 1 constituting a positive screen (U.S. Department of

Health and Human Services 2007). Many other measures are also available that may be useful for specific practice settings or individual patients (see Deady 2009 for review).

Balancing of Potential Benefits and Harms in Rating the Strength of the Guideline Statement

Benefits

Use of a quantitative behavioral measure as part of the initial evaluation can establish baseline information on the patient's reported use of alcohol and on symptoms and impairment associated with alcohol use. As compared with a clinical interview, use of a quantitative behavioral measure may improve the consistency with which this information is obtained. When administered through paper-based or electronic self-report, use of quantitative behavioral measures may allow routine questions to be asked more efficiently.

Harms

The harms of using a quantitative behavioral measure include the time required for administration and review. Overreliance on quantitative measures may lead to other aspects of the patient's symptoms and clinical presentation being overlooked. In addition, some patients may have difficulty completing self-report scales or may interpret questions incorrectly. Patients may also provide inaccurate information about their alcohol use, minimizing consumption and leading to an underestimate of the severity of their use. Reliance on inaccurate information can have a negative impact on clinical decision-making, including recommendations for treatment. Some patients may view quantitative measures as impersonal or may feel annoyed by having to complete detailed questionnaires. Changes in the workflow of clinical practices may be needed to incorporate quantitative behavioral measures into routine care.

Patient Preferences

Clinical experience suggests that the majority of patients are cooperative with and accepting of quantitative behavioral measures as part of an initial assessment.

Balancing of Benefits and Harms

The potential benefits of this recommendation were viewed as far outweighing the potential harms. (For additional discussion of the research evidence, see Appendix B, Statement 2.) This recommendation is also consistent with Guideline VII, "Quantitative Assessment," as part of the APA *Practice Guidelines for the Psychiatric Evaluation of Adults* (American Psychiatric Association 2016). The level of research evidence for this recommendation is rated as low. Evidence suggests that quantitative behavioral measures have good sensitivity and specificity in identifying risky drinking behaviors and AUD, but data come predominantly from hospital-based, emergency department, and primary care settings rather than from psychiatric settings. There is minimal research on the harms of using quantitative behavioral measures as part of the psychiatric evaluation as compared with assessment as usual. However, expert opinion suggests that harms of assessment are minimal compared with the benefits of such assessments in improving identification and assessment of AUD. (For additional details, see the APA *Practice Guidelines for the Psychiatric Evaluation of Adults*; American Psychiatric Association 2016.)

Differences of Opinion Among Writing Group Members

Eight writing group members voted to recommend this statement, and one writing group member voted to suggest this statement.

Quality Measurement Considerations

It is not known how frequently psychiatrists and other health professionals use a quantitative behavioral measure to detect the presence of alcohol misuse and assess its severity in ambulatory settings. Anecdotal observations suggest variability in the routine use of such measures, and even when such measures are used routinely, there can be variability in results (Bradley et al. 2011).

Use of quantitative behavioral measures to assess individuals with AUD could be one approach to meeting a measure on assessing past and current use of alcohol. As described in Statement 1, a measure could consider the presence or absence of scoring from a relevant measurement tool but should avoid endorsing the use of a specific scale.

One example measure is the NQF-endorsed Measure 2152, "Preventive Care and Screening: Unhealthy Alcohol Use: Screening & Brief Counseling." The measure specifies the use of the AUDIT, the AUDIT-C, or the NIAAA one-question screen. Brief counseling is described as at least one session of "a minimum of 5–15 minutes, which may include: feedback on alcohol use and harms; identification of high risk situations for drinking and coping strategies; increased motivation and the development of a personal plan to reduce drinking" (National Quality Measures Clearinghouse 2016). An expert panel convened by the RAND Corporation has suggested a number of potential AUD-related quality measures that would be appropriate for detailed specification development and pilot testing; many of these use specific threshold scores on the AUDIT-C as a method for identifying individuals who are appropriate for the use of the measure (Hepner et al. 2017).

A process-focused internal or health system–based quality improvement measure could also determine rates of quantitative behavioral measure use and implement quality improvement initiatives to increase the frequency with which such measures are used in individuals with AUD.

STATEMENT 3: Use of Physiological Biomarkers

APA *suggests* (2C) that physiological biomarkers be used to identify persistently elevated levels of alcohol consumption as part of the initial evaluation of patients with alcohol use disorder or in the treatment of individuals who have an indication for ongoing monitoring of their alcohol use.

Implementation

Alcohol consumption can also be evaluated and monitored using alcohol biomarkers (see reviews by the Substance Abuse and Mental Health Services Administration 2012, Dasgupta 2015, and Litten and colleagues 2010).

Biomarkers for alcohol consumption are not intended to replace the clinical interview and quantitative behavioral measures but may augment these assessments (do Amaral and Malbergier 2008; Miller et al. 2004) along with input from collateral informants. Alcohol consumption biomarkers may be particularly useful in certain patient populations, such as those with co-occurring psychiatric illness or cognitive impairment that limits the ability to self-report alcohol use. Biomarker testing may also be of particular use when a clinician suspects a patient to be minimizing reported use of alcohol (e.g., due to concerns about employment or insurance termination), when heavy drinking requires verification (e.g., forensic liability and custody cases), or when abstinence is needed (e.g., in court-mandated alcohol treatment). In addition, some biomarkers can help to evaluate for alcohol-related organ damage, which may prompt treatment referral for medical complications of alcohol use. When biomarkers are used, results should be discussed with patients in ways that encourage open and honest communication about alcohol consumption (Miller et al. 2004).

Biomarkers may be obtained from a variety of sources (e.g., blood, urine, hair). Direct biomarkers measure alcohol or alcohol metabolites over a time course of hours (blood ethanol level) to months (hair ethyl glucuronide [EtG]) and generally are more sensitive to any alcohol consumption. Other direct biomarkers, such as phosphatidylethanol (PEth), detect steady low to heavy drinking over a period of weeks. Carbohydrate-deficient transferrin (CDT), an indirect marker, detects only heavy drinking (e.g., four or more drinks per day for women and five or more per day for men consumed frequently in the weeks prior to testing). In contrast, other indirect biomarkers, such as gamma-glutamyl transferase (GGT), alanine transaminase (ALT), aspartate transaminase (AST), and mean corpuscular volume (MCV), typically reflect organ damage or physiological dysfunction resulting from more chronic, heavy alcohol consumption. Using a combination of biomarkers should improve sensitivity and increase specificity (e.g., a less specific positive GGT would be confirmed as alcohol related by a positive %CDT).

There are several other factors to consider when choosing a biomarker. It is important to evaluate for co-occurring medical conditions or medications that may interfere with biomarker testing (see reviews by the Substance Abuse and Mental Health Services Administration 2012, Dasgupta 2015, and Litten and colleagues 2010). Interpreting biomarker levels is further complicated by variations in assay techniques and threshold values for a positive test (Weykamp et al. 2013). Different thresholds may also be necessary depending on the patient's therapeutic goal (e.g., abstinence vs. moderation) (Balldin et al. 2010). Access to urine (with risk for obfuscation), blood (e.g., availability of phlebotomy services), and insurance coverage for specific biomarkers can also influence test selection.

Serum Ethanol Level

Serum ethanol level is a direct biomarker commonly used in the acute intoxication phase. Depending on the amount of alcohol ingested, serum ethanol normalizes within hours of cessation of drinking and typically follows zero-order kinetics (Jones 2011), with one standard drink being metabolized per hour. Regulatory alcohol limits (e.g., for driving) are commonly based on the serum ethanol level.

Ethyl Glucuronide

EtG is a conjugation product of alcohol and naturally occurring glucuronide; therefore, it is a direct biomarker. In contrast to serum ethanol, ethyl glucuronide can be detected in urine or hair up to 2–5 days after the last drink depending on the extent of alcohol consumption (Jatlow et al. 2014; McDonell et al. 2015). It is recommended that a 100–200 ng/mL cutoff be used clinically but, typically, a 500 ng/mL cutoff be used for forensic work. EtG can also be measured in hair samples, but difficulty in obtaining a sample and concerns about reliability limit its use. Although not common, a false-positive EtG result can occur with incidental exposure to products that contain alcohol (Kelly and Mozayani 2012; Walsham and Sherwood 2014), so ideally, patients should be counseled to avoid alcohol-containing products prior to testing. Co-occurring urinary tract bacterial infection can result in either a false-positive test due to in vitro fermentation of glucose to ethanol (especially in diabetics) or a false-negative test due to accelerated elimination of urine EtG (Helander et al. 2007).

Phosphatidylethanol (PEth)

Ethanol interacts with phosphatidylcholine on erythrocyte cell membranes to form PEth. As a result, PEth serves as a whole blood biomarker of recent consumption of alcohol. As a direct biomarker, PEth differs from serum ethanol level in two ways. First, PEth requires a longer duration of alcohol use in order to become elevated (at least 20–50 g or two to four standard drinks daily for several weeks) and remains elevated for 2–3 weeks after cessation of drinking (Isaksson et al. 2011; Stewart et al. 2014). It is believed to have nearly 100% sensitivity for alcohol consumption, making it more sensitive to a range of consumption than many other biomarkers (Isaksson et al. 2011; Walther et al. 2015; Wurst et al. 2015), but it cannot discriminate between low to moderate and heavy consumption.

Carbohydrate-Deficient Transferrin

CDT was the first FDA-approved alcohol biomarker and now refers to an isoform of transferrin (an iron-transporting protein synthesized by the liver) that specifically lacks one of two glycan side chains. This specific isoform is now called disialotransferrin and is accepted as the analyte of choice by the International Federation of Clinical Chemistry and Laboratory Medicine (IFCC) (Jeppsson et al. 2007). With sustained heavy alcohol consumption, the serum concentration of disialo CDT increases through a mechanism that is not fully understood (Niemelä 2016), but it is likely genetically based because not all individuals have abnormal CDT after heavy drinking.

The value reported as disialotransferrin is the fraction of total transferrin (%CDT). Although a number of commercial assays report different values and cutoffs for CDT, the IFCC has recommended a reference high-performance liquid chromatography (HPLC) assay for %CDT measurement (Schellenberg et al. 2017). All other assays will now be expected to be calibrated to this HPLC assay, with a threshold value of 1.7% being standard. At this cutoff value, the sensitivity for detection of heavy alcohol consumption is 50%–70%, with approximately 95%–98% specificity. In responders, %CDT increases after just 1 week of heavy alcohol consumption and slowly returns to normal with abstinence (half-life=14 days). It also can be used over time to monitor relapse to heavy drinking (Anton et al. 2002). False-positive CDT findings can result from end-stage liver disease (Stewart et al. 2014) or genetic variants of CDT (Helander et al. 2003). Women in the last trimester of pregnancy might have higher %CDT values, but, unlike with older assays, sex should not otherwise influence results with the HPLC assay (Bergström and Helander 2008b). With this IFCC standard for measurement, the use of CDT should become more efficient and widespread, enhancing the value of testing.

Liver Enzymes

Over time, heavy alcohol consumption damages hepatocytes. Such damage can be measured with indirect serum biomarkers such as ALT and AST, but elevations in these enzymes are not specific for alcohol-induced liver injury and may reflect hepatic damage due to other conditions (Conigrave et al. 2003).

GGT is among the most commonly used alcohol biomarkers (Whitfield 2001). Elevations in GGT reflect both altered hepatic metabolism and hepatocyte damage in the setting of sustained heavy alcohol consumption (at least 60 g or more per day for 3–6 weeks but usually after many years of prior consumption). However, the relationship between alcohol consumption and GGT elevation can vary among individuals, with significant variability in the sensitivity and specificity of GGT to detect heavy drinking depending on the setting and patient characteristics such as sex (Anton et al. 2002; Bertholet et al. 2014; Conigrave et al. 2002; Gough et al. 2015). Therefore, a normal GGT level does not rule out heavy alcohol consumption (Conigrave et al. 2003). Additionally, adolescents and young adults who drink alcohol heavily do not usually have elevations in GGT. Obesity, smoking, diabetes mellitus, and viral hepatitis C can also lead to elevated levels of GGT (Puukka et al. 2007). False-positive elevations of GGT have also been associated with certain medications (e.g., barbiturates, phenytoin, monoamine oxidase inhibitors, tricyclic antidepressants, warfarin, thiazide diuretics, anabolic steroids; Dasgupta 2015). False negative results can occur with excessive caffeine consumption (>4 cups per day), which may lower GGT levels (Dasgupta 2015).

Mean Corpuscular Volume

MCV is increased with heavy alcohol use, even in the presence of normal folate and vitamin B_{12} levels, and can remain increased for 3–4 months after abstaining from alcohol. MCV, however, has a low sensitivity as an indirect biomarker of alcohol consumption (<50%) (Conigrave et al. 2003), and other causes of macrocytosis are possible (e.g., vitamin B_{12} or folate deficiency).

Trait Markers

Trait biomarkers (e.g., genetic polymorphisms) are under investigation as a means to help clinicians assess a patient's risk of developing AUD or likelihood of responding to a particular treatment. This research has yielded promising results but requires further confirmation before trait biomarkers can be recommended for routine clinical use (Jonas et al. 2014).

Balancing of Potential Benefits and Harms in Rating the Strength of the Guideline Statement

Benefits

Physiological biomarkers can complement the findings of self-report with an objective measure of alcohol use. Evidence suggests that some physiological biomarkers have adequate sensitivity, specificity, and positive predictive values; however, the interpretation of the results will depend on the amount and duration of alcohol consumption prior to testing, the setting in which the biomarker is used, the specific physiological biomarker being tested, the threshold values used to define a positive test result, and other test characteristics that influence biomarker detection. Biomarker results can be helpful in determining the initial severity of AUD and in identifying relapses into drinking or heavy drinking that require adjustments to the plan of treatment. Some indirect biomarkers (e.g., AST, ALT, GGT, CDT, MCV) can also reflect physiological damage related to alcohol consumption and may signal a need for further medical monitoring or intervention. Use of laboratory monitoring of AUD may help to emphasize the medical nature of AUD and potentially reduce stigma.

Harms

False-positive results can occur with physiological biomarkers, although the rate varies with the test, the testing method, and the threshold values for a positive test result. Co-occurring medical conditions and use of specific medications can generate false-positive test results and may require more expensive confirmatory testing. A false-positive biomarker result can be particularly problematic if a patient is having abstinence monitored as part of employment, legal obligations, or other treatment requirements. Discussions with patients about false-positive results can also affect the therapeutic relationship if a patient feels that he or she is not trusted by the clinician. Similarly, false-negative results can be problematic by conveying an incorrect picture of the patient's actual use of alcohol, which may lead to inappropriate clinical decisions. Costs of physiological biomarkers can be a barrier for some patients, depending on insurance status and the frequency of biomarker use. Patients may also experience anxiety about having blood drawn or while awaiting test results. Pain, bruising, or other side effects can occur with phlebotomy for blood-based biomarkers. If phlebotomy occurs at a separate laboratory testing center, practical barriers may include time spent in going for testing, time off from work, or issues with transportation.

Patient Preferences

Information from primary care and substance use disorder treatment programs suggests that the majority of patients are positive about and accepting of blood and urine tests to evaluate their alcohol use (Barrio et al. 2017; Miller et al. 2006). However, some patients may not wish to undergo phlebotomy for assessment of blood biomarkers. Patient preferences may also be affected by testing costs, anxiety related to laboratory testing, or practical barriers. Patients who are ambivalent about abstinence from alcohol use may also prefer to avoid physiological biomarker testing even though verification of the patient's self-reported alcohol use may be needed to ensure effective treatment.

Balancing of Benefits and Harms

The potential benefits of this statement were viewed as likely to outweigh the harms of the statement, although patient preferences may differ and additional research evidence may influence the strength of the guideline statement. (See Appendix B, Statement 3 for additional discussion of the research evidence.) Although there are demonstrated benefits to the use of physiological biomarkers, some patients may experience harms related to false-positive or false-negative test results. Patient preferences about testing may vary, and there are costs and practical barriers that may be associated with physiological biomarker use.

Differences of Opinion Among Writing Group Members

There were no differences of opinion. The writing group voted unanimously in favor of this suggestion.

Quality Measurement Considerations

As a suggestion, this statement is inappropriate for use as a quality measure.

STATEMENT 4: Assessment of Co-occurring Conditions

APA *recommends* **(1C)** that patients be assessed for co-occurring conditions (including substance use disorders, other psychiatric disorders, and other medical disorders) that may influence the selection of pharmacotherapy for alcohol use disorder.

Implementation

AUD frequently co-occurs with other psychiatric disorders, particularly mood or anxiety disorders (Hasin et al. 2005). Identifying co-occurring conditions can aid treatment planning and help in providing integrated care for AUD and other psychiatric conditions. The relationship between alcohol use and psychiatric symptoms is complex and likely bidirectional (Grant et al. 2004; Kenneson et al. 2013; Martins and Gorelick 2011). Alcohol may exacerbate some symptoms (e.g., depressed mood) during periods of use or withdrawal but may reduce the patient's experience of other symptoms (e.g., anxiety, psychosis), contributing to ongoing alcohol use. Problematic alcohol use may also occur in the context of certain disorders that result in impaired impulse control (e.g., bipolar disorder, borderline personality disorder) or may itself lead to worsening behavioral disinhibition. Therefore, it is important to screen for other co-occurring psychiatric disorders. It is also important to assess a patient's risk for suicide and aggressive behaviors (American Psychiatric Association 2016; Buchanan et al. 2011) because heavy alcohol use is a known risk factor for both suicide (Norström and Rossow 2016) and violence (Abramsky et al. 2011; Branas et al. 2016). Such assessments can be accomplished through clinical interview, mental status examination, or use of quantitative measures. Additionally, as described above, screening for other substance use disorders is important for treatment planning because co-occurring disorders may influence medication considerations. For example, an individual with comorbid AUD and opioid use disorder might benefit from extended-release naltrexone to treat both disorders after an informed consent discussion that includes the risk of precipitated opioid withdrawal. More detailed recommendations about screening for co-occurring conditions can be found in the APA *Practice Guidelines for the Psychiatric Evaluation of Adults* (American Psychiatric Association 2016).

It is also important to screen for nonpsychiatric medical conditions that may have arisen as sequelae of or independent from heavy alcohol use. Such assessments include, but are not limited to, measuring serum creatinine and hepatic transaminase levels. One should also evaluate for other causes of hepatic (e.g., viral hepatitis) or renal (e.g., diabetes mellitus, hypertension, HIV) impairment because this may influence the choice of AUD pharmacotherapy. For example, acamprosate is contraindicated in severe renal disease (creatinine clearance [CrCl] <30 mL/min or estimated glomerular filtration rate (eGFR) <30 mL/min/1.73 m^2), and naltrexone must be used cautiously in individuals with hepatic impairment (see Statement 17: Implementation).

Balancing of Potential Benefits and Harms in Rating the Strength of the Guideline Statement

Benefits

Individuals with AUD often have other co-occurring disorders. When such conditions are present, they are important to identify. Pharmacotherapies for AUD may interact with treatments for other disorders, and specific medical conditions may be contraindications for the use of specific pharmacotherapies for AUD. In addition, some medications are indicated for more than one condition, and knowledge of all relevant diagnoses can aid in treatment choice.

Harms

Some individuals may have difficulty concentrating or may become annoyed if asked multiple questions during the evaluation. This could interfere with the therapeutic relationship between the patient and the clinician. Another potential consequence is that time used to focus on assessment of co-occurring disorders could reduce time available to address other issues of importance to the patient or of relevance to diagnosis and treatment planning.

Patient Preferences

Clinical experience suggests that the majority of patients are cooperative with and accepting of assessments for other conditions that may influence treatment options.

Balancing of Benefits and Harms

The potential benefits of this recommendation were viewed as far outweighing the potential harms. (See Appendix B, Statement 4 for additional discussion of the research evidence.) This recommendation is also consistent with Guideline I, "Review of Psychiatric Symptoms, Trauma History, and Psychiatric Treatment History," and with Guideline VI, "Assessment of Medical Health," as part of the APA *Practice Guidelines for the Psychiatric Evaluation of Adults* (American Psychiatric Association 2016). The level of research evidence is rated as low because there is minimal research on the benefits and harms of assessing for co-occurring conditions as part of the psychiatric evaluation as compared with not conducting such assessments. However, expert opinion suggests that such assessments improve the identification and diagnosis of other psychiatric disorders and other medical disorders that can influence treatment planning. (For additional details, see the APA *Practice Guidelines for the Psychiatric Evaluation of Adults*; American Psychiatric Association 2016.)

Differences of Opinion Among Writing Group Members

There were no differences of opinion. The writing group voted unanimously in favor of this recommendation.

Quality Measurement Considerations

As described in the APA *Practice Guidelines for the Psychiatric Evaluation of Adults* (American Psychiatric Association 2016), individuals who were identified by peers as experts in psychiatric evaluation reported high rates of inquiring about co-occurring conditions. The typical practices of other psychiatrists and mental health professionals are unknown. There are many challenges in developing a quality measure from assessment-related recommendations (American Psychiatric Association 2016). There are no NQF-endorsed recommendations on this topic. However, some unendorsed measures exist related to co-occurring conditions in individuals with psychiatric illness. These would be useful to review before considering development of a new measure. In addition, an expert panel convened by the RAND Corporation has suggested screening for liver disease in individuals with an AUD diagnosis or an AUDIT-C score of greater than or equal to 8 (Hepner et al. 2017), and the American Society of Addiction Medicine has proposed a measure on documenting diagnoses of co-occurring psychiatric disorders (American Society of Addiction Medicine 2014). With the increasing use of electronic medical record systems and associated recording of problems and diagnoses using structured terminology, it may be possible to develop electronic measures from this recommendation that could be used for process-focused internal or health system–based quality improvement initiatives.

Statement 5: Determination of Initial Treatment Goals

APA *suggests* **(2C)** that the initial goals of treatment of alcohol use disorder (e.g., abstinence from alcohol use, reduction or moderation of alcohol use, other elements of harm reduction) be agreed on between the patient and clinician and that this agreement be documented in the medical record.

Implementation

Clinicians should collaborate with patients to identify specific treatment goals regarding their alcohol use. With the patient's permission, involvement of family members in developing treatment goals can be helpful. Options for treatment goals might include abstinence, reduction in alcohol use, or eliminating drinking in particularly high-risk situations (e.g., at work, before driving, when responsible for caring for children). Data have shown that having explicit drinking goals at baseline may be associated with improved AUD treatment outcomes (Dunn and Strain 2013). Abstinence as a pretreatment goal has been associated with greater rates of abstinence or moderation, but all groups with an explicit pretreatment goal showed some reduction in alcohol use. Abstinent and nonabstinent drinking goals can include controlled or occasional use, abstinence with the recognition that slips may occur, or total abstinence on a short- or long-term basis (Dunn and Strain 2013).

Motivational interviewing (MI) is one model for having discussions about goals with patients (Levounis et al. 2017; Miller and Rollnick 2013). In MI, the clinician first asks permission to discuss alcohol use. After the patient consents, the goal is to help the patient articulate his or her ambivalence about drinking by asking about positive and negative aspects of alcohol use along with assessments of readiness to reduce drinking and confidence in his or her ability to do so. Such discussions are facilitated by a clinician stance that is curious and nonjudgmental, while also expressing concern for the patient's well-being.

Clinicians should clearly document the agreed-on treatment goals in the medical record (e.g., a brief notation as part of a progress note). Additional documentation may be needed when the goals of the patient and the clinician are not in agreement. For example, a patient may only agree to a reduction in drinking but continue to drink in situations that place him or her at risk of legal involvement (e.g., DUIs, DWIs) or of significant medical sequelae from alcohol use (e.g., hepatic injury). Progress note documentation should reflect that both the clinician and patient understand these risks and have engaged in a discussion about them. As the evaluation and treatment of the patient proceed, the patient and clinician can adjust these initial goals on the basis of factors such as responses to treatment, additional history, family input, or education about treatment options and potential treatment effects (e.g., reduced craving).

Balancing of Potential Benefits and Harms in Rating the Strength of the Guideline Statement

Benefits

Discussing and agreeing on the initial goals of treatment facilitates treatment planning in several respects by eliciting patient preferences and motivations, permitting individualized education on the potential value of harm reduction and abstinence, setting expectations for treatment, and establishing a framework for shared decision-making. It may also assist in forming a therapeutic relationship between the patient and clinician. For some pharmacotherapies, particularly disulfiram, the patient's treatment goal(s) may influence the choice of a pharmacotherapy. Documentation of treatment goals promotes accurate communication among all those caring for the patient and can serve as a reminder of initial discussions about treatment goals.

Harms

The only identifiable harm from this recommendation relates to the time spent in discussion and documentation that may reduce the opportunity to focus on other aspects of the evaluation.

Patient Preferences

Clinical experience suggests that patients are cooperative with and accepting of efforts to establish initial goals of treatment.

Balancing of Benefits and Harms

The potential benefits of this statement were viewed as likely to outweigh the potential harms. (See Appendix B, Statement 5 for additional discussion of the research evidence.) The advantages of specifically setting and documenting goals as compared with assessment as usual are less clear (low strength of research evidence), which influenced the strength of the guideline statement (suggestion). No information is available on the harms of such an approach.

Differences of Opinion Among Writing Group Members

There were no differences of opinion. The writing group voted unanimously in favor of this suggestion.

Quality Measurement Considerations

As a suggestion, this statement is inappropriate for use as a quality measure. A process-focused internal or health system–based quality improvement measure could determine rates at which initial treatment goals are documented. Quality improvement initiatives could be implemented to increase the frequency at which such discussions and documentation occur in individuals with AUD.

STATEMENT 6: Discussion of Legal Obligations

APA *suggests* **(2C)** that the initial goals of treatment of alcohol use disorder include discussion of the patient's legal obligations (e.g., abstinence from alcohol use, monitoring of abstinence) and that this discussion be documented in the medical record.

Implementation

Some patients come to treatment as a consequence of legal involvement, and their engagement in treatment may be court mandated. The initial assessment of AUD should include inquiry about legal involvement and legal obligations, if any, that the patient may have in relation to alcohol use. For individuals in mandated treatment, reporting requirements will vary with the local jurisdiction but should be discussed with the patient. Mandated treatment situations may also influence the treatment goals (e.g., abstinence) and the monitoring of abstinence, such as with serum ethanol levels, ethanol breath tests, or other alcohol-related biomarkers. It is important to document any such legal obligations in the medical record (e.g., as a brief notation as part of a progress note) along with a discussion of the treatment plan and therapeutic goals.

Balancing of Potential Benefits and Harms in Rating the Strength of the Guideline Statement

Benefits

Identifying and discussing the patient's legal obligations as part of the initial goals of treatment facilitates treatment planning and setting of expectations for treatment. Documentation of any legal obligations promotes accurate communication among all those caring for the patient and can serve as a reminder of initial discussions about treatment goals.

Harms

A potential harm of this recommendation relates to the time spent in discussion and documentation that may reduce the opportunity to focus on other aspects of the evaluation. If legal obligations and related details of legal history are documented in a patient's chart, other health care team members who read those details may treat the patient differently, and the patient's privacy could also be compromised.

Patient Preferences

Clinical experience suggests that patients recognize the importance of meeting their legal obligations for treatment and wish to have these addressed by the treating clinician. Some patients may be anxious or uncomfortable about discussing legal issues. They may also have concerns about the privacy of information about their legal history in the medical record.

Balancing of Benefits and Harms

The potential benefits of this statement were viewed as likely to outweigh the harms. (See Appendix B, Statement 6 for additional discussion of the research evidence.) The level of research evidence is rated as low because there is minimal research on whether discussing and documenting patients' legal obligations improves outcomes. No information is available on the harms of such an approach. The strength of the statement (suggestion) was influenced by the potential variations in patient preferences as well as the uncertainty that benefits of the statement would outweigh harms for the majority of patients.

Differences of Opinion Among Writing Group Members

There were no differences of opinion. The writing group voted unanimously in favor of this suggestion.

Quality Measurement Considerations

As a suggestion, this statement is inappropriate for use as a quality measure. A process-focused internal or health system–based quality improvement measure could determine rates at which initial treatment goals are documented, including discussion of legal obligations, if any. Quality improvement initiatives could then be implemented to increase the frequency at which such discussions and documentation occur in individuals with AUD.

STATEMENT 7: Review of Risks to Self and Others

APA *suggests* **(2C)** that the initial goals of treatment of alcohol use disorder include discussion of risks to self (e.g., physical health, occupational functioning, legal involvement) and others (e.g., impaired driving) from continued use of alcohol and that this discussion be documented in the medical record.

Implementation

Discussion of risks to self and others from continued alcohol use will be a natural outgrowth of the assessment. Most individuals who are seeking treatment will already have experienced some negative consequences of alcohol use, which they will typically mention in the context of describing current motivations for treatment. Additional risks can be explored with the patient and documented (e.g., a brief notation as part of a progress note), with the aim of reducing harms associated with drinking. Health risks can include increases in all-cause mortality (Laramée et al. 2015); injury (Cherpitel et al. 2017) or physical or psychological problems (Borges et al. 2017; Rehm et al. 2013, 2017; Shield et al. 2013) related to alcohol use; or interactions between alcohol and other medications that the patient is taking (Breslow et al. 2015). Other common risks include difficulties in occupational, academic, family, social, or other interpersonal functioning; legal involvement; or use of alcohol in physically hazardous situations. When discussing potential harms of alcohol use, it is also important to consider that risk may vary with factors such as concomitant health conditions, age (Moore et al. 2006), and sex and gender (Erol and Karpyak 2015). Materials available through NIAAA may also be helpful in discussing risks of AUD with patients and families (U.S. Department of Health and Human Services 2007). Screening instruments, such as the Drinker Inventory of Consequences (Miller et al. 1995) or the shortened version, the Short Index of Problems (SIP; Feinn et al. 2003; Forcehimes et al. 2007), may also aid clinicians in identifying and supporting discussions of negative consequences of alcohol use.

Balancing of Potential Benefits and Harms in Rating the Strength of the Guideline Statement

Benefits

Discussing potential risks to self and to others from continued use of alcohol can have a number of benefits. Such risks will often contribute to the patient's motivation for treatment, and knowledge of the patient's concerns, preferences, and motivations can facilitate treatment planning. Discussion of such risks permits education on the value of harm reduction and abstinence and helps set expectations for treatment. Documentation of such discussions promotes accurate communication among all those caring for the patient and can serve as a reminder of initial treatment goals.

Harms

A possible harm of this statement relates to the time spent in discussion and documentation that may reduce the opportunity to focus on other aspects of the evaluation. Some patients may be reluctant to discuss risks to self or others or may become anxious while discussing such risks. If the tone of the discussion is perceived as moralizing or judgmental, it may have a negative impact on the therapeutic relationship.

Patient Preferences

Clinical experience suggests that patients are cooperative with and accepting of discussions about harms of alcohol use, although some individuals may minimize the possibility of harms, particularly if they are ambivalent about reducing or abstaining from alcohol use.

Balancing of Benefits and Harms

The potential benefits of this statement were viewed as likely to outweigh the harms. (See Appendix B, Statement 7 for additional discussion of the research evidence.) The strength of the statement (suggestion) was influenced by the uncertainty of whether a discussion of risks to self and others and documentation improve outcomes relative to a more general discussion of goals with the patient. Studies of motivational interviewing offer some support for this suggestion, but the level of research evidence is rated as low because there is minimal research on the benefits or harms of specifically discussing and documenting the risks to self and others of continued alcohol use.

Differences of Opinion Among Writing Group Members

There were no differences of opinion. The writing group voted unanimously in favor of this suggestion.

Quality Measurement Considerations

As a suggestion, this statement is inappropriate for use as a quality measure. A process-focused internal or health system–based quality improvement measure could determine rates at which the risks of alcohol use have been discussed and documented. Quality improvement initiatives could be implemented to increase the frequency at which such discussions and documentation occur in individuals with AUD.

STATEMENT 8: Evidence-Based Treatment Planning

APA *recommends* **(1C)** that patients with alcohol use disorder have a documented comprehensive and person-centered treatment plan that includes evidence-based nonpharmacological and pharmacological treatments.

Implementation

In treating individuals with AUD, a person-centered treatment plan should be developed, documented in the medical record (e.g., as part of a progress note), and updated at appropriate intervals. Such a plan may require tailoring based on sociocultural factors such as gender and age (Erol and Karpyak 2015; Kerr-Corrêa et al. 2007; Sudhinaraset et al. 2016). A person-centered treatment plan can be recorded as part of an evaluation note or progress note and does not need to adhere to a defined development process (e.g., face-to-face multidisciplinary team meeting) or format (e.g., time-specified goals and objectives). However, it should give an overview of the identified clinical and psychosocial issues along with a specific plan for addressing factors such as acute intoxication or alcohol-related medical issues (if present), further history and mental status examination, physical examination (either by the evaluating clinician or another health professional), laboratory testing (as needed, based on the history, examination, and planned treatments), ongoing monitoring, and nonpharmacological and pharmacological interventions, as indicated (Substance Abuse and Mental Health Services Administration and National Institute on Alcohol Abuse and Alcoholism 2015). Plans can also include educating patients about treatment options, engaging family members, collaborating with other treating clinicians, or providing integrated care. Depending on the urgency of the initial clinical presentation, the availability of laboratory results, or collateral informants, the initial treatment plan may need to be augmented over several visits and as more details of history and treatment response are obtained. Collateral informants such as family members, friends, or other treating health professionals may express specific concerns about the individual's alcohol use or related behaviors or concerns or biases about specific treatment approaches. If present, such concerns should be documented and addressed as part of the treatment plan. Additionally, the patient's goals and readiness to change his or her alcohol consumption may evolve over time and necessitate changes to the treatment plan. Changes to the treatment plan will also be needed if a patient has not tolerated or responded to a specific treatment or if he or she chooses to switch treatment approaches. For example, if a patient does not wish to receive further nonpharmacological treatment, a reconsideration of AUD pharmacotherapy would be warranted if such medications are not already prescribed.

As part of a person-centered treatment plan, it is important to consider both nonpharmacological and pharmacological treatment approaches. Although recommending a particular nonpharmacological approach is outside the scope of this practice guideline, there are several evidence-based options for the treatment of AUD. These include MET (Lenz et al. 2016) and CBT for AUD (Epstein and McCrady 2009). MET is a manualized psychotherapy based on the principles of motivational interviewing that has been shown in multiple studies to have a small to medium effect size on achieving abstinence (Dieperink et al. 2014; Lenz et al. 2016). This treatment is designed to help patients develop intrinsic motivation to reduce or abstain from alcohol use by helping them explore their own ambivalence about alcohol use and its sequelae. Motivational interviewing principles can also be used to foster shared-decision making regarding AUD pharmacotherapy and in promoting medication adherence (Levounis et al. 2017). CBT focuses on the relationships between thoughts, feelings, and behaviors (Epstein and McCrady 2009). Particular attention is paid to strategies that help the patient manage urges and triggers (i.e., cues) to drink. Medical management (MM) is also a manualized treatment (Pettinati et al. 2004) that was developed for use in the Combined Pharmacotherapies and Behavioral Interventions for Alcohol Dependence (COMBINE) study. It provides education and strategies to support abstinence and promote medication adherence. Community-based peer support groups such as Alcoholics Anonymous (AA) and other 12-step programs have been helpful for many patients. In fact, TSF relies on the utility of community-based peer supports (Kaskutas 2009; Kaskutas et al. 2009; Kowinski et al. 1992; Project MATCH Research Group 1998a, 1998b). Nevertheless, the focus and structure of groups can vary considerably, and there is a paucity of research on these modalities (Ferri et al. 2006). For these reasons, community-based peer support programs can assist many individuals in achieving long-term remission from AUD but cannot substitute for formal medical treatment in the management of AUD.

When an individual with AUD also has other psychiatric conditions (including other substance use disorders), the treatment plan should assure that each of the co-occurring disorders is addressed, either individually (with appropriate care coordination) or using an integrated model of care. The statements in this guideline should generally be applicable to individuals with co-occurring conditions, although the evidence base in individuals with co-occurring disorders remains limited (Tiet and Mausbach 2007; see Appendix B).

Balancing of Potential Benefits and Harms in Rating the Strength of the Guideline Statement

Benefits

Development and documentation of a comprehensive treatment plan assures that the clinician has considered the available nonpharmacological and pharmacological options for treatment and has identified those treatments that are best suited to the needs of the individual patient, with a goal of improving overall outcome. It may also assist in forming a therapeutic relationship, eliciting patient preferences, permitting education about possible treatments, setting expectations for treatment, and establishing a framework for shared decision-making. Documentation of a treatment plan promotes accurate communication among all those caring for the patient and can serve as a reminder of prior discussions about treatment.

Harms

The only identifiable harm from this recommendation relates to the time spent in discussion and documentation that may reduce the opportunity to focus on other aspects of the evaluation.

Patient Preferences

Clinical experience suggests that patients are cooperative with and accepting of efforts to establish treatment plans.

Balancing of Benefits and Harms

The potential benefits of this recommendation were viewed as far outweighing the potential harms. (See Appendix B, Statement 8 for additional discussion of the research evidence.) The level of research evidence is rated as low because no information is available on the harms of such an approach. There is also minimal research on whether developing and documenting a specific treatment plan improves outcomes as compared with assessment and documentation as usual. However, the majority of studies of pharmacotherapy for AUD included nonpharmacological treatments aimed at providing supportive counseling, enhancing coping strategies, and promoting adherence. This indirect evidence supports the benefits of comprehensive treatment planning.

Differences of Opinion Among Writing Group Members

There were no differences of opinion. The writing group voted unanimously in favor of this recommendation.

Quality Measurement Considerations

It is not known whether psychiatrists and other mental health professionals typically develop and document a comprehensive and person-centered treatment plan that includes evidence-based nonpharmacological and pharmacological treatments, and there is likely to be variability. Among individuals who were identified with AUD via screening in general ambulatory settings, only a small fraction received any information about treatment (Glass et al. 2016). Some specific elements of a comprehensive treatment plan, including counseling about treatment options, offer of psychotherapy, receipt of AUD pharmacotherapy, referral to community-based recovery support, and integrated treatment of co-occurring disorders, have been suggested for detailed development of quality measure specifications and pilot testing by an expert panel convened by the RAND Corporation on AUD-related quality measures (Hepner et al. 2017). Nevertheless, an overarching performance measure derived from this recommendation is not recommended because of the associated burdens and practical challenges. Clinical judgment would be needed to determine whether a documented treatment plan was comprehensive and person centered, even if listed treatments were evidence based. If a performance measure assessed for the presence or absence of specific text in the medical record, increased documentation burden could result. Such an approach could also foster overuse of standardized language that would not accurately reflect what has occurred in practice.

Selection of a Pharmacotherapy

STATEMENT 9: Naltrexone or Acamprosate

APA *recommends* **(1B)** that naltrexone or acamprosate be offered to patients with moderate to severe alcohol use disorder who

- have a goal of reducing alcohol consumption or achieving abstinence,
- prefer pharmacotherapy or have not responded to nonpharmacological treatments alone, and
- have no contraindications to the use of these medications.

Implementation

Naltrexone and acamprosate have the best available evidence as pharmacotherapy for patients with AUD (Center for Substance Abuse and Treatment 2009; Jonas et al. 2014). In most studies, participants were included on the basis of a DSM-IV diagnosis of alcohol dependence, which roughly corresponds to moderate to severe AUD in DSM-5 (Compton et al. 2013; Hasin et al. 2013; Peer et al. 2013). Use of these medications may also be appropriate to consider on an individualized basis for patients with mild AUD, particularly if the patient prefers this treatment modality.

Acamprosate is efficacious in the treatment of AUD when administered at a mean dose of 1998 mg per day, typically 666 mg three times per day (Jonas et al. 2014). Although its exact mechanism of action is unclear, it may act by modulating glutamate, with indirect effects on other neurotransmitters or ion channels (Kalk and Lingford-Hughes 2014). Individuals who were randomly assigned to take acamprosate were significantly less likely to return to drinking after attaining abstinence and had a significant reduction in the number of drinking days, although data on the number of heavy drinking days were mixed. Most experts recommend starting treatment as soon as abstinence is attained and continuing even if the patient relapses (Jonas et al. 2014). The most positive data for acamprosate efficacy comes from outside the United States, where it is typically started in the hospital after detoxification and a period of abstinence.

The lack of metabolism of acamprosate through the liver and the lack of reported hepatotoxicity with acamprosate (National Library of Medicine 2017a) are often important considerations in its use given the significant rates of hepatic dysfunction in individuals with AUD (O'Shea et al. 2010). However, because of the excretion of acamprosate through the kidneys, serum creatinine should be measured at baseline and, in individuals with a history of renal impairment, results should be reviewed before initiating treatment. Acamprosate is contraindicated if estimated CrCl is less than 30 mL/min or eGFR is less than 30 mL/min/1.73 m^2; dose reduction may be necessary for CrCl values between 30 and 50 mL/min or eGFR values between 30 and 59 mL/min/1.73 m^2. Common side effects include diarrhea (17% compared with 10% in placebo; Micromedex 2017a).

Naltrexone is an opioid receptor antagonist that has efficacy in the treatment of both AUD and opioid use disorder. It has greatest affinity for μ opioid receptors, next highest affinity for δ opioid receptors, and lowest affinity for κ opioid receptors (Ashenhurst et al. 2012). This medication has been associated with a reduced likelihood of return to drinking and with fewer drinking days overall. Naltrexone is also thought to decrease the subjective experience of "craving" (Maisel et al. 2013). Naltrexone is available in both a daily oral and monthly depot intramuscular (im) injection. Although long-acting injectable naltrexone may improve adherence (Hartung et al. 2014), there have been no head-to-head comparisons of oral versus injectable naltrexone for AUD, and both formulations appear to be effective. Engaging family members or others to assist with adherence can be particularly helpful if the oral formulation of naltrexone is used. The recommended dose of oral naltrexone is 50 mg daily; however, some patients may require doses up to 100 mg daily to achieve efficacy, which was the dose of naltrexone used in the COMBINE trial (Anton et al. 2006; Garbutt et al. 2005; McCaul et al. 2000a, 2000b). For long-acting naltrexone, the dose is 380 mg im every 4 weeks. There is limited information on use of naltrexone in individuals with co-occurring disorders, but some studies suggest benefit for combined treatment with naltrexone and an antidepressant in depression (Pettinati et al. 2010) and in posttraumatic stress disorder (PTSD; Petrakis et al. 2012) that co-occurs with AUD. Also, smokers with AUD may respond better than nonsmokers to naltrexone (Fucito et al. 2012), which could also influence treatment selection.

Naltrexone is generally well tolerated in clinical trials. Potential gastrointestinal side effects of naltrexone may occur more often among women than men (Herbeck et al. 2016) and include abdominal pain (11% vs. 8% in placebo), diarrhea (13% vs. 10% in placebo), nausea (29% vs. 11% in placebo), and vomiting (12% vs. 6% in placebo; Micromedex 2017c). Dizziness also appears to be more frequent with naltrexone (13% vs. 4% in placebo; Micromedex 2017c). In clinical trials of oral and long-acting injectable naltrexone, rates of anxiety and depression were comparable for naltrexone-treated individuals as compared with placebo. Suicide, suicide attempts, and suicidal ideation were reported in postmarketing surveillance but were infrequent in clinical trials (1% with long-acting injectable naltrexone vs. 0% with placebo; 0%–1% with oral naltrexone vs. 0%–3% with placebo in an open-label trial; Micromedex 2017c). For individuals treated with long-acting injectable naltrexone, pain or induration can occur at the injection site. The potential for bleeding at the injection site should be taken into consideration for patients who have coagulopathy or are taking anticoagulants.

Hepatic functioning can also be affected by naltrexone, and the labeling includes a warning about use of this medication in patients with acute hepatitis or liver failure. With naltrexone, assessment of liver chemistries is appropriate prior to treatment with additional evaluation or consultation and follow-up liver chemistries obtained, as indicated, depending on the extent of any abnormalities (Kwo et al. 2017). The American College of Gastroenterology Clinical Guideline Evaluation of Abnormal Liver Chemistries suggests additional history, physical examination, and laboratory assessment for elevations of AST and ALT that are borderline (less than twice the upper limit of normal) or mild (two to five times the upper limit of normal), with assessment for signs of acute liver failure at values of AST and ALT that are more than five times the upper limit of normal (Kwo et al. 2017). In clinical trials, individuals were generally excluded if hepatic enzyme levels were more than three times the upper limit of normal. In the COMBINE study (Anton et al. 2006), there was an increase in AST or ALT to more than five times the upper limit in 0 of 309 placebo subjects (0%) and 1 of 303 (0%) acamprosate subjects as compared with 6 of 309 naltrexone-treated subjects (2%) and 5 of 305 subjects (2%) treated with acamprosate and naltrexone ($p=0.02$). However, other studies have suggested comparable rates of elevations in hepatic enzymes with naltrexone as with placebo, even in patient populations at increased risk for hepatic dysfunction due to co-occurring hepatitis C or HIV infection (Croop et al. 1997; Lucey et al. 2008; M.C. Mitchell et al. 2012; Tetrault et al. 2012; Vagenas et al. 2014).

Because naltrexone is an opioid receptor antagonist, naltrexone may lead to reduced effectiveness of opioids taken for analgesia. Additionally, depending on the half-life of the opioid consumed, outpatients must be abstinent from opioids for 7–14 days prior to starting naltrexone and should be informed of the risk for precipitating opioid withdrawal if naltrexone is used in conjunction with an opioid. If prescription-related information is available through an electronic medical record or prescription drug monitoring program, it should be checked for current or recent opioid prescriptions. Coordinating care with other clinicians is also important. Some clinicians suggest obtaining urine toxicology screening to confirm the absence of opioids before starting naltrexone, particularly if use of the long-acting injectable formulation is planned. It is also advisable for patients to carry a wallet card noting that they are taking naltrexone so this information will be available to emergency personnel. A template for wallet cards and sample templates for documenting medication management visits are available through NIAAA (U.S. Department of Health and Human Services 2007).

In choosing between acamprosate and naltrexone for an individual patient, selection of a medication is likely to be guided by factors such as ease of administration, available formulations, side effect profile, potential risks in women who are pregnant or breastfeeding (see guideline Statement 14), the presence of co-occurring conditions (e.g., hepatic or renal disease), or the presence of specific features of AUD (e.g., craving). In the COMBINE study, patients who received naltrexone and medical management had a greater proportion of days abstinent and a reduced risk of having a heavy drinking day, whereas acamprosate did not affect drinking outcomes in any of the treatment arms (Anton et al. 2006). However, the German PREDICT study (Mann et al. 2013) found no difference among naltrexone, acamprosate, and placebo groups on the time to first heavy drinking. Consistent with this, the AHRQ systematic review and meta-analysis (Jonas et al. 2014) found no statistically significant difference between naltrexone and acamprosate in the percent with a return to any drinking, the percent with a return to heavy drinking, or the number of drinking days, suggesting that neither of these medications was superior to the other. Thus, either naltrexone or acamprosate could be viewed as an appropriate initial treatment choice, depending on other patient-specific considerations. Decisions about the duration of treatment with these medications will also be based on individual factors such as patient preference, disorder severity, history of relapses, potential consequences of relapse, clinical response, and tolerability. There is insufficient evidence available on concomitant use of acamprosate and naltrexone to determine the benefits and harms of combined treatment or to make any statement about using these medications together.

Balancing of Potential Benefits and Harms in Rating the Strength of the Guideline Statement

Benefits

Acamprosate is associated with a small benefit on the outcomes of returning to any drinking and on the number of drinking days (moderate strength of research evidence). Naltrexone is associated with a small benefit on the outcomes of returning to any drinking, returning to heavy drinking, frequency of drinking days, and frequency of heavy drinking days (moderate strength of research evidence). Evidence is limited, but the use of long-acting injectable naltrexone may have benefits for adherence as compared with oral formulations of naltrexone. In the AHRQ meta-analysis of head-to-head comparisons, neither acamprosate nor naltrexone showed superiority to the other medication in terms of return to heavy drinking (moderate strength of research evidence), return to any drinking (moderate strength of research evidence), or percentage of drinking days (low strength of research evidence). However, in the U.S. COMBINE study (but not the German PREDICT study), naltrexone was associated with better outcomes than acamprosate.

Harms

The harms of acamprosate are small in magnitude, with slight overall increases in diarrhea and vomiting as compared with placebo (moderate strength of research evidence). The harms of naltrexone are small in magnitude, with slight overall increases in dizziness, nausea, and vomiting relative to placebo (moderate strength of research evidence). Alterations in hepatic function are also possible with naltrexone, but changes in liver chemistries were not assessed in the AHRQ review. Individuals taking naltrexone would not be able to take opioids for pain, and other treatments for acute pain would be needed. For individuals treated with long-acting injectable naltrexone, pain or induration can occur at the injection site, and access to the medication can be an issue because of geographic- or payment-related issues. With long durations of naltrexone use, individuals lose tolerance to opioids. This can result in overdose and death if large but previously tolerated opioid doses are taken after naltrexone is discontinued. For many other potential harms, including mortality, evidence was not available or was rated by the AHRQ review as insufficient. However, withdrawals from the studies due to adverse events did not differ from placebo for acamprosate (low strength of research evidence) and were only slightly greater than placebo for naltrexone although statistically significant (moderate strength of research evidence).

Patient Preferences

Some patients prefer to avoid the use of medication, whereas others prefer to combine pharmacological and nonpharmacological treatment approaches or take a medication rather than use nonpharmacological treatment approaches alone. Some patients may also prefer one medication over another medication on the basis of prior treatment experiences or other factors. With naltrexone, the availability of a long-acting injectable formulation may be viewed positively by patients in terms of helping to assure medication adherence, but other individuals may prefer to avoid the minor discomfort associated with im injections. However, clinical experience suggests that the majority of patients would want to be offered the option of these pharmacotherapies for AUD.

Balancing of Benefits and Harms

The potential benefits of this recommendation were viewed as far outweighing the potential harms. (See Appendix B, Statement 9 for additional discussion of the research evidence.) For both acamprosate and naltrexone, the harms of treatment were considered minimal, particularly compared with the harms of continued alcohol use, as long as there was no contraindication to the use of the medication. The positive effects of acamprosate and naltrexone were small overall, and not all studies showed a statistically significant benefit from these medications. In addition, European studies showed greater benefit of acamprosate than did U.S. studies, and naltrexone exhibited greater effect than acamprosate in the COMBINE trial. Nevertheless, the potential benefit of each medication was viewed as far outweighing the harms of continued alcohol use, particularly when nonpharmacological approaches have not produced an effect or when patients prefer to use one of these medications as an initial treatment option. In addition, it was noted that even small effect sizes may be clinically meaningful because of the significant morbidity associated with AUD. Patients with mild AUD rarely participated in clinical trials of naltrexone and acamprosate pharmacotherapy. Therefore, although they might respond to these medications, patients with mild AUD are not included in this recommendation because of the limited amount of research evidence.

Differences of Opinion Among Writing Group Members

There were no differences of opinion. The writing group voted unanimously in favor of this recommendation.

Quality Measurement Considerations

Information from the Veterans Health Administration suggests low rates of pharmacotherapy for AUD. Approximately 3% of patients with AUD received a prescription for naltrexone, with less than 10% of those treated with naltrexone receiving long-acting injectable naltrexone (Iheanacho et al. 2013; Marienfeld et al. 2014).

Given the clinical considerations associated with the selection of a pharmacotherapy for a patient with AUD, a performance measure derived from this recommendation is not recommended. Clinical judgment would be needed to assess whether contraindications to treatment are present and to determine if there was a lack of response to nonpharmacological treatments alone. Increased documentation burden could result if each element of the recommendation needed to be recorded as standardized or structured text. Alternatively, if information was recorded as free text, additional time would be needed in reviewing documentation and determining if measure criteria were met. However, this recommendation could be used as a process-focused internal or health system–based quality improvement measure by tracking rates of prescribing for naltrexone and acamprosate in individuals with AUD. A quality measure could also examine receipt of AUD pharmacotherapy more broadly, as has been suggested by an expert panel convened by the RAND Corporation on AUD-related quality measures (Hepner et al. 2017). The American Society of Addiction Medicine (ASAM) Performance Measures for the Addiction Specialist Physician also include a suggested measure related to receipt of AUD pharmacotherapy (American Society of Addiction Medicine 2014). Changes in prescribing rates could be determined after initiatives to educate clinicians or reduce barriers to pharmacotherapy use (Abraham et al. 2011; Harris et al. 2016). Electronic decision support could identify individuals with a new diagnosis of moderate to severe AUD (as documented as a problem or diagnosis) and provide information on acamprosate and naltrexone for consideration by the clinician through a passive alert or "infobutton" (Del Fiol et al. 2012).

STATEMENT 10: Disulfiram

APA *suggests* **(2C)** that disulfiram be offered to patients with moderate to severe alcohol use disorder who

- have a goal of achieving abstinence,
- prefer disulfiram or are intolerant to or have not responded to naltrexone and acamprosate,
- are capable of understanding the risks of alcohol consumption while taking disulfiram, and
- have no contraindications to the use of this medication.

Implementation

Disulfiram is an inhibitor of the enzyme aldehyde dehydrogenase, which breaks down the ethanol byproduct acetaldehyde. Disulfiram is appropriate only for individuals seeking abstinence and is contraindicated in patients who are actively using alcohol or products containing alcohol. When a patient consumes alcohol within 12–24 hours of taking disulfiram, the accumulation of acetaldehyde produces a response that includes tachycardia, flushing, headache, nausea, and vomiting. The anticipatory fear of this response acts as a deterrent to alcohol use. However, this benefit of disulfiram requires consistent adherence to the medication (Allen and Litten 1992; Krampe and Ehrenreich 2010), and involving a family member or roommate as a direct observer of daily medication adherence is helpful (O'Farrell et al. 1995).

Given the physiological consequences of drinking in combination with disulfiram and the evidence for efficacy of naltrexone and acamprosate, disulfiram is not generally chosen as an initial therapy. However, there may be circumstances in which an individual patient prefers disulfiram or has a clear goal of abstinence for which disulfiram would be indicated. Although results have been mixed, disulfiram has also been used in individuals with cocaine use disorder, either as a primary diagnosis (Carroll et al. 2000; Higgins et al. 1993; Pettinati et al. 2008a) or co-occurring with AUD (Carroll et al. 2012; Kosten et al. 2013; Oliveto et al. 2011; Pani et al. 2010). There is no evidence available regarding the duration of treatment with disulfiram; therefore, decisions are likely to be based on individual factors such as patient preference, disorder severity, history of relapses, potential consequences of relapse, clinical response, and tolerability.

Before disulfiram is prescribed, patients should be fully informed of the physiological consequences of consuming alcohol while taking disulfiram and should agree to taking the medication. They should be instructed to abstain from drinking alcohol for at least 12 hours before taking a dose of the medication and be advised that reactions with alcohol can occur up to 14 days after taking disulfiram. It is important to caution patients that a reaction can be provoked by any product containing alcohol (e.g., certain mouthwashes and cold remedies, alcohol-based hand sanitizer, some foods or beverages, some formulations of medications). For example, the oral concentrate formulation of sertraline contains 12% alcohol, and the oral solution of ritonavir contains 43% alcohol. Ritonavir and other antiretroviral medications can also interact with disulfiram and affect disulfiram levels through cytochrome P450 3A4 isoenzymes (McCance-Katz et al. 2014). In addition, the combination of disulfiram and metronidazole has been associated with psychosis and a confusional state (Rothstein and Clancy 1969), although psychosis has also been reported with disulfiram independent of concomitant metronidazole use (Larson et al. 1992).

In general, disulfiram is well tolerated (Chick 1999) at a usual dose of 250 mg daily (range 125–500 mg daily). Before starting disulfiram, baseline liver chemistries are important to assess with follow-up testing during the initial month of disulfiram therapy. Disulfiram treatment has been associated with mild increases in hepatic enzymes in about one-quarter of patients, but acute and potentially fatal hepatotoxicity has been reported in 1 per 10,000–30,000 years of disulfiram treatment (Björnsson et al. 2006; National Library of Medicine 2017c). For this reason, patients should be warned about potential symptoms and signs of liver toxicity and instructed to seek medical attention immediately if these symptoms or signs occur.

Assessment of cardiac function may also be indicated before initiating disulfiram treatment, depending on the patient's clinical history. The risk of tachycardia with concomitant consumption of alcohol may preclude use of disulfiram in individuals with a recent myocardial infarction, coronary artery disease, or other significant cardiovascular issue. Alcohol consumption during disulfiram treatment for cocaine dependence has been associated with QTc prolongation (Roache et al. 2011). Disulfiram has also been reported to cause reversible increases in blood pressure, perhaps through actions on the enzyme dopamine-β-hydroxylase (Rogers et al. 1979; Volicer and Nelson 1984).

Disulfiram is not generally recommended in patients with a seizure disorder because of the possibility of accidental disulfiram-alcohol reactions. A seizure in the absence of a prior seizure disorder or disulfiram-alcohol reaction has also been reported with disulfiram use (Kulkarni and Bairy 2015; McConchie et al. 1983). In diabetes and other disorders with significant autonomic dysregulation, disulfiram should be used with caution. In addition, neuropathy has been reported with disulfiram (Frisoni and Di Monda 1989), and disulfiram may augment neuropathy associated with diabetes. For discussion of the use of disulfiram in women who are pregnant or breastfeeding, see guideline Statement 14.

Given the potential for disulfiram inducing medical emergencies and possible drug-drug interactions with specific medications, it is important to advise patients to carry a wallet card noting that they are taking disulfiram so this information will be available to emergency personnel (U.S. Department of Health and Human Services 2007).

Balancing of Potential Benefits and Harms in Rating the Strength of the Guideline Statement

Benefits

Benefits of disulfiram on alcohol-related outcomes were not reported in the AHRQ review. However, a subsequent meta-analysis (Skinner et al. 2014) that included randomized open-label studies (low strength of research evidence) showed a moderate effect of disulfiram as compared with no disulfiram as well as compared with acamprosate, naltrexone, and topiramate. In studies where medication adherence was assured through supervised administration, the effect of disulfiram was large (Skinner et al. 2014).

Harms

There were insufficient data on harms of disulfiram to conduct a meta-analysis in the AHRQ report. When randomized open-label studies were included (low strength of research evidence; Skinner et al. 2014), there was a significantly greater number of adverse events with disulfiram than with control conditions. Significant harms have been reported if alcohol-containing products are ingested concomitantly with disulfiram use.

Patient Preferences

Because of the aversive effects of disulfiram, some patients may prefer to take it as compared with other AUD pharmacotherapies or nonpharmacological treatments to help strengthen their motivation to abstain from alcohol. Other patients may prefer not to take disulfiram because of the potential for significant adverse events if it is ingested concomitantly with alcohol.

Balancing of Benefits and Harms

The potential benefits of this statement were viewed as likely to outweigh the harms. (See Appendix B, Statement 10 for additional discussion of the research evidence.) The strength of research evidence is rated as low because there were insufficient data from double-blind randomized controlled trials (RCTs), and the bulk of the research evidence for benefits and harms was from randomized open-label studies. With carefully selected patients in clinical trials, adverse events were somewhat greater with disulfiram. However, serious adverse events were few and comparable in numbers to serious adverse events in comparison groups consistent with the long history of safe use of disulfiram in clinical practice. Consequently, the potential benefits of disulfiram were viewed as likely to outweigh the harms for most patients given the medium to large effect size for the benefit of disulfiram when open-label studies are considered and particularly compared with the harms of continued alcohol use. In addition, it was noted that even small effect sizes may be clinically meaningful because of the significant morbidity associated with AUD. The strength of the guideline statement (suggestion) was influenced both by the strength of research evidence and by patient preferences related to disulfiram as compared with other interventions.

Differences of Opinion Among Writing Group Members

There were no differences of opinion. The writing group voted unanimously in favor of this suggestion.

Quality Measurement Considerations

As a suggestion, this statement is inappropriate for use as a quality measure. However, a quality measure could examine receipt of AUD pharmacotherapy more broadly, as has been suggested by an expert panel convened by the RAND Corporation to identify potential AUD-related quality measures (Hepner et al. 2017). The ASAM Performance Measures for the Addiction Specialist Physician also include a suggested measure related to receipt of AUD pharmacotherapy (American Society of Addiction Medicine 2014).

STATEMENT 11: Topiramate or Gabapentin

APA *suggests* **(2C)** that topiramate or gabapentin be offered to patients with moderate to severe alcohol use disorder who

- have a goal of reducing alcohol consumption or achieving abstinence,
- prefer topiramate or gabapentin or are intolerant to or have not responded to naltrexone and acamprosate, and
- have no contraindications to the use of these medications.

Implementation

Several additional medications may be efficacious in the treatment of moderate to severe AUD. These include topiramate and gabapentin. Although these medications will typically be used after trials of naltrexone and acamprosate, patient preference may lead to earlier use. Other factors that can guide medication selection include ease of administration, side effect profile, and the presence of co-occurring conditions that would affect treatment with a specific medication. There is no specific evidence on the optimal duration of treatment with these medications; such decisions are likely to be based on individual factors such as patient preference, disorder severity, history of relapses, potential consequences of relapse, clinical response, and tolerability. For discussion of the use of these medications in women who are pregnant or breastfeeding, see guideline Statement 14.

In clinical trials, topiramate was associated with significant reductions in the percent of heavy drinking days and the percent of drinking days in most (Johnson et al. 2003, 2007; Knapp et al. 2015; Kranzler et al. 2014a), but not all (Kampman et al. 2013; Likhitsathian et al. 2013), studies. Some studies also showed improvements in other drinking outcomes, such as drinks per drinking day and abstinence (Knapp et al. 2015; Kranzler et al. 2014a), the subjective experience of "craving" (Johnson et al. 2003; Kranzler et al. 2014b; Martinotti et al. 2014), and quality of life and well-being (Johnson et al. 2004a). Topiramate was typically administered at doses of 200–300 mg daily, but gradual dose titration may minimize some of the medication's adverse effects. Because of its association with weight loss in 4%–21% of patients (Micromedex 2017d), topiramate may be a medication to consider in patients with obesity. Other common side effects of topiramate include sedation, cognitive dysfunction (e.g., effects on short-term memory, 3%–12%), dizziness (4%–25%), paresthesias (1%–51%), and gastrointestinal side effects (2%–11% vs. 6% in placebo) (Micromedex 2017d). In AUD patients, clinical trials most often reported dizziness, paresthesias, taste abnormalities, decreased appetite or weight loss, and cognitive or memory effects as occurring more often with topiramate than with placebo (Johnson et al. 2003, 2007; Kampman et al. 2013; Knapp et al. 2015; Kranzler et al. 2014a; Likhitsathian et al. 2013). Less common but notable side effects include metabolic acidosis, nephrolithiasis, and precipitation of acute angle-closure glaucoma. When initiating treatment with topiramate, it may be appropriate to assess cognitive status at baseline and renal function. In individuals with renal impairment, the dose of topiramate will need a reduction. Caution is also warranted in patients at risk for falls, including the elderly.

Gabapentin, at doses between 900 and 1800 mg/day, was associated with an increased rate of abstinence (number needed to treat [NNT]=8 for 1800 mg daily) and a reduction in heavy drinking days (NNT=5 for 1800 mg daily) in a 12-week double-blind, randomized, placebo-controlled, dose-ranging study (Mason et al. 2014). Reductions were also noted in drinking quantity and frequency, GGT, craving, mood, and insomnia. Several small randomized trials of shorter duration also showed benefit of gabapentin on alcohol-related outcomes (Anton et al. 2009, 2011; Furieri and Nakamura-Palacios 2007). In patients with AUD treated with gabapentin, there were no differences in the number, severity, or type of reported adverse effects (Mason et al. 2014). Fatigue (23%), insomnia (18%), and headache (14%) were noted most often, but rates with gabapentin did not differ from placebo. Some individuals have been noted to misuse gabapentin (Mersfelder and Nichols 2016), and attention for possible misuse may be warranted if prescribing gabapentin for treatment of AUD (Evoy et al. 2017). In individuals with renal impairment, the dose of gabapentin requires adjustment because gabapentin does not undergo metabolism and is excreted unchanged, predominantly in urine (Micromedex 2017b).

Other medications are being investigated for use in the treatment of AUD; however, the evidence for their use is more limited. Examples include zonisamide and ondansetron. Alcohol-related outcomes were also reduced by varenicline in several studies (de Bejczy et al. 2015; Litten et al. 2013), suggesting that varenicline may be a promising treatment of AUD, particularly for individuals with co-occurring nicotine dependence (Litten et al. 2016). Aripiprazole has been studied in a large multisite trial of AUD, and treatment was associated with reduced secondary endpoints of harm and reduced drinking, although the primary endpoint of abstinence did not differ from placebo (Anton et al. 2008a). However, aripiprazole could be considered in a patient with AUD and another indication for this medication. Findings with baclofen are mixed, and recent RCTs have found no benefit of its use in treatment for AUD (Beraha et al. 2016; Garbutt et al. 2010; Hauser et al. 2017; Ponizovsky et al. 2015). Nalmefene has also been studied in AUD in multiple European trials but is not available in the United States or Canada (Rösner et al. 2010).

Balancing of Potential Benefits and Harms in Rating the Strength of the Guideline Statement

Benefits

Topiramate is associated with moderate benefit on drinks per drinking day, percentage of heavy drinking days, and percentage of drinking days (moderate strength of research evidence). Gabapentin is associated with moderate benefit on rates of abstinence from drinking and abstinence from heavy drinking (low strength of research evidence).

Harms

Topiramate is associated with an increased likelihood of cognitive dysfunction and numbness, tingling, or paresthesias relative to placebo (moderate strength of research evidence). Dizziness, taste abnormalities, and decreased appetite or weight loss were also reported more often with topiramate in placebo-controlled trials in AUD. Metabolic acidosis has been reported when topiramate is used to treat other conditions. Less often, topiramate has been associated with the development of nephrolithiasis or acute angle-closure glaucoma. Gabapentin was not associated with an increased likelihood of adverse events relative to placebo (low strength of research evidence). In studies that examined side effects of gabapentin in other conditions reported, side effects have included dizziness and somnolence but are typically mild.

Patient Preferences

Clinical experience suggests that many patients would want to be offered the option of these pharmacotherapies for AUD, particularly if therapies such as naltrexone or acamprosate were not helpful or had contraindications. Some patients may also prefer one medication over another medication on the basis of factors such as prior treatment experiences, available medication formulations, or side effect profiles.

Balancing of Benefits and Harms

The potential benefits of this statement were viewed as likely to outweigh the harms. (See Appendix B, Statement 11 for additional discussion of the research evidence.) Gabapentin had a small positive effect, but the harm of treatment was seen as being minimal, particularly compared with the harms of continued alcohol use, as long as there was no contraindication to the use of the medication. In addition, it was noted that even small effect sizes may be clinically meaningful because of the significant morbidity associated with AUD. With topiramate, benefits were moderate, but some patients might express concern about associated cognitive effects. The role of patient preference in being offered potentially helpful medications was also taken into consideration in rating the strength of the guideline statement (suggestion). There was no evidence that directly compared these medications with each other, which also supports a role for patient preference based on factors such as medication availability or side effect profiles.

Differences of Opinion Among Writing Group Members

There were no differences of opinion. The writing group voted unanimously in favor of this suggestion.

Quality Measurement Considerations

As a suggestion, this statement is inappropriate for use as a quality measure. However, a quality measure could also examine receipt of AUD pharmacotherapy more broadly, as has been suggested by an expert panel convened by the RAND Corporation on AUD-related quality measures (Hepner et al. 2017). The ASAM Performance Measures for the Addiction Specialist Physician also include a suggested measure related to receipt of AUD pharmacotherapy (ASAM 2014).

Recommendations Against Use of Specific Medications

STATEMENT 12: Antidepressants

APA *recommends* **(1B)** that antidepressant medications not be used for treatment of alcohol use disorder unless there is evidence of a co-occurring disorder for which an antidepressant is an indicated treatment.

Implementation

Antidepressant medications are not recommended for treating AUD unless a co-occurring disorder such as a depressive or anxiety disorder is present that would warrant such treatment. When antidepressant medications have been studied in individuals with AUD and no co-occurring disorders, minimal efficacy was noted for alcohol-related outcomes for samples as a whole, and, in some studies, outcomes worsened. Individuals with specific patterns of high-risk or severe drinking or early onset of problem drinking may be more prone to exhibiting an increase in alcohol consumption (Dundon et al. 2004; Kranzler et al. 1996, 2012a; Pettinati et al. 2000), whereas a small subgroup of individuals with later onset and low risk or severity may show some benefit from antidepressants (Dundon et al. 2004; Kranzler et al. 1996, 2012a; Pettinati et al. 2000). Genetic factors (e.g., SLC6A4 genotype) may modulate these responses (Kranzler et al. 2011).

AUD often co-occurs with other psychiatric disorders, and individuals with AUD have increased odds of having a mood or anxiety disorder as compared with those without AUD (Lai et al. 2015). Among individuals with a 12-month prevalence of any AUD, the 12-month prevalence of any mood disorder is 18.9%, and the 12-month prevalence of any anxiety disorder (including specific phobia) is 17.1% (Grant et al. 2004). The 12-month prevalence of a mood or anxiety disorder is even larger in individuals with moderate to severe AUD and in individuals who seek treatment for AUD (Grant et al. 2004; Kaufmann et al. 2014). Thus, about one-third of individuals who seek treatment for AUD will have a major depressive disorder that is independent of alcohol intoxication or withdrawal (Grant et al. 2004). When AUD co-occurs with a mood disorder or an anxiety disorder, it can affect access to care and reduces treatment outcomes for both types of disorders (Drake et al. 2001). Consequently, the initial evaluation of a patient with AUD should include assessment for co-occurring psychiatric disorders. (See guideline Statement 4.) In determining whether an antidepressant medication is indicated for a co-occurring diagnosis, it is essential to keep in mind that use of alcohol or withdrawal from alcohol can be associated with mood or anxiety symptoms that can mimic a mood or anxiety disorder. In addition, AUD can be associated with psychosocial stressors (e.g., family issues, employment or financial difficulties, legal problems) that can also influence mood or be associated with anxiety. Thus, a careful consideration of differential diagnostic possibilities (American Psychiatric Association 2013) is important before embarking on treatment. Research is limited, but with depression, symptoms that appear to be independent of alcohol may respond better to antidepressant medications than do symptoms of substance-induced depression (Foulds et al. 2015). If an antidepressant medication is indicated for a co-occurring condition, it can be used in combination with other AUD pharmacotherapies. For example, in one randomized placebo-controlled trial conducted in individuals with AUD and major depressive disorder, a combination of sertraline plus naltrexone produced a higher rate of abstinence and a longer time to relapse to heavy drinking than naltrexone alone, sertraline alone, or placebo, with fewer serious adverse events with combination treatment as compared with other treatment groups (Pettinati et al. 2010). In another study of predominantly male veterans with co-occurring AUD and PTSD, all groups showed reductions in PTSD symptoms, but combination treatment with naltrexone and an antidepressant was associated with reduced craving as compared with groups treated with antidepressant plus placebo (Petrakis et al. 2012).

Balancing of Potential Benefits and Harms in Rating the Strength of the Guideline Statement

Benefits

The benefits of this statement are that patients would not be exposed to antidepressant medications (with the associated possibility of side effects) or increased alcohol consumption when a therapeutic response to those medications would be unlikely in terms of alcohol-related outcomes (moderate strength of research evidence).

Harms

The harms of this statement are that some individuals may not be offered a medication that could be useful to them in reducing drinking behaviors.

Patient Preferences

Clinical experience suggests that few patients would want to receive a medication that may have side effects and that is unlikely to improve alcohol-related outcomes.

Balancing of Benefits and Harms

The potential benefits of avoiding side effects from a treatment that is likely to be ineffective for AUD was viewed as far outweighing the potential harms of restricting access to antidepressants to a small number of patients whose AUD may show some response. In addition, in a subset of individuals, alcohol-related outcomes appear to worsen with antidepressant treatment when used for AUD alone. (See Appendix B, Statement 12 for additional discussion of the research evidence.) Individuals with other indications for treatment with an antidepressant agent for co-occurring depressive disorders, anxiety disorders, or PTSD would still be able to receive an antidepressant for those conditions. The strength of the guideline statement (recommendation) was influenced both by the strength of research evidence and by patient preferences for avoiding medication side effects and avoiding ineffective therapies.

Differences of Opinion Among Writing Group Members

There were no differences of opinion. The writing group voted unanimously in favor of this recommendation.

Quality Measurement Considerations

This statement is not likely to be appropriate for use as a quality measure because the recommendation would not pertain to the majority of individuals with AUD. However, this recommendation may be appropriate for use in the Choosing Wisely initiative. It could also be used as an internal or health system–based quality improvement measure if prescribing of antidepressant medications appears to be frequent among patients with AUD. Furthermore, this recommendation could be integrated into electronic clinical decision support. If an order for an antidepressant is entered for an individual with AUD, the clinicians could be alerted to consider whether or not antidepressant therapy is indicated. The alert could be configured so that it would not be presented to the clinician for patients with a documented problem or diagnosis of major depressive disorder, obsessive-compulsive disorder, PTSD, or panic disorder with or without agoraphobia.

STATEMENT 13: Benzodiazepines

APA *recommends* **(1C)** that in individuals with alcohol use disorder, benzodiazepines not be used unless treating acute alcohol withdrawal or unless a co-occurring disorder exists for which a benzodiazepine is an indicated treatment.

Implementation

There is no evidence for the use of benzodiazepines in the primary treatment of AUD, except for alcohol detoxification or the treatment of alcohol withdrawal, which are outside the scope of this practice guideline. Similarly, there is no evidence related to the use of other sedative-hypnotic medications such as barbiturates, meprobamate, or nonbenzodiazepine hypnotics (zolpidem, eszopiclone, zaleplon) in individuals with AUD. Clinicians should exercise caution because the use of benzodiazepines or other sedative-hypnotic agents in the setting of alcohol intoxication carries with it an increased risk for sedation, behavioral impairment, respiratory depression, and death in severe cases (Bachhuber et al. 2016). Clinicians should discuss this risk with patients who are actively drinking alcohol and consider other treatments or medications when possible. For example, in a patient with an anxiety disorder and AUD, use of psychotherapy or an antidepressant medication would be indicated before considering a benzodiazepine or other sedating medication with addictive potential. Although there may still be limited circumstances in which prescribing a benzodiazepine or sedative-hypnotic agent is appropriate for treating a co-occurring disorder, if a benzodiazepine is prescribed, one might consider prescribing only a limited quantity at the lowest possible dose in order to mitigate potential risks.

Balancing of Potential Benefits and Harms in Rating the Strength of the Guideline Statement

Benefits

The benefits of this statement are that patients would not be exposed to medication that would be unlikely to treat AUD. In avoiding the use of benzodiazepines or other sedative-hypnotic medications, the patient also would be less susceptible to developing misuse of or tolerance to these medications and would not be exposed to the increased risk of a potentially lethal overdose when these medications are taken in combination with alcohol or other substances.

Harms

The harms of this statement are that some individuals may not be offered a medication that could be useful to them as an individual.

Patient Preferences

Some patients may request treatment with a benzodiazepine on the basis of short-term anxiolytic effects or beliefs that it may serve as a substitute for alcohol. However, generally, patients do not want to receive a medication that may have side effects and that is unlikely to improve outcomes for their condition.

Balancing of Benefits and Harm

The potential benefits of avoiding side effects from a treatment that is likely to be ineffective for AUD was viewed as far outweighing the potential harms of restricting access to benzodiazepines to a small number of patients whose AUD or other symptoms may show some response. (See Appendix B, Statement 13 for additional discussion of the research evidence.) The potential for developing tolerance to or misuse of benzodiazepines was given additional weight in the recommendation to avoid using this class of medications in a patient with AUD except for the acute treatment of alcohol withdrawal. Individuals with other indications for treatment with a benzodiazepine would still be able to receive the medication after consideration of the advantages and disadvantages for the individual and after considering using other pharmacotherapies or nonpharmacological treatment options. In determining the strength of the guideline statement (recommendation), the fact that some patients may desire treatment with a benzodiazepine was given less weight than the potential for side effects, misuse, or developing tolerance to benzodiazepines, particularly because no studies have examined whether benzodiazepines or other sedative-hypnotic medications have any efficacy in reducing drinking behaviors.

Differences of Opinion Among Writing Group Members

There were no differences of opinion. The writing group voted unanimously in favor of this recommendation.

Quality Measurement Considerations

This statement is not likely to be appropriate for use as a quality measure. Most clinicians are already aware of the potential difficulties in using benzodiazepines to treat an individual with AUD unless acute alcohol withdrawal or another appropriate indication is present. However, this recommendation may be appropriate for use in the Choosing Wisely initiative. In addition, this recommendation may be appropriate for integration into electronic clinical decision support. Clinicians could be alerted to consider whether an appropriate indication exists for benzodiazepine treatment if a benzodiazepine order is entered for an individual with a documented problem with or diagnosis of AUD.

STATEMENT 14: Pharmacotherapy in Pregnant or Breastfeeding Women

APA *recommends* (1C) that for pregnant or breastfeeding women with alcohol use disorder, pharmacological treatments not be used unless treating acute alcohol withdrawal with benzodiazepines or unless a co-occurring disorder exists that warrants pharmacological treatment.

Implementation

Alcohol use during pregnancy can contribute to an increased risk of congenital malformations or later intellectual disability (Harris et al. 2017; Huang et al. 2016) as well as an increased risk of fetal alcohol spectrum disorders (Gupta et al. 2016; Riley et al. 2011). With pharmacotherapies for AUD, there is limited evidence regarding the potential risks to an exposed fetus or infant (Briggs and

Freeman 2015). As with other medications, however, the risks to the fetus are likely to be greatest during the first trimester (Mitchell et al. 2011). On the basis of data in pregnant women, there does appear to be an increased risk of malformation associated with the use of topiramate (Alsaad et al. 2015; Briggs and Freeman 2015; Tennis et al. 2015; Weston et al. 2016). Data in pregnant animals are not available for disulfiram but suggest a moderate risk for use of naltrexone, high risk for use of acamprosate, and possible risks for use of gabapentin and topiramate (Briggs and Freeman 2015). For these reasons, it is recommended that nonpharmacological interventions be used preferentially for treating AUD during pregnancy. For individuals who become pregnant while taking a medication to treat AUD, the risk of continuing or stopping pharmacological treatment should be individualized to the patient and discussed with the patient, her obstetrician, and, if applicable, her partner. Potential risk to the fetus from medication should be balanced against the risk of relapse to alcohol use, which itself carries teratogenic risk.

Decisions about breastfeeding and use of these medications in breastfeeding women also require individualized discussion with the patient and the infant's pediatrician in balancing the benefits of breastfeeding and potential harms of exposure to medication in breast milk. Again, data are limited, but there may be potential for toxicity with disulfiram, naltrexone, and topiramate (Briggs and Freeman 2015), whereas acamprosate and gabapentin are noted to be "probably compatible" with breast-feeding (Briggs and Freeman 2015).

Balancing of Potential Benefits and Harms in Rating the Strength of the Guideline Statement

Benefits

The benefits of this statement are that a fetus or infant would not be exposed to medication used to treat AUD, and the potential for adverse events (including malformations) from such an exposure would be minimized.

Harms

The potential harms of this statement are that a woman might not receive treatment with medication for AUD and would not experience any associated reductions in drinking behavior from AUD pharmacotherapy. This could also contribute to harms for the fetus or infant due to the effects of ongoing alcohol use.

Patient Preferences

Clinical experience suggests that most women who are pregnant or breastfeeding prefer to use nonpharmacological treatment approaches as compared with pharmacotherapy to minimize the risk of possible malformations or side effects in their child.

Balancing of Benefits and Harms

The potential benefits of avoiding medications for AUD treatment while pregnant or breastfeeding were viewed as far outweighing the potential harms of restricting access to these medications. (See Appendix B, Statement 14 for additional discussion of the research evidence.) In determining the strength of the guideline statement (recommendation), the relatively small magnitude of clinical benefit with naltrexone and acamprosate was considered (moderate strength of research evidence), as well as the uncertainty of knowledge about teratogenic effects of these medications. The balance of benefits and harms was less clear for topiramate and gabapentin. The guideline statement also considers the preference of most women and their partners to avoid medications if pregnant or breastfeeding as far as possible.

Differences of Opinion Among Writing Group Members

There were no differences of opinion. The writing group voted unanimously in favor of this is recommendation.

Quality Measurement Considerations

This statement is not likely to be appropriate for use as a quality measure. The recommendation would not pertain to the majority of individuals with AUD, and adherence with this recommendation is already likely to be high as a result of the patient and clinician concern about use of medication while the patient is pregnant or breastfeeding. However, this recommendation may be appropriate for integration into electronic clinical decision support. In women who are pregnant or breastfeeding, clinicians could be alerted to avoid pharmacotherapy for AUD except under the circumstances noted in the recommendation.

STATEMENT 15: Acamprosate in Severe Renal Impairment

APA *recommends* (1C) that acamprosate not be used by patients who have severe renal impairment.

Implementation

Because of the excretion of acamprosate through the kidneys, serum creatinine should be measured at baseline, and in individuals with a history of renal impairment, results should be reviewed before initiating treatment. A CrCl less than 30 mL/min or an eGFR less than 30 mL/min/1.73 m^2 is a contraindication to the use of acamprosate, and a different medication such as naltrexone should be used.

Balancing of Potential Benefits and Harms in Rating the Strength of the Guideline Statement

Benefits

Avoiding use of acamprosate in patients with severe renal impairment is beneficial because the patient would also avoid experiencing toxicity from excessive drug levels as a result of reduced clearance of acamprosate.

Harms

The potential harm of this recommendation is that it could restrict access to acamprosate for a patient who might otherwise benefit from it.

Patient Preferences

Clinical experience suggests that few patients would want to receive a medication that may have significant increases in potential toxicity in the presence of severe co-occurring renal impairment.

Balancing of Benefits and Harms

The potential benefits of this recommendation were viewed as far outweighing the potential harms. (See Appendix B, Statement 15 for additional discussion of the research evidence.) This recommendation is rated as having a low strength of evidence because it was based on a single pharmacokinetic study in individuals with renal impairment (Sennesael 1992). The strength of the guideline statement (recommendation) was influenced by the value placed on the FDA recommendation, the availability of other effective medications, and the desire of clinicians and patients to avoid known toxicities of medication.

Differences of Opinion Among Writing Group Members

There were no differences of opinion. The writing group voted unanimously in favor of this recommendation.

Quality Measurement Considerations

This statement is not likely to be appropriate for use as a quality measure. Adherence to this recommendation is already likely to be high as a result of the FDA warning about use of acamprosate in individuals with severe renal impairment. However, this recommendation may be appropriate for integration into electronic clinical decision support. Clinicians could be alerted to use a different pharmacotherapy for AUD in individuals with a documented problem or diagnosis of severe renal impairment.

STATEMENT 16: Acamprosate in Mild to Moderate Renal Impairment

APA *recommends* (1C) that for individuals with mild to moderate renal impairment, acamprosate not be used as a first-line treatment and, if used, the dose of acamprosate be reduced compared with recommended doses in individuals with normal renal function.

Implementation

Because of the excretion of acamprosate through the kidneys, serum creatinine should be measured at baseline, and in individuals with a history of renal impairment, results should be reviewed before initiating treatment. For a CrCl between 30 and 50 mL/min or eGFR between 30 and 59 mL/min/1.73 m^2, a reduced dose of 333 mg three times per day is suggested. Alternatively, a different medication such as naltrexone could be used.

Balancing of Potential Benefits and Harms in Rating the Strength of the Guideline Statement

Benefits

Avoiding first-line use of acamprosate in patients with mild to moderate renal impairment is beneficial because the patient would avoid experiencing toxicity from excessive drug levels as a result of reduced clearance of acamprosate. Similarly, if acamprosate were used in patients with mild to moderate renal impairment, reducing the administered dose would also reduce the likelihood of experiencing toxicity.

Harms

The potential harm of this statement is that it could restrict access to acamprosate for a patient who might otherwise benefit from it.

Patient Preferences

Clinical experience suggests that when efficacy is otherwise comparable, most patients would prefer to begin treatment with a medication that is less likely to be associated with side effects. In addition, virtually all patients would want to have doses of medication adjusted to reduce the possibility of medication-related toxicity.

Balancing of Benefits and Harms

The potential benefits of this statement were viewed as far outweighing the potential harms. (See Appendix B, Statement 16 for additional discussion of the research evidence.) The benefits of this statement were expected to be greatest for individuals with moderate renal impairment, but the statement was also viewed as applicable to those with mild renal impairment because there were linear increases in acamprosate levels with reductions in CrCl (Sennesael 1992). This recommendation is rated as having a low strength of evidence because it was based on a single pharmacokinetic study (Sennesael 1992). This finding was sufficient for the FDA to include information in the package insert about reducing acamprosate doses in the presence of moderate renal impairment (Forest Pharmaceuticals 2005). The strength of the guideline statement (recommendation) was influenced by both the value placed on the FDA recommendation and the availability of other effective medications, as well as the desire of clinicians and patients to avoid known toxicities of medication.

Differences of Opinion Among Writing Group Members

There were no differences of opinion. The writing group voted unanimously in favor of this recommendation.

Quality Measurement Considerations

This statement is not likely to be appropriate for use as a quality measure. Although clinicians may be less aware of the need to adjust the dosing of acamprosate in mild to moderate renal impairment, the recommendation would not pertain to the majority of individuals with AUD. However, this recommendation may be appropriate for integration into electronic clinical decision support. Clinicians could be alerted to consider a different pharmacotherapy for AUD in individuals with a documented problem or diagnosis of renal impairment. If an order for acamprosate is placed after review of the preceding alert, clinical decision support could advise adjusting the dose of the medication in proportion to the degree of renal impairment.

STATEMENT 17: Naltrexone in Acute Hepatitis or Hepatic Failure

APA *recommends* (1C) that naltrexone not be used by patients who have acute hepatitis or hepatic failure.

Implementation

On the basis of data from clinical trials, a fraction of individuals treated with naltrexone exhibit increases in hepatic enzyme levels or other signs of hepatocellular injury (Anton et al. 2006). However, other studies have suggested that rates of elevated hepatic enzymes with naltrexone are comparable to rates with placebo, even in patient populations at increased risk for hepatic dysfunction due to co-occurring hepatitis C or HIV infection (Croop et al. 1997; Lucey et al. 2008; M.C. Mitchell et al. 2012; Tetrault et al. 2012; Vagenas et al. 2014). Nevertheless, it seems prudent to avoid exposure to naltrexone in individuals who are already experiencing significant evidence of liver damage such as acute hepatitis or hepatic failure. Acamprosate could be considered in these individuals because of its lack of hepatic effects.

Liver chemistries are appropriate to obtain before treating a patient with naltrexone, with additional evaluation or consultation and follow-up liver chemistries, as indicated, depending on the extent of any abnormalities (Kwo et al. 2017). In making a determination about use of naltrexone in an individual with some elevations in liver chemistries, it is important to recognize that individuals with AUD will often have hepatic enzyme abnormalities due to alcohol use, other medications, infectious etiologies (e.g., hepatitis C), or obesity. In clinical trials, individuals were generally not excluded unless hepatic enzyme levels were more than 3 times the upper limit of normal. For comparison, the case definition of acute hepatitis C includes a peak elevated serum ALT level >200 IU/L (Centers for Disease Control and Prevention 2016), and the definition of drug-induced hepatitis includes peak ALT levels above 800 IU/L, or about 20 times the upper limit of normal (National Library of Medicine 2017b). Furthermore, decisions about whether or not to use naltrexone will balance an infrequent but potentially negative effect of naltrexone on liver function with the improvements in liver chemistries that are associated with successful treatment of AUD.

Balancing of Potential Benefits and Harms in Rating the Strength of the Guideline Statement

Benefits

Because of initial reports that naltrexone treatment may be associated with hepatic changes, including increases in liver chemistries, in a small fraction of AUD patients, it is beneficial to minimize the risk of additional hepatic damage by avoiding the use of naltrexone in patients with significant hepatic dysfunction such as acute hepatitis or hepatic failure.

Harms

The potential harm of this recommendation is that it could restrict access to naltrexone for a patient who might otherwise benefit from it.

Patient Preferences

Clinical experience suggests that few patients would want to receive a medication that may have significant increases in potential toxicity in the presence of acute hepatitis or hepatic failure.

Balancing of Benefits and Harms

The potential benefits of this recommendation were viewed as far outweighing the potential harms. (See Appendix B, Statement 17 for additional discussion of the research evidence.) The evidence for naltrexone-associated hepatoxicity is relatively weak (low strength of research evidence). Early studies of other conditions (e.g., obesity, dementia) showed severalfold elevations in hepatic transaminase levels in some patients (Knopman and Hartman 1986; Malcolm et al. 1985; Mitchell et al. 1987; Pfohl et al. 1986; Verebey and Mulé 1986), and this finding was sufficient for the FDA to include a warning that naltrexone should not be used in individuals with acute hepatitis or hepatic failure. Subsequent studies such as the COMBINE trial (Anton et al. 2006) show a small fraction of individuals (2%) with hepatic transaminase levels that reached at least five times the upper limit of normal. The strength of the guideline statement (recommendation) was influenced by both the value placed on the FDA recommendation and the availability of other effective medications, as well as the desire of clinicians and patients to avoid toxicities of medication.

Differences of Opinion Among Writing Group Members

There were no differences of opinion. The writing group voted unanimously in favor of this recommendation.

Quality Measurement Considerations

This statement is not likely to be appropriate for use as a quality measure. Adherence to this recommendation is already likely to be high as a result of the FDA warning about use of naltrexone in individuals with acute hepatitis or hepatic failure. However, this recommendation may be appropriate for integration into electronic clinical decision support. Clinicians could be alerted to consider a different pharmacotherapy for AUD in individuals with a documented problem with or diagnosis of acute hepatitis or hepatic failure.

STATEMENT 18: Naltrexone With Concomitant Opioid Use

APA *recommends* **(1C)** that naltrexone not be used as a treatment for alcohol use disorder by individuals who use opioids or who have an anticipated need for opioids.

Implementation

Because naltrexone is an opioid receptor antagonist, it is efficacious in treating both AUD and opioid use disorder. However, before starting naltrexone in either its oral or long-acting injectable formulation, outpatients must be abstinent from opioids for 7–14 days (depending on the duration of action of the opioid) because of the risk for precipitating opioid withdrawal. It is also important that patients understand the risk of precipitated withdrawal if they continue to use opioids during treatment initiation with naltrexone. Strategies for minimizing the risk of opioid withdrawal might include starting with a small test dose of oral naltrexone (e.g., 25 mg) and/or obtaining a urine drug screen for opioids before initiating treatment.

Balancing of Potential Benefits and Harms in Rating the Strength of the Guideline Statement

Benefits

It is beneficial to avoid using naltrexone in individuals who are currently using opioids because the addition of naltrexone to an opioid will produce a withdrawal syndrome. It is also beneficial to avoid using naltrexone in an individual who may need opioid medications in the near future because those medications would not have their usual efficacy if naltrexone had been previously administered.

Harms

The potential harm of this statement is that it could restrict access to naltrexone for a patient who might otherwise benefit from it. However, an individual with co-occurring AUD and opioid use disorder could receive naltrexone to treat both disorders if he or she is able to maintain abstinence for a clinically appropriate period of time before starting on naltrexone.

Patient Preferences

Clinical experience suggests that patients do not wish to experience the significant opioid withdrawal syndrome that is precipitated by giving an opioid antagonist in the presence of an opioid.

Patients also would not wish to forego adequate pain control because of a prior use of naltrexone if their anticipated pain needs cannot be adequately controlled using nonopioid medications.

Balancing of Benefits and Harms

The potential benefits of this statement were viewed as far outweighing the potential harms. (See Appendix B, Statement 18 for additional discussion of the research evidence.) Although there is no research evidence that addresses the precise clinical circumstances described in the statement, the clinical use of opioid antagonists to reverse the effects of opioid intoxication produces a predictable syndrome of opioid withdrawal that is consistent with the neurobiological mechanisms of opioid antagonists such as naltrexone. Product labeling for naltrexone warns that abruptly precipitating opioid withdrawal by administering an opioid antagonist to an opioid-dependent patient can result in severe withdrawal that in some individuals may require hospital admission and intensive care unit management. The strength of the guideline statement (recommendation) was influenced by these clinical observations as well as by patient preferences.

Differences of Opinion Among Writing Group Members

There were no differences of opinion. The writing group voted unanimously in favor of this recommendation.

Quality Measurement Considerations

This statement is not likely to be appropriate for use as a quality measure because among individuals who present for treatment of AUD, the fraction of patients who use or have an anticipated need for opioids is likely to be small. However, this recommendation may be appropriate for integration into electronic clinical decision support. At the time of placing an initial order for naltrexone, clinicians could be alerted to consider whether the individual is currently using opioids or has an anticipated need for opioids.

Treatment of Alcohol Use Disorder and Co-occurring Opioid Use Disorder

STATEMENT 19: Naltrexone for Co-occurring Opioid Use Disorder

APA *recommends* (1C) that in patients with alcohol use disorder and co-occurring opioid use disorder, naltrexone be prescribed to individuals who

- wish to abstain from opioid use and either abstain from or reduce alcohol use and
- are able to abstain from opioid use for a clinically appropriate time prior to naltrexone initiation.

Implementation

Because naltrexone is an opioid receptor antagonist, it is efficacious in treating both AUD and opioid use disorder; however, it can be considered only in individuals who wish to abstain from opioid use. Methadone and buprenorphine exhibit the best efficacy for treatment of opioid use disorder (Kampman and Jarvis 2015; Mattick et al. 2014), and acamprosate or other pharmacotherapies can be given concomitantly to address AUD. If naltrexone is used for individuals with co-occurring AUD and opioid use disorder, adherence can be assured more readily by the use of a long-acting formulation of naltrexone. Studies of oral naltrexone in individuals with opioid use disorder suggest that with poor adherence, efficacy is limited and mortality is greater than with long-acting injectable or implantable preparations (Degenhardt et al. 2015; Kelty and Hulse 2012; Krupitsky et al. 2011, 2012). (See guideline Statement 9 for additional details on treatment of patients with naltrexone.)

Before starting naltrexone, outpatients must be abstinent from opioids for 7–14 days (depending on the duration of action of the opioid) because of the risk of precipitating opioid withdrawal. For patients being treated with an opioid agonist (e.g., methadone, buprenorphine), protocols have been developed for transitioning to antagonist therapy with naltrexone (Mannelli et al. 2012). In addition, strategies for minimizing the risk of opioid withdrawal might include starting with a small test dose of oral naltrexone (e.g., 25 mg) and/or obtaining a urine drug screen for opioids before initiating treatment. If prescription-related information is available through an electronic medical record or prescription drug monitoring program, it should be checked for current or recent opioid prescriptions. Coordinating care with other clinicians is also important. Patients should be warned about returning to opioid use after being on naltrexone because tolerance will be much reduced and the risk of a fatal overdose is greater. It is also advisable for patients to carry a wallet card noting that they are taking naltrexone so this information will be available to emergency personnel. A template for wallet cards as well as sample templates for documenting medication management visits are available through NIAAA (U.S. Department of Health and Human Services 2007).

Balancing of Potential Benefits and Harms in Rating the Strength of the Guideline Statement

Benefits

Naltrexone has benefits in treating AUD (see Statement 9), and evidence from some studies supports the efficacy of naltrexone in individuals with opioid use disorder (Larney et al. 2014; Minozzi et al. 2011; Timko et al. 2016). It is also beneficial to treat both disorders with a single medication in order to reduce the potential for some side effects and for medication interactions. Adherence to treatment may also be improved by less complicated medication regimens.

Harms

The harms of treating AUD and co-occurring opioid use disorder with naltrexone are that a patient may not experience therapeutic benefits from naltrexone for both disorders. Alterations in hepatic function are also possible with naltrexone. In addition, individuals taking naltrexone would not be able to take opioids for pain, so other treatments for acute pain would be needed. For individuals treated with long-acting injectable naltrexone, which is the preferred formulation for those with opioid use disorder, pain or induration can occur at the injection site. Also, with long durations of naltrexone use, individuals become more sensitive to doses of opioids that they would have previously tolerated, which can result in overdose and death if large opioid doses are taken.

Patient Preferences

Most patients prefer to take the smallest number of medications that will address all their symptoms and diagnoses, with the goals of minimizing side effects, cost, and inconvenience in taking multiple medications or doses.

Balancing of Benefits and Harms

The potential benefits of this statement were viewed as far outweighing the potential harms. (See Appendix B, Statement 19 for additional discussion of the research evidence.) Clinical experience supports the value of prescribing the smallest number of medications and medication doses that will address the patient's clinical condition. Although there is no research evidence that addresses the precise clinical circumstances described in the recommendation, the strength of the guideline statement (recommendation) was influenced by the evidence for naltrexone efficacy in both AUD and opioid use disorder for individuals who wish to abstain from opioid use as well as by clinical experience and patient preferences.

Differences of Opinion Among Writing Group Members

There were no differences of opinion. The writing group voted unanimously in favor of this recommendation.

Quality Measurement Considerations

This statement is not likely to be appropriate for use as a quality measure because the fraction of patients who have AUD and a co-occurring opioid use disorder is likely to be small. However, this recommendation may be appropriate for integration into electronic clinical decision support. Clinicians could be alerted to consider whether naltrexone would be an appropriate pharmacotherapy for individuals with documented AUD and opioid use disorder as a problem or diagnosis.

Areas for Further Research

This practice guideline incorporates available evidence on the treatment of AUD; however, additional research is essential (Jonas et al. 2014; Litten et al. 2014). More knowledge is needed about the basic neurobiology and genetics of AUD if we are to understand the etiology of this disorder and develop novel treatments. In terms of clinical practice, most knowledge of assessment and documentation is based on clinical consensus. Well-designed studies can be difficult to conduct when they include topics such as the following:

- Developing and documenting a comprehensive, person-centered, evidence-based plan of treatment
- Discussing, gaining patient agreement to, and documenting initial goals of treatment, including legal obligations and risks to self or others
- Assessing current and past tobacco, alcohol, and other substance use
- Assessing for co-occurring conditions that are common in individuals with AUD or that would influence treatment choices

In terms of other means of assessing individuals with AUD, additional research is needed on topics such as the following:

- Optimizing selection and use of quantitative measures for initial evaluation and for longitudinal monitoring
- Individualizing selection of a physiological biomarker for initial evaluation and for longitudinal monitoring, based on the goals of treatment, goals of monitoring, and test performance (including predictive value)
- Determining the appropriate frequency of longitudinal monitoring with quantitative measures and with physiological biomarkers

Although naltrexone and acamprosate have been well studied in placebo-controlled and some head-to-head trials, other pharmacotherapies for AUD require additional study with adequately powered sample sizes and appropriate methods for analysis of missing data. We also need more knowledge on the efficacy, effectiveness, and adverse events of available and novel pharmacotherapies for AUD in individuals with

- Other co-occurring psychiatric conditions (including other substance use disorders)
- Co-occurring medical conditions, including obesity, significant cardiac disease, chronic kidney disease, and significant hepatic disease (including cirrhosis) and in individuals who have had a liver transplant
- Differing severities of AUD, including mild AUD
- Different settings for treatment, including primary care, general ambulatory psychiatry, and specialized alcohol treatment programs

Measured outcomes should focus on quality of life, including physical and mental health, as well as outcomes related to alcohol consumption. In addition, studies need to identify the magnitude of reduction in alcohol consumption that is associated with a clinically meaningful effect on outcomes.

In terms of specific subgroups of patients, additional information is needed on the following:

- Comparative effectiveness of naltrexone versus combination therapy (e.g., acamprosate plus opioid agonist) for individuals with AUD and opioid use disorder

- Effects of alcohol pharmacotherapy in women who have become pregnant while taking one of these medications, as measured through registry studies
- Differential treatment responses that would allow personalized medication selection and dose based on factors such as the following:
  - Patient sex/gender
  - Patient age
  - Patient preferences for treatment goals or approaches
  - Pattern and amount of alcohol consumption
  - Age of onset of AUD
  - Duration of AUD
  - Family history of AUD
  - Pharmacogenetic alleles and other biomarkers identified through genomics, epigenomics, transcriptomics, proteomics, and metabolomics
  - Biomarkers identified through brain imaging
  - Prior response (or lack of response) to treatment
  - Concomitant treatments
  - Presence or absence of specific co-occurring disorders or symptoms (e.g., suicidal ideas, aggressive behaviors, anxiety)

Other aspects of clinical pharmacotherapy for AUD that require head-to-head comparison studies and additional research include the following:

- Optimal period of abstinence (if any) before initiating treatment with a specific pharmacotherapy
- Use of AUD pharmacotherapy, such as disulfiram or naltrexone, on a short-term basis to reduce initial risk of relapse after hospitalization or detoxification
- Initiation of treatment while the patient is still consuming alcohol
- Optimal type, frequency, and duration of nonpharmacological treatments used in combination with pharmacotherapies for AUD
- Duration of treatment needed once the patient has achieved abstinence or a reduction in alcohol consumption
- Duration of treatment needed before changing to a different medication in a patient with a lack of response or a partial response to treatment
- Sequence with which treatment options (including pharmacological and nonpharmacological approaches) should be used
- Impact of different medication formulations (e.g. oral, long-acting injectable, implantable) on treatment outcomes, including adverse events

Finally, we need more studies on ways to improve the quality of care that is received by individuals with AUD, including the following:

- Developing educational initiatives or health care delivery system changes to enhance guideline adherence
- Identifying approaches to address underuse of guideline-concordant pharmacotherapy of AUD
- Addressing disparities in access to and receipt of guideline-concordant treatment for AUD
- Developing improved approaches to reduce treatment dropouts and maintain adherence to pharmacotherapy
- Developing and testing of additional quality measures aimed at assuring improved patient outcomes and receipt of evidence-based care, including pharmacotherapy

Together with the already sizable evidence base on AUD and its treatment, additional research on these and other topics could lead to significant improvements in outcomes for patients with AUD.

Guideline Development Process

This guideline was developed using a process intended to meet standards of the Institute of Medicine (2011) (now known as the National Academy of Medicine). The process is fully described in a document available on the APA Web site at: www.psychiatry.org/psychiatrists/practice/clinical-practice-guidelines/guideline-development-process.

Management of Potential Conflicts of Interest

Members of the Guideline Writing Group (GWG) are required to disclose all potential conflicts of interest before appointment, before and during guideline development, and on publication. If any potential conflicts are found or disclosed during the guideline development process, the member must recuse himself or herself from any related discussion and voting on a related recommendation. The members of both the GWG and the Systematic Review Group (SRG), as well as the two consultants, reported no conflicts of interest. The Disclosures section includes more detailed disclosure information for each GWG and SRG member and for the consultants involved in the guideline's development.

Guideline Writing Group Composition

The GWG was initially composed of seven psychiatrists and one registered nurse with general research and clinical expertise. This non-topic-specific group was intended to provide diverse and balanced views on the guideline topic to minimize potential bias. For subject matter expertise, two experts on AUD were added, one of whom is board-certified in both internal medicine and addiction medicine and the other of whom is board-certified in psychiatry, with subspecialty certification in child and adolescent psychiatry. One consultant (J.M.) was also added to the GWG to provide input on quality measure considerations. An additional consultant (J.K.) assisted with drafting of guideline text. The vice-chair of the GWG (L.J.F.) provided methodological expertise on such topics as appraising the strength of research evidence. The GWG was also diverse and balanced with respect to other characteristics, such as geographical location and demographic background.

Mental Health America reviewed the draft and provided perspective from patients, families, and other care partners.

Systematic Review Methodology

The AHRQ's systematic review, *Pharmacotherapy for Adults With Alcohol-Use Disorders in Outpatient Settings* (Jonas et al. 2014), served as the predominant source of information for this guideline. Both the AHRQ review and the guideline are based on a systematic search of available research evidence using MEDLINE (PubMed), Cochrane Library, PsycINFO, CINAHL, and EMBASE databases (Table 1). The search terms and limits used are available in Appendix A. Results were limited to English-language, adult (18 and older), and human-only studies. The search that informed the

TABLE 1. Literature search results

	AHRQ search	APA search	Total
Articles identified	5844	2927	8771
PubMed	1226	124	1350
EMBASE	1730	545	2275
Cochrane	958	1838	2796
CINAHL	467	239	706
PsycINFO	1010	181	1191
Other sources	453	–	453
Duplicates removed	2423	2007	4430
Records screened	3460	920	4380
Records excluded	2924	772	3696
Articles assessed for eligibility	536	148	684
Articles excluded	369	94	463
Non-English	11	0	11
Wrong publication type	23	34	57
Wrong population	38	5	43
Wrong intervention	20	23[a]	43
Wrong comparator	52	1	53
Wrong outcome	64	4	68
Wrong setting	18	0	18
Wrong study design	90	32	122
Duration <12 weeks	46	23[b]	69
Outdated systematic review	2	0	2
Studies in qualitative synthesis	135	14	149
Articles in qualitative synthesis	167	17	184
Studies in quantitative synthesis	96	0	96

[a]Includes 19 articles on nalmefene, which is not marketed in the United States or Canada.
[b]Includes meta-analyses in which the majority of studies had a duration of less than 12 weeks.

AHRQ review (Jonas et al. 2014) was from January 1, 1970 to October 11, 2013, and the subsequent search of the literature by APA staff was from September 1, 2013 through April 24, 2016. Literature from the updated search was screened by two reviewers (L.J.F. and S.-H.H.) according to APA's general screening criteria: RCT, systematic review or meta-analysis, or observational study with a sample of at least 50 individuals; human; study of the effects of a specific intervention or psychiatric disorder or symptoms. Abstracts were then reviewed by one individual (L.J.F.), with verification by a second reviewer (S.-H.H.) to determine whether they met eligibility criteria.

Studies were included if subjects were adults (age 18 years or older) with AUD, including alcohol abuse or alcohol dependence as defined in DSM-IV-TR (American Psychiatric Association 2000), who received treatment with medications approved by the FDA for treating alcohol dependence (acamprosate, disulfiram, naltrexone) or with medications that have been used off-label or are under investigation for treatment of AUD (e.g., amitriptyline, aripiprazole, atomoxetine, baclofen, buspirone, citalopram, desipramine, escitalopram, fluoxetine, fluvoxamine, gabapentin, imipramine, nalmefene, olanzapine, ondansetron, paroxetine, prazosin, quetiapine, sertraline, topiramate, valproate, varenicline, viloxazine). Outcomes could include consumption-related outcomes (e.g., return to any drinking, return to heavy drinking, drinking days, heavy drinking days, drinks per drinking day, time to lapse or relapse), health outcomes (e.g., accidents, injuries, quality of life, function, mortality), and adverse events (including study withdrawal). Studies also needed to be published in English and to include at least 12 weeks of outpatient follow-up from the time of treatment initiation.

Exclusion criteria were studies of children and adolescents under 18 years of age, trials in which the purpose of pharmacotherapy was to treat alcohol withdrawal, trials with craving or cue reactivity as primary outcomes, studies that were conducted predominantly in inpatient settings or with follow-up of less than 12 weeks, and those that were published in languages other than English.

For each trial identified for inclusion from the updated search, risk of bias was determined (Agency for Healthcare Research and Quality 2014; Viswanathan et al. 2012) on the basis of information from each study that was extracted by one reviewer (L.J.F.) and checked for accuracy by another reviewer (S.-H.H.). In addition to specific information about each reported outcome, extracted information included citation; study design; treatment arms (including doses, sample sizes); co-intervention, if applicable; trial duration and follow-up duration, if applicable; country; setting; funding source; recruitment method; sample characteristics (mean age, percent nonwhite, percent female, percent with co-occurring condition); methods for randomization and allocation concealment; similarity of groups at baseline; overall and differential attrition; cross-overs or other contamination in group composition; adequacy of intervention fidelity; adequacy of adherence; appropriate masking of patients, outcome assessors, and care providers; validity and reliability of outcome measures; appropriateness of statistical methods and handling of missing data; appropriate methods for assessing harms (e.g., well-defined, pre-specified, well-described valid/reliable ascertainment); and adequate follow-up period for assessing harms.

Summary tables (see Appendices B and C) include specific details for each study identified for inclusion from the updated literature search and also include data on studies identified for inclusion in the AHRQ review. For studies from the AHRQ review, study details were obtained from tables published with the AHRQ review by one reviewer (S.-H.H.) and double-checked by a second reviewer (L.J.F.). Data on elements that were not included in the AHRQ review were extracted from the original articles as described above for articles from the updated search.

Available guidelines from other organizations were also reviewed (National Collaborating Centre for Mental Health 2011; Rolland et al. 2016; U.S. Department of Veterans Affairs, U.S. Department of Defense 2015).

Additional targeted searches were conducted in MEDLINE (PubMed) on alcohol biomarkers, patient preferences in AUD pharmacotherapy, and use of pharmacotherapy for AUD during pregnancy and while breastfeeding. The search terms, limits used, and dates of these searches are available in Appendix A. Results were limited to English-language, adult (18 and older), and human-only studies. These titles and abstracts were reviewed for relevance by one individual (L.J.F.).

Rating the Strength of Supporting Research Evidence

Strength of supporting research evidence describes the level of confidence that findings from scientific observation and testing of an effect of an intervention reflect the true effect. Confidence is enhanced by such factors as rigorous study design and minimal potential for study bias.

Ratings were determined, in accordance with the AHRQ's *Methods Guide for Effectiveness and Comparative Effectiveness Reviews* (Agency for Healthcare Research and Quality 2014), by the methodologist (L.J.F.) and reviewed by members of the SRG and GWG. Available clinical trials were assessed across four primary domains: risk of bias, consistency of findings across studies, directness of the effect on a specific health outcome, and precision of the estimate of effect.

The ratings are defined as follows:

- **High** (denoted by the letter *A*)=High confidence that the evidence reflects the true effect. Further research is very unlikely to change our confidence in the estimate of effect.
- **Moderate** (denoted by the letter *B*)=Moderate confidence that the evidence reflects the true effect. Further research may change our confidence in the estimate of effect and may change the estimate.
- **Low** (denoted by the letter *C*)=Low confidence that the evidence reflects the true effect. Further research is likely to change our confidence in the estimate of effect and is likely to change the estimate.

The AHRQ has an additional category of *insufficient* for evidence that is unavailable or does not permit estimation of an effect. The APA uses the *low* rating when evidence is insufficient because there is low confidence in the conclusion and further research, if conducted, would likely change the estimated effect or confidence in the estimated effect.

Rating the Strength of Recommendations

Each guideline statement is separately rated to indicate strength of recommendation and strength of supporting research evidence. *Strength of recommendation* describes the level of confidence that potential benefits of an intervention outweigh potential harms. This level of confidence is informed by available evidence, which includes evidence from clinical trials as well as expert opinion and patient values and preferences. As described in the section "Rating the Strength of Supporting Research Evidence"), this rating is a consensus judgment of the authors of the guideline and is endorsed by the APA Board of Trustees.

There are two possible ratings: recommendation or suggestion. A *recommendation* (denoted by the numeral 1 after the guideline statement) indicates confidence that the benefits of the intervention clearly outweigh harms. A *suggestion* (denoted by the numeral 2 after the guideline statement) indicates greater uncertainty. Although the benefits of the statement are still viewed as outweighing the harms, the balance of benefits and harms is more difficult to judge, or either the benefits or the harms may be less clear. With a suggestion, patient values and preferences may be more variable, and this can influence the clinical decision that is ultimately made. These strengths of recommendation correspond to ratings of *strong* or *weak* (also termed *conditional*) as defined under the GRADE method for rating recommendations in clinical practice guidelines (described in publications such as Guyatt et al. 2008 and others available on the Web site of the GRADE Working Group at http://www.gradeworkinggroup.org/).

When a negative statement is made, ratings of strength of recommendation should be understood as meaning the inverse of the above (e.g., *recommendation* indicates confidence that harms clearly outweigh benefits).

The GWG determined ratings of strength of recommendation by a modified Delphi method using blind, iterative voting and discussion. In order for the GWG members to be able to ask for clarifications about the evidence, the wording of statements, or the process, the vice-chair of the GWG served as a resource and did not vote on statements. All other formally appointed GWG members, including the chair, voted.

In weighing potential benefits and harms, GWG members considered the strength of supporting research evidence, their own clinical experiences and opinions, and patient preferences. For recommendations, at least eight out of nine members must have voted to recommend the intervention or assessment after two rounds of voting, and at most one member was allowed to vote other than "recommend" the intervention or assessment. On the basis of the discussion among the GWG members, adjustments to the wording of recommendations could be made between the voting rounds. If this level of consensus was not achieved, the GWG could have agreed to make a suggestion rather than a recommendation. No suggestion or statement could have been made if three or more members voted "no statement." Differences of opinion within the group about ratings of strength of recommendation, if any, are described in the subsection "Balancing of Potential Benefits and Harms in Rating the Strength of the Guideline Statement" for each statement.

Use of Guidelines to Enhance Quality of Care

Clinical practice guidelines can help enhance quality by synthesizing available research evidence and delineating recommendations for care on the basis of the available evidence. In some circumstances, practice guideline recommendations will be appropriate to use in developing quality measures. Guideline statements can also be used in other ways, such as educational activities or electronic clinical decision support, to enhance the quality of care that patients receive.

Typically, guideline recommendations that are chosen for development into quality measures will advance one or more aims of the Institute of Medicine's (2001) report on "Crossing the Quality Chasm" and the ongoing work guided by the multistakeholder-integrated AHRQ-led National Quality Strategy by facilitating care that is safe, effective, patient-centered, timely, efficient, and equitable. To achieve these aims, a broad range of quality measures (Watkins et al. 2015) is needed that spans the entire continuum of care (e.g., prevention, screening, assessment, treatment, continuing care), addresses the different levels of the health system hierarchy (e.g., system-wide, organization, program/department, individual clinicians), and includes measures of different types (e.g., process, outcome, patient-centered experience). Emphasis is also needed on factors that influence the dissemination and adoption of evidence-based practices (Drake et al. 2008; Greenhalgh et al. 2004; Horvitz-Lennon et al. 2009).

Measure development is complex and requires detailed development of specification and pilot testing (Center for Health Policy/Center for Primary Care and Outcomes Research and Battelle Memorial Institute 2011; Fernandes-Taylor and Harris 2012; Iyer et al. 2016; Pincus et al. 2016; Watkins et al. 2011). Generally, however, measure development should be guided by the available evidence and focused on measures that are broadly relevant, feasible to implement, and meaningful to patients, clinicians, and policy makers. Often, quality measures will focus on gaps in care or on care processes and outcomes that have significant variability across specialties, health care settings, geographic areas, or patients' demographic characteristics. Administrative databases, registries, and data from electronic health records can help to identify gaps in care and key domains that would benefit from performance improvements (Acevedo et al. 2015; Patel et al. 2015; Watkins et al. 2016). Nevertheless, for some guideline statements, evidence of practice gaps or variability will be based on anecdotal observations if the typical practices of psychiatrists and other health professionals are unknown. Variability in the use of guideline-recommended approaches may reflect appropriate differences that are tailored to the patient's preferences, treatment of co-occurring illnesses, or other clinical circumstances that may not have been studied in the available research. On the other hand, variability may indicate a need to strengthen clinician knowledge or address other barriers to adoption of best practices (Drake et al. 2008; Greenhalgh et al. 2004; Horvitz-Lennon et al. 2009). When performance is compared among organizations, variability may reflect a need for quality improvement initiatives to improve overall outcomes but could also reflect case-mix differences such as socioeconomic factors or the prevalence of co-occurring illnesses.

When a guideline recommendation is considered for development into a quality measure, it must be possible to define the applicable patient group (i.e., the denominator) and the clinical action or outcome of interest that is measured (i.e., the numerator) in validated, clear, and quantifiable terms. Furthermore, the health system's or clinician's performance on the measure must be readily ascertained from chart review, patient-reported outcome measures, registries, or administrative data. Documentation of quality measures can be challenging, and, depending on the practice setting, can pose practical barriers to meaningful interpretation of quality measures based on guideline recommendations.

For example, when recommendations relate to patient assessment or treatment selection, clinical judgment may need to be used to determine whether the clinician has addressed the factors that merit emphasis for an individual patient. In other circumstances, standardized instruments can facilitate quality measurement reporting, but it is difficult to assess the appropriateness of clinical judgment in a validated, standardized manner. Furthermore, utilization of standardized assessments remains low (Fortney et al. 2017), and clinical findings are not routinely documented in a standardized format. Many clinicians appropriately use free text prose to describe symptoms, response to treatment, discussions with family, plans of treatment, and other aspects of care and clinical decision making. Reviewing these free text records for measurement purposes would be impractical, and it would be inappropriate to hold clinicians accountable to such measures without significant increases in electronic medical record use and advances in natural language processing technology.

Conceptually, quality measures can be developed for purposes of accountability, for internal or health system–based quality improvement, or both. Accountability measures require clinicians to report their rate of performance of a specified process, intermediate outcome, or outcome in a specified group of patients. Because these data are used to determine financial incentives or penalties based on performance, accountability measures must be scientifically validated, have a strong evidence base, and fill gaps in care. In contrast, internal or health system–based quality improvement measures are typically designed by and for individual providers, health systems, or payers. They typically focus on measurements that can suggest ways for clinicians or administrators to improve efficiency and delivery of services within a particular setting. Internal or health system–based quality improvement programs may or may not link performance with payment, and, in general, these measures are not subject to strict testing and validation requirements. Quality improvement activities, including performance measures derived from these guidelines, should yield improvements in quality of care to justify any clinician burden (e.g., documentation burden) or related administrative costs (e.g., for manual extraction of data from charts, for modifications of electronic medical record systems to capture required data elements). Possible unintended consequences of any derived measures would also need to be addressed in testing of a fully specified measure in a variety of practice settings. For example, highly specified measures may lead to overuse of standardized language that does not accurately reflect what has occurred in practice. If multiple discrete fields are used to capture information on a paper or electronic record form, data will be easily retrievable and reportable, but oversimplification is a possible unintended consequence of measurement. Just as guideline developers must balance the benefits and harms of a particular guideline recommendation, developers of performance measures must weigh the potential benefits, burdens, and unintended consequences in optimizing quality measure design and testing.

External Review

This guideline was made available for review in February 2017 by stakeholders, including the APA membership, scientific and clinical experts, allied organizations, and the public. In addition, a number of patient advocacy organizations were invited for input. Forty-eight individuals and 12 organizations submitted comments on the guideline (see the section "Individuals and Organizations That Submitted Comments" for a list of the names). Dr. Raymond Anton provided significant helpful input on the implementation section of Statement 3 (Use of Physiological Biomarkers). The Chair and Co-chair of the GWG reviewed and addressed all comments received; substantive issues were reviewed by the GWG.

Funding and Approval

This guideline development project was funded and supported by the APA without any involvement of industry or external funding. The guideline was submitted to the APA Assembly and APA Board of Trustees and approved on May 20, 2017 and July 16, 2017, respectively.

Glossary of Terms

Abstinence   Avoiding or refraining from the intake of alcohol.

Acute hepatitis   An acute illness characterized by inflammation of the liver. Although hepatitis is most commonly due to viral infection, it can also result from other infections, heavy alcohol use, toxins, certain medications, and autoimmune disease. In addition to a pattern of hepatocellular injury, individuals with hepatitis have either jaundice or elevated serum alanine aminotransferase (ALT) or aspartate aminotransferase (AST) levels. Hepatitis can be asymptomatic or associated with fatigue, anorexia, nausea, and abdominal pain. Depending on the cause of the hepatitis, fever, headache, vomiting, or diarrhea can also be present (National Institute of Allergy and Infectious Disease 2017; National Library of Medicine 2017b).

Alcohol misuse   Behaviors including risky or harmful alcohol use (U.S. Preventive Services Task Force 2013).

Alcohol withdrawal   A characteristic syndrome that develops within several hours to a few days after the cessation of (or reduction in) heavy and prolonged alcohol use. See DSM-5 (American Psychiatric Association 2013) for the full criteria for alcohol withdrawal.

Assessment   The process of obtaining information about a patient through any of a variety of methods, including face-to-face interview, review of medical records, physical examination (by the psychiatrist, another physician, or a medically trained clinician), diagnostic testing, or history taking from collateral sources (American Psychiatric Association 2016).

Biomarker   A defined characteristic that is measured as an indicator of normal biological processes, pathogenic processes, or responses to an exposure or intervention, including therapeutic interventions. Molecular, histologic, radiographic, or physiological characteristics are types of biomarkers. A biomarker is not an assessment of how an individual feels, functions, or survives (FDA-NIH Biomarker Working Group 2016).

Comprehensive and person-centered treatment plan   A plan of treatment that is developed as an outgrowth of the psychiatric evaluation and is modified as clinically indicated. A comprehensive treatment plan can include nonpharmacological treatments, pharmacological treatments, or both. It is individualized to the patient's clinical presentation, safety-related needs, concomitant medical conditions, personal background, relationships, life circumstances, and strengths and vulnerabilities. There is no prescribed format that a comprehensive treatment plan must follow. The breadth and depth of the initial treatment plan will depend on the amount of time and extent of information that are available, as well as the needs of the patients and the care setting. Additions and modifications to the treatment plan are made as additional information accrues (e.g., from family, staff, medical records, and other collateral sources) and the patient's responses to clinical interventions are observed.

Contraindication   A situation in which a drug or procedure should not be used because it may be harmful to the patient.

Harm reduction   A strategy that aims to reduce or minimize the adverse health, social, and economic consequences related to the use of alcohol and other substances.

Hepatic failure   Deterioration of liver function that results in coagulation abnormality (usually an international normalized ratio [INR] greater than or equal to 1.5) and any degree of mental alteration (encephalopathy). Although there is no identifiable cause in approximately 15% of cases of acute hepatic failure, typical etiologies include drug-induced liver injury, viral hepatitis, autoimmune liver disease, and shock or hypoperfusion (Lee et al. 2011).

I^2 A statistical estimate of the proportion of the variance that is due to heterogeneity.

Initial psychiatric evaluation   A comprehensive assessment of a patient that has the following aims: identify the reason that the patient is presenting for evaluation; establish rapport with the patient; understand the patient's background, relationships, current life circumstances, and strengths and vulnerabilities; establish whether the patient has a psychiatric condition; collect information needed to develop a differential diagnosis and clinical formulation; identify immediate concerns for patient safety; and develop an initial treatment plan or revise an existing plan in collaboration with the patient. Relevant information may be obtained by interviewing the patient; reviewing prior records; or obtaining collateral information from treating clinicians, family members, or others involved in the patient's life. Physical examination, laboratory studies, imaging, psychological or neuropsychological testing, or other assessments may also be included. The psychiatric evaluation may occur in a variety of settings, including inpatient or outpatient psychiatric settings and other medical settings. The evaluation is usually time intensive. The amount of time spent depends on the complexity of the problem, the clinical setting, and the patient's ability and willingness to cooperate with the assessment. Several meetings with the patient (and family or others) over time may be necessary. Psychiatrists may conduct other types of evaluations that have other goals (e.g., forensic evaluations) or that may be more focused and circumscribed than a psychiatric evaluation as defined here. Guidelines are not intended to address such evaluations (American Psychiatric Association 2016).

Moderate to severe alcohol use disorder   An alcohol use disorder as defined by DSM-5 criteria that is associated with the presence of 4–5 symptoms for moderate AUD and 6 or more symptoms for severe AUD (American Psychiatric Association 2013).

Nonpharmacological treatments   Any of a wide variety of interventions other than medications. Some of the nonpharmacological treatments for alcohol use disorder include motivational enhancement therapy, cognitive-behavioral therapy, 12-step facilitation therapy, and community-based peer support groups such as Alcoholics Anonymous.

Over-the-counter medications or supplements   Drugs or supplements that can be bought without a prescription.

Quantitative behavioral measures   Clinician- or patient-administered tests or scales that provide a numerical rating of features such as symptom severity, level of functioning, or quality of life and have been shown to be valid and reliable (American Psychiatric Association 2016).

Renal impairment   Inability of the kidney(s) to function normally, typically described in terms of reductions in creatinine clearance or estimated glomerular filtration rate (eGFR). An eGFR of 60–89 mL/min/1.73 m^2 indicates mildly reduced kidney function, an eGFR of 30–59 mL/min/ 1.73 m^2 indicates moderately reduced kidney function, an eGFR of 15–29 mL/min/1.73 m^2 indicates severely reduced kidney function, and an eGFR of less than 15 mL/min/1.73 m^2 indicates a very severe reduction in kidney function or end-stage renal disease (Kidney Disease: Improving Global Outcomes (KDIGO) CKD Work Group 2013).

References

Abraham AJ, Knudsen HK, Roman PM: A longitudinal examination of alcohol pharmacotherapy adoption in substance use disorder treatment programs: patterns of sustainability and discontinuation. J Stud Alcohol Drugs 72(4):669–677, 2011 21683049

Abramsky T, Watts CH, Garcia-Moreno C, et al: What factors are associated with recent intimate partner violence? Findings from the WHO multi-country study on women's health and domestic violence. BMC Public Health 11:109, 2011 21324186

Acevedo A, Garnick DW, Dunigan R, et al: Performance measures and racial/ethnic disparities in the treatment of substance use disorders. J Stud Alcohol Drugs 76(1):57–67, 2015 25486394

Adamson SJ, Heather N, Morton V, Raistrick D; UKATT Research Team: Initial preference for drinking goal in the treatment of alcohol problems: II. Treatment outcomes. Alcohol Alcohol 45(2):136–142, 2010 20130150

Adamson SJ, Sellman JD, Foulds JA, et al: A randomized trial of combined citalopram and naltrexone for non-abstinent outpatients with co-occurring alcohol dependence and major depression. J Clin Psychopharmacol 35(2):143–149, 2015 25679122

Agency for Healthcare Research and Quality: Methods Guide for Effectiveness and Comparative Effectiveness Reviews. AHRQ Publ No 10(14)-EHC063-EF. Rockville, MD, Agency for Healthcare Research and Quality. January 2014. Available at: www.effectivehealthcare.ahrq.gov/search-for-guides-reviews-and-reports/?pageaction=displayproduct&productid=318. Accessed February 15, 2017.

Ahmadi J, Ahmadi N: A double blind, placebo-controlled study of naltrexone in the treatment of alcohol dependence. German Journal of Psychiatry 5(4):85–89, 2002

Ahmadi J, Babaeebeigi M, Maany I, et al: Naltrexone for alcohol-dependent patients. Ir J Med Sci 173(1):34–37, 2004 15732235

Alatalo P, Koivisto H, Puukka K, et al: Biomarkers of liver status in heavy drinkers, moderate drinkers and abstainers. Alcohol Alcohol 44(2):199–203, 2009 19054785

Allen JP, Litten RZ: Techniques to enhance compliance with disulfiram. Alcohol Clin Exp Res 16(6):1035–1041, 1992 1471757

Al-Otaiba Z, Worden BL, McCrady BS, Epstein EE: Accounting for self-selected drinking goals in the assessment of treatment outcome. Psychol Addict Behav 22(3):439–443, 2008 18778138

Alsaad AM, Chaudhry SA, Koren G: First trimester exposure to topiramate and the risk of oral clefts in the offspring: a systematic review and meta-analysis. Reprod Toxicol 53:45–50, 2015 25797654

American College of Obstetricians and Gynecologists. Committee on Health Care for Underserved Women: Committee opinion no. 496: At-risk drinking and alcohol dependence: obstetric and gynecologic implications. Obstet Gynecol 118(2 Pt 1):383–388, 2011 21775870

American Psychiatric Association: Diagnostic and Statistical Manual of Mental Disorders, 4th Edition, Text Revision. Washington, DC, American Psychiatric Association, 2000

American Psychiatric Association: Diagnostic and Statistical Manual of Mental Disorders, 5th Edition. Arlington, VA, American Psychiatric Publishing, 2013

American Psychiatric Association: Practice Guidelines for the Psychiatric Evaluation of Adults, 3rd Edition. Arlington, VA, American Psychiatric Association Publishing, 2016

American Society of Addiction Medicine: The ASAM Performance Measures for the Addiction Specialist Physician, 2014. Available at: www.asam.org/docs/default-source/advocacy/performance-measures-for-the-addiction-specialist-physician.pdf?sfvrsn=0. Accessed March 28, 2017.

Andréasson S, Danielsson AK, Wallhed-Finn S: Preferences regarding treatment for alcohol problems. Alcohol Alcohol 48(6):694–699, 2013 23842842

Andrews JC, Schünemann HJ, Oxman AD, et al: GRADE guidelines: 15. Going from evidence to recommendation-determinants of a recommendation's direction and strength. J Clin Epidemiol 66(7):726–735, 2013 23570745

Anton RF; COMBINE Study Research Group: Testing combined pharmacotherapies and behavioral interventions for alcohol dependence (the COMBINE study): a pilot feasibility study. Alcohol Clin Exp Res 27(7):1123–1131, 2003 12878918

Anton RF, Moak DH, Waid LR, et al: Naltrexone and cognitive behavioral therapy for the treatment of outpatient alcoholics: results of a placebo-controlled trial. Am J Psychiatry 156(11):1758–1764, 1999 10553740

Anton RF, Moak DH, Latham PK, et al: Posttreatment results of combining naltrexone with cognitive-behavior therapy for the treatment of alcoholism. J Clin Psychopharmacol 21(1):72–77, 2001 11199951

Anton RF, Lieber C, Tabakoff B; CDTect Study Group: Carbohydrate-deficient transferrin and gamma-glutamyltransferase for the detection and monitoring of alcohol use: results from a multisite study. Alcohol Clin Exp Res 26(8):1215–1222, 2002 12198396

Anton RF, Moak DH, Latham P, et al: Naltrexone combined with either cognitive behavioral or motivational enhancement therapy for alcohol dependence. J Clin Psychopharmacol 25(4):349–357, 2005 16012278

Anton RF, O'Malley SS, Ciraulo DA, et al; COMBINE Study Research Group: Combined pharmacotherapies and behavioral interventions for alcohol dependence: the COMBINE study: a randomized controlled trial. JAMA 295(17):2003–2017, 2006 16670409

Anton RF, Kranzler H, Breder C, et al: A randomized, multicenter, double-blind, placebo-controlled study of the efficacy and safety of aripiprazole for the treatment of alcohol dependence. J Clin Psychopharmacol 28(1):5–12, 2008a 18204334

Anton RF, Oroszi G, O'Malley S, et al: An evaluation of mu-opioid receptor (OPRM1) as a predictor of naltrexone response in the treatment of alcohol dependence: results from the Combined Pharmacotherapies and Behavioral Interventions for Alcohol Dependence (COMBINE) study. Arch Gen Psychiatry 65(2):135–144, 2008b 18250251

Anton RF, Myrick H, Baros AM, et al: Efficacy of a combination of flumazenil and gabapentin in the treatment of alcohol dependence: relationship to alcohol withdrawal symptoms. J Clin Psychopharmacol 29(4):334–342, 2009 19593171

Anton RF, Myrick H, Wright TM, et al: Gabapentin combined with naltrexone for the treatment of alcohol dependence. Am J Psychiatry 168(7):709–717, 2011 21454917

Arias AJ, Gelernter J, Gueorguieva R, et al: Pharmacogenetics of naltrexone and disulfiram in alcohol dependent, dually diagnosed veterans. Am J Addict 23(3):288–293, 2014 24724887

Ashenhurst JR, Bujarski S, Ray LA: Delta and kappa opioid receptor polymorphisms influence the effects of naltrexone on subjective responses to alcohol. Pharmacol Biochem Behav 103(2):253–259, 2012 22954510

Bachhuber MA, Hennessy S, Cunningham CO, Starrels JL: Increasing Benzodiazepine Prescriptions and Overdose Mortality in the United States, 1996-2013. Am J Public Health 106(4):686–688, 2016 26890165

Balldin J, Berglund M, Borg S, et al: A 6-month controlled naltrexone study: combined effect with cognitive behavioral therapy in outpatient treatment of alcohol dependence. Alcohol Clin Exp Res 27(7):1142–1149, 2003 12878920

Balldin J, Berggren U, Berglund K, et al: Gamma-glutamyltransferase in alcohol use disorders: modification of decision limits in relation to treatment goals? Scand J Clin Lab Invest 70(2):71–74, 2010 19929269

Balshem H, Helfand M, Schünemann HJ, et al: GRADE guidelines: 3. Rating the quality of evidence. J Clin Epidemiol 64(4):401–406, 2011 21208779

Baltieri DA, De Andrade AG: Acamprosate in alcohol dependence: a randomized controlled efficacy study in a standard clinical setting. J Stud Alcohol 65(1):136–139, 2004 15000513

Baltieri DA, Daró FR, Ribeiro PL, de Andrade AG: Comparing topiramate with naltrexone in the treatment of alcohol dependence. Addiction 103(12):2035–2044, 2008 18855810

Baltieri DA, Daró FR, Ribeiro PL, Andrade AG: Effects of topiramate or naltrexone on tobacco use among male alcohol-dependent outpatients. Drug Alcohol Depend 105(1–2):33–41, 2009 19595518

Barrio P, Gual A: Patient-centered care interventions for the management of alcohol use disorders: a systematic review of randomized controlled trials. Patient Prefer Adherence 10:1823–1845, 2016 27695301

Barrio P, Teixidor L, Ortega L, et al: Patients' knowledge and attitudes towards regular alcohol urine screening: a survey study. J Addict Med 11(4):300–307, 2017 28358755

Batki SL, Pennington DL, Lasher B, et al: Topiramate treatment of alcohol use disorder in veterans with posttraumatic stress disorder: a randomized controlled pilot trial. Alcohol Clin Exp Res 38(8):2169–2177, 2014 25092377

Beraha EM, Salemink E, Goudriaan AE, et al: Efficacy and safety of high-dose baclofen for the treatment of alcohol dependence: a multicentre, randomised, double-blind controlled trial. Eur Neuropsychopharmacol 26(12):1950–1959, 2016 27842939

Berger L, Fisher M, Brondino M, et al: Efficacy of acamprosate for alcohol dependence in a family medicine setting in the United States: a randomized, double-blind, placebo-controlled study. Alcohol Clin Exp Res 37(4):668–674, 2013 23134193

Berger L, Brondino M, Fisher M, et al: Alcohol use disorder treatment: the association of pretreatment use and the role of drinking goal. J Am Board Fam Med 29(1):37–49, 2016 26769876

Bergström JP, Helander A: Clinical characteristics of carbohydrate-deficient transferrin (%disialotransferrin) measured by HPLC: sensitivity, specificity, gender effects, and relationship with other alcohol biomarkers. Alcohol Alcohol 43(4):436–441, 2008a 18411243

Bergström JP, Helander A: Influence of alcohol use, ethnicity, age, gender, BMI and smoking on the serum transferrin glycoform pattern: implications for use of carbohydrate-deficient transferrin (CDT) as alcohol biomarker. Clin Chim Acta 388(1–2):59–67, 2008b 17980706

Bertholet N, Winter MR, Cheng DM, et al: How accurate are blood (or breath) tests for identifying self-reported heavy drinking among people with alcohol dependence? Alcohol Alcohol 49(4):423–429, 2014 24740846

Besson J, Aeby F, Kasas A, et al: Combined efficacy of acamprosate and disulfiram in the treatment of alcoholism: a controlled study. Alcohol Clin Exp Res 22(3):573–579, 1998 9622434

Björnsson E, Nordlinder H, Olsson R: Clinical characteristics and prognostic markers in disulfiram-induced liver injury. J Hepatol 44(4):791–797, 2006 16487618

Bogenschutz MP, Bhatt S, Bohan J, et al: Coadministration of disulfiram and lorazepam in the treatment of alcohol dependence and co-occurring anxiety disorder: an open-label pilot study. Am J Drug Alcohol Abuse 42(5):490–499, 2016 27184605

Book SW, Thomas SE, Randall PK, Randall CL: Paroxetine reduces social anxiety in individuals with a co-occurring alcohol use disorder. J Anxiety Disord 22(2):310–318, 2008 17448631

Borges G, Bagge CL, Cherpitel CJ, et al: A meta-analysis of acute use of alcohol and the risk of suicide attempt. Psychol Med 47(5):949–957, 2017 27928972

Bouchery EE, Harwood HJ, Sacks JJ, et al: Economic costs of excessive alcohol consumption in the U.S., 2006. Am J Prev Med 41(5):516–524, 2011 22011424

Bradley KA, Kivlahan DR: Bringing patient-centered care to patients with alcohol use disorders. JAMA 311(18):1861–1862, 2014 24825640

Bradley KA, Lapham GT, Hawkins EJ, et al: Quality concerns with routine alcohol screening in VA clinical settings. J Gen Intern Med 26(3):299–306, 2011 20859699

Brady KT, Sonne S, Anton RF, et al: Sertraline in the treatment of co-occurring alcohol dependence and posttraumatic stress disorder. Alcohol Clin Exp Res 29(3):395–401, 2005 15770115

Branas CC, Han S, Wiebe DJ: Alcohol use and firearm violence. Epidemiol Rev 38(1):32–45, 2016 26811427

Breslow RA, Dong C, White A: Prevalence of alcohol-interactive prescription medication use among current drinkers: United States, 1999 to 2010. Alcohol Clin Exp Res 39(2):371–379, 2015 25597432

Brewer C, Wong VS: Naltrexone: report of lack of hepatotoxicity in acute viral hepatitis, with a review of the literature. Addict Biol 9(1):81–87, 2004 15203443

Briggs GG, Freeman RK: Drugs in Pregnancy and Lactation: A Reference Guide to Fetal and Neonatal Risk. Philadelphia, PA, Wolters Kluwer/Lippincott Williams & Wilkins Health, 2015

Brito JP, Domecq JP, Murad MH, et al: The Endocrine Society guidelines: when the confidence cart goes before the evidence horse. J Clin Endocrinol Metab 98(8):3246–3252, 2013 23783104

Brown ES, Carmody TJ, Schmitz JM, et al: A randomized, double-blind, placebo-controlled pilot study of naltrexone in outpatients with bipolar disorder and alcohol dependence. Alcohol Clin Exp Res 33(11):1863–1869, 2009 19673746

Buchanan A, Binder R, Norko M, Swartz M: American Psychiatric Association resource document on psychiatric violence risk assessment. Washington, DC, American Psychiatric Association, 2011. Available at: www.psychiatry.org/File%20Library/Psychiatrists/Directories/Library-and-Archive/resource_documents/rd2011_violencerisk.pdf. Accessed March 22, 2017.

Bujarski S, O'Malley SS, Lunny K, Ray LA: The effects of drinking goal on treatment outcome for alcoholism. J Consult Clin Psychol 81(1):13–22, 2013 23231573

Burns E, Gray R, Smith LA: Brief screening questionnaires to identify problem drinking during pregnancy: a systematic review. Addiction 105(4):601–614, 2010 20403013

Bush K, Kivlahan DR, McDonell MB, et al: The AUDIT alcohol consumption questions (AUDIT-C): an effective brief screening test for problem drinking: Ambulatory Care Quality Improvement Project (ACQUIP) Alcohol Use Disorders Identification Test. Arch Intern Med 158(16):1789–1795, 1998 9738608

Carroll K, Ziedonis D, O'Malley SS, et al: Pharmacologic interventions for alcohol- and cocaine-abusing individuals: A pilot study of disulfiram vs. naltrexone. Am J Addict 2(1):77–79, 1993

Carroll KM, Nich C, Ball SA, et al: One-year follow-up of disulfiram and psychotherapy for cocaine-alcohol users: sustained effects of treatment. Addiction 95(9):1335–1349, 2000 11048353

Carroll KM, Nich C, Shi JM, et al: Efficacy of disulfiram and twelve step facilitation in cocaine-dependent individuals maintained on methadone: a randomized placebo-controlled trial. Drug Alcohol Depend 126(1–2):224–231, 2012 22695473

Center for Health Policy/Center for Primary Care and Outcomes Research and Battelle Memorial Institute: Quality Indicator Measure Development, Implementation, Maintenance, and Retirement (Prepared by Battelle, under Contract No 290-04-0020). Rockville, MD: Agency for Healthcare Research and Quality, May 2011. Available at: www.qualityindicators.ahrq.gov/Downloads/Resources/Publications/2011/QI_Measure_Development_Implementation_Maintenance_Retirement_Full_5-3-11.pdf. Accessed April 2, 2017.

Center for Substance Abuse and Treatment: Incorporating Alcohol Pharmacotherapies Into Medical Practice. (Treatment Improvement Protocol [TIP] No 49). Rockville, MD, Substance Abuse and Mental Health Services Administration (SAMHSA), 2009

Centers for Disease Control and Prevention (CDC): Quitting smoking among adults—United States, 2001–2010. MMWR Morb Mortal Wkly Rep 60(44):1513–1519, 2011 22071589

Centers for Disease Control and Prevention: Hepatitis C, Acute 2016 Case Definition. Atlanta, GA, Centers for Disease Control and Prevention, 2016. Available at: www.cdc.gov/nndss/conditions/hepatitis-c-acute/case-definition/2016/. Accessed March 31, 2017.

Chang G, McNamara TK, Orav EJ, Wilkins-Haug L: Brief intervention for prenatal alcohol use: the role of drinking goal selection. J Subst Abuse Treat 31(4):419–424, 2006 17084796

Chapman C, Slade T, Hunt C, Teesson M: Delay to first treatment contact for alcohol use disorder. Drug Alcohol Depend 147:116–121, 2015 25533894

Charlet K, Heinz A: Harm reduction—a systematic review on effects of alcohol reduction on physical and mental symptoms. Addict Biol 22(5):1119–1159, 2017 27353220

Charney DA, Heath LM, Zikos E, et al: Poorer drinking outcomes with citalopram treatment for alcohol dependence: a randomized, double-blind, placebo-controlled trial. Alcohol Clin Exp Res 39(9):1756–1765, 2015 26208048

Chavez LJ, Williams EC, Lapham G, Bradley KA: Association between alcohol screening scores and alcohol-related risks among female Veterans Affairs patients. J Stud Alcohol Drugs 73(3):391–400, 2012 22456244

Chen AC, Davis CM, Kahler CW, et al: 5-HTTLPR moderates naltrexone and psychosocial treatment responses in heavy drinking men who have sex with men. Alcohol Clin Exp Res 38(9):2362–2368, 2014 25070809

Cherpitel CJ: Screening for alcohol problems in the U.S. general population: comparison of the CAGE, RAPS4, and RAPS4-QF by gender, ethnicity, and service utilization: Rapid Alcohol Problems Screen. Alcohol Clin Exp Res 26(11):1686–1691, 2002 12436057

Cherpitel CJ, Ye Y, Andreuccetti G, et al: Risk of injury from alcohol, marijuana and other drug use among emergency department patients. Drug Alcohol Depend 174:121–127, 2017 28324814

Chick J: Safety issues concerning the use of disulfiram in treating alcohol dependence. Drug Saf 20(5):427–435, 1999 10348093

Chick J, Anton R, Checinski K, et al: A multicentre, randomized, double-blind, placebo-controlled trial of naltrexone in the treatment of alcohol dependence or abuse. Alcohol Alcohol 35(6):587–593, 2000a 11093966

Chick J, Howlett H, Morgan MY, Ritson B: United Kingdom Multicentre Acamprosate Study (UKMAS): a 6-month prospective study of acamprosate versus placebo in preventing relapse after withdrawal from alcohol. Alcohol Alcohol 35(2):176–187, 2000b 10787394

Chick J, Aschauer H, Hornik K; Investigators' Group: Efficacy of fluvoxamine in preventing relapse in alcohol dependence: a one-year, double-blind, placebo-controlled multicentre study with analysis by typology. Drug Alcohol Depend 74(1):61–70, 2004 15072808

Chou R, Gordon DB, de Leon-Casasola OA, et al: Management of Postoperative Pain: a clinical practice guideline from the American Pain Society, the American Society of Regional Anesthesia and Pain Medicine, and the American Society of Anesthesiologists' Committee on Regional Anesthesia, Executive Committee, and Administrative Council. J Pain 17(2):131–157, 2016b 26827847 Correction: Pain 17(4):508–510, 2016

Chou SP, Goldstein RB, Smith SM, et al: The epidemiology of DSM-5 nicotine use disorder: results from the National Epidemiologic Survey on Alcohol and Related Conditions-III. J Clin Psychiatry 77(10):1404–1412, 2016 27135834

Coller JK, Cahill S, Edmonds C, et al: OPRM1 A118G genotype fails to predict the effectiveness of naltrexone treatment for alcohol dependence. Pharmacogenet Genomics 21(12):902–905, 2011 21946895

Collins SE, Grazioli VS, Torres NI, et al: Qualitatively and quantitatively evaluating harm-reduction goal setting among chronically homeless individuals with alcohol dependence. Addict Behav 45:184–190, 2015 25697724

Compton WM, Dawson DA, Goldstein RB, Grant BF: Crosswalk between DSM-IV dependence and DSM-5 substance use disorders for opioids, cannabis, cocaine and alcohol. Drug Alcohol Depend 132(1–2):387–390, 2013 23642316

Conigrave KM, Degenhardt LJ, Whitfield JB, et al; WHO/ISBRA Study Group: CDT, GGT, and AST as markers of alcohol use: the WHO/ISBRA collaborative project. Alcohol Clin Exp Res 26(3):332 339, 2002 11923585

Conigrave KM, Davies P, Haber P, Whitfield JB: Traditional markers of excessive alcohol use. Addiction 98(Suppl 2):31–43, 2003 14984240

Cornelius JR, Salloum IM, Cornelius MD, et al: Preliminary report: double-blind, placebo-controlled study of fluoxetine in depressed alcoholics. Psychopharmacol Bull 31(2):297–303, 1995 7491382

Cornelius JR, Salloum IM, Ehler JG, et al: Fluoxetine in depressed alcoholics: a double-blind, placebo-controlled trial. Arch Gen Psychiatry 54(8):700–705, 1997 9283504

Coskunol H, Gökden O, Ercan ES, et al: Long-term efficacy of sertraline in the prevention of alcoholic relapses in alcohol-dependent patients: a single-center, double-blind, randomized, placebo-controlled, parallel-group study. Current Therapeutic Research 63(11):759–771, 2002

Council of Medical Specialty Societies: Principles for the Development of Specialty Society Clinical Guidelines. Chicago, IL, Council of Medical Specialty Societies, 2012

Croop RS, Faulkner EB, Labriola DF; The Naltrexone Usage Study Group: The safety profile of naltrexone in the treatment of alcoholism: results from a multicenter usage study. Arch Gen Psychiatry 54(12):1130–1135, 1997 9400350

Darvishi N, Farhadi M, Haghtalab T, Poorolajal J: Alcohol-related risk of suicidal ideation, suicide attempt, and completed suicide: a meta-analysis. PLoS One 10(5):e0126870, 2015 25993344

Dasgupta A: Alcohol biomarkers: an overview, in Alcohol and Its Biomarkers: Clinical Aspects and Laboratory Determination. San Diego, CA, Elsevier, 2015, pp 91–120

Dawson DA, Grant BF, Stinson FS, Chou PS: Estimating the effect of help-seeking on achieving recovery from alcohol dependence. Addiction 101(6):824–834, 2006 16696626

Dawson DA, Goldstein RB, Grant BF: Rates and correlates of relapse among individuals in remission from DSM-IV alcohol dependence: a 3-year follow-up. Alcohol Clin Exp Res 31(12):2036–2045, 2007 18034696

Dawson DA, Smith SM, Saha TD, et al: Comparative performance of the AUDIT-C in screening for DSM-IV and DSM-5 alcohol use disorders. Drug Alcohol Depend 126(3):384–388, 2012 22728044

de Bejczy A, Löf E, Walther L, et al: Varenicline for treatment of alcohol dependence: a randomized, placebo-controlled trial. Alcohol Clin Exp Res 39(11):2189–2199, 2015 26414337

De Sousa A, De Sousa A: A one-year pragmatic trial of naltrexone vs disulfiram in the treatment of alcohol dependence. Alcohol Alcohol 39(6):528–531, 2004 15525790

De Sousa A, De Sousa A: An open randomized study comparing disulfiram and acamprosate in the treatment of alcohol dependence. Alcohol Alcohol 40(6):545–548, 2005 16043433

De Sousa AA, De Sousa J, Kapoor H: An open randomized trial comparing disulfiram and topiramate in the treatment of alcohol dependence. J Subst Abuse Treat 34(4):460–463, 2008 17629442

Deady M: A review of screening, assessment and outcome measures for drug and alcohol settings. Woolloomooloo, NSW, Australia, Network of Alcohol and Other Drugs Agencies, 2009. Available at: www.nada.org.au/media/7678/review_of_measures_09.pdf. Accessed March 27, 2017.

Degenhardt L, Larney S, Kimber J, et al: Excess mortality among opioid-using patients treated with oral naltrexone in Australia. Drug Alcohol Rev 34(1):90–96, 2015 25302627

Del Fiol G, Huser V, Strasberg HR, et al: Implementations of the HL7 Context-Aware Knowledge Retrieval ("Infobutton") Standard: challenges, strengths, limitations, and uptake. J Biomed Inform 45(4):726–735, 2012 22226933

Delker E, Brown Q, Hasin DS: Alcohol consumption in demographic subpopulations: an epidemiologic overview. Alcohol Res 38(1):7–15, 2016 27159807

Dhalla S, Kopec JA: The CAGE questionnaire for alcohol misuse: a review of reliability and validity studies. Clin Invest Med 30(1):33–41, 2007 17716538

Dieperink E, Fuller B, Isenhart C, et al: Efficacy of motivational enhancement therapy on alcohol use disorders in patients with chronic hepatitis C: a randomized controlled trial. Addiction 109(11):1869–1877, 2014 25040898

Djulbegovic B, Trikalinos TA, Roback J, et al: Impact of quality of evidence on the strength of recommendations: an empirical study. BMC Health Serv Res 9:120, 2009 19622148

do Amaral RA, Malbergier A: Effectiveness of the CAGE questionnaire, gamma-glutamyltransferase and mean corpuscular volume of red blood cells as markers for alcohol-related problems in the workplace. Addict Behav 33(6):772–781, 2008 18337017

Donovan DM, Kivlahan DR, Doyle SR, et al: Concurrent validity of the Alcohol Use Disorders Identification Test (AUDIT) and AUDIT zones in defining levels of severity among out-patients with alcohol dependence in the COMBINE study. Addiction 101(12):1696–1704, 2006 17156168

Donovan DM, Anton RF, Miller WR, et al; COMBINE Study Research Group: Combined pharmacotherapies and behavioral interventions for alcohol dependence (The COMBINE Study): examination of posttreatment drinking outcomes. J Stud Alcohol Drugs 69(1):5–13, 2008 18080059

Drake RE, Essock SM, Shaner A, et al: Implementing dual-diagnosis services for clients with severe mental illness. Psychiatr Serv 52(4):469–476, 2001 11274491

Drake R, Skinner J, Goldman HH: What explains the diffusion of treatments for mental illness? Am J Psychiatry 165(11):1385–1392, 2008 18981070

Dundon W, Lynch KG, Pettinati HM, Lipkin C: Treatment outcomes in type A and B alcohol dependence 6 months after serotonergic pharmacotherapy. Alcohol Clin Exp Res 28(7):1065–1073, 2004 15252293

Dunlap LJ, Zarkin GA, Bray JW, et al: Revisiting the cost-effectiveness of the COMBINE study for alcohol dependent patients: the patient perspective. Med Care 48(4):306–313, 2010 20355261

Dunn KE, Strain EC: Pretreatment alcohol drinking goals are associated with treatment outcomes. Alcohol Clin Exp Res 37(10):1745–1752, 2013 23800222

Durand MA, Carpenter L, Dolan H, et al: Do interventions designed to support shared decision-making reduce health inequalities? A systematic review and meta-analysis. PLoS One 9(4):e94670, 2014 24736389

Epstein EE, McCrady BS: A Cognitive-Behavioral Treatment Program for Overcoming Alcohol Problems. Oxford, UK, Oxford University Press, 2009

Erol A, Karpyak VM: Sex and gender-related differences in alcohol use and its consequences: contemporary knowledge and future research considerations. Drug Alcohol Depend 156:1–13, 2015 26371405

Evoy KE, Morrison MD, Saklad SR: Abuse and misuse of pregabalin and gabapentin. Drugs 77(4):403–426, 2017 28144823

Ewing JA: Detecting alcoholism: the CAGE questionnaire. JAMA 252(14):1905–1907, 1984 6471323

FDA-NIH Biomarker Working Group: BEST (Biomarkers, EndpointS, and other Tools) Resource. Silver Spring, MD, U.S. Food and Drug Administration; Bethesda, MD, National Institutes of Health, 2016. Available at: www.ncbi.nlm.nih.gov/books/NBK326791/. Accessed March 8, 2017.

Feinn R, Tennen H, Kranzler HR: Psychometric properties of the short index of problems as a measure of recent alcohol-related problems. Alcohol Clin Exp Res 27(9):1436–1441, 2003 14506404

Fernandes-Taylor S, Harris AH: Comparing alternative specifications of quality measures: access to pharmacotherapy for alcohol use disorders. J Subst Abuse Treat 42(1):102–107, 2012 21839604

Ferri M, Amato L, Davoli M: Alcoholics Anonymous and other 12-step programmes for alcohol dependence. Cochrane Database Syst Rev (3):CD005032, 2006 16856072

Flórez G, García-Portilla P, Alvarez S, et al: Using topiramate or naltrexone for the treatment of alcohol-dependent patients. Alcohol Clin Exp Res 32(7):1251–1259, 2008 18482157

Flórez G, Saiz PA, García-Portilla P, et al: Topiramate for the treatment of alcohol dependence: comparison with naltrexone. Eur Addict Res 17(1):29–36, 2011 20975274

Foa EB, Williams MT: Methodology of a randomized double-blind clinical trial for comorbid posttraumatic stress disorder and alcohol dependence. Ment Health Subst Use 3(2):131–147, 2010 22942892

Foa EB, Yusko DA, McLean CP, et al: Concurrent naltrexone and prolonged exposure therapy for patients with comorbid alcohol dependence and PTSD: a randomized clinical trial. JAMA 310(5):488–495, 2013 23925619

Fogaça MN, Santos-Galduróz RF, Eserian JK, Galduróz JC: The effects of polyunsaturated fatty acids in alcohol dependence treatment—a double-blind, placebo-controlled pilot study. BMC Clin Pharmacol 11:10, 2011 21787433

Forcehimes AA, Tonigan JS, Miller WR, et al: Psychometrics of the Drinker Inventory of Consequences (DrInC). Addict Behav 32(8):1699–1704, 2007 17182194

Forest Pharmaceuticals: CAMPRAL® (acamprosate calcium) [package insert], 2005. Available at: www.accessdata.fda.gov/drugsatfda_docs/label/2010/021431s013lbl.pdf. Accessed April 3, 2017.

Fortney JC, Unützer J, Wrenn G, et al: A tipping point for measurement-based care. Psychiatr Serv 68(2):179–188, 2017 27582237

Foulds JA, Adamson SJ, Boden JM, et al: Depression in patients with alcohol use disorders: systematic review and meta-analysis of outcomes for independent and substance-induced disorders. J Affect Disord 185:47–59, 2015 26143404

Fridberg DJ, Cao D, Grant JE, King AC: Naltrexone improves quit rates, attenuates smoking urge, and reduces alcohol use in heavy drinking smokers attempting to quit smoking. Alcohol Clin Exp Res 38(10):2622–2629, 2014 25335648

Frisoni GB, Di Monda V: Disulfiram neuropathy: a review (1971–1988) and report of a case. Alcohol Alcohol 24(5):429–437, 1989 2554935

Fucito LM, Park A, Gulliver SB, et al: Cigarette smoking predicts differential benefit from naltrexone for alcohol dependence. Biol Psychiatry 72(10):832–838, 2012 22541040

Fuller RK, Roth HP: Disulfiram for the treatment of alcoholism: an evaluation in 128 men. Ann Intern Med 90(6):901–904, 1979 389121

Fuller RK, Branchey L, Brightwell DR, et al: Disulfiram treatment of alcoholism: a Veterans Administration cooperative study. JAMA 256(11):1449–1455, 1986 3528541

Furieri FA, Nakamura-Palacios EM: Gabapentin reduces alcohol consumption and craving: a randomized, double-blind, placebo-controlled trial. J Clin Psychiatry 68(11):1691–1700, 2007 18052562

Garbutt JC, Kranzler HR, O'Malley SS, et al; Vivitrex Study Group: Efficacy and tolerability of long-acting injectable naltrexone for alcohol dependence: a randomized controlled trial. JAMA 293(13):1617–1625, 2005 15811981

Garbutt JC, Kampov-Polevoy AB, Gallop R, et al: Efficacy and safety of baclofen for alcohol dependence: a randomized, double-blind, placebo-controlled trial. Alcohol Clin Exp Res 34(11):1849–1857, 2010 20662805

Gastpar M, Bonnet U, Böning J, et al: Lack of efficacy of naltrexone in the prevention of alcohol relapse: results from a German multicenter study. J Clin Psychopharmacol 22(6):592–598, 2002 12454559

Geerlings PJ, Ansoms C, Van Den Brink W: Acamprosate and prevention of relapse in alcoholics: results of a randomized, placebo-controlled, double-blind study in out-patient alcoholics in the Netherlands, Belgium and Luxembourg. Eur Addict Res 3(3):129–137, 1997

Gelernter J, Gueorguieva R, Kranzler HR, et al; VA Cooperative Study #425 Study Group: Opioid receptor gene (OPRM1, OPRK1, and OPRD1) variants and response to naltrexone treatment for alcohol dependence: results from the VA Cooperative Study. Alcohol Clin Exp Res 31(4):555–563, 2007 17374034

Glass JE, Bohnert KM, Brown RL: Alcohol screening and intervention among United States adults who attend ambulatory healthcare. J Gen Intern Med 31(7):739–745, 2016 26862079

Gough G, Heathers L, Puckett D, et al: The utility of commonly used laboratory tests to screen for excessive alcohol use in clinical practice. Alcohol Clin Exp Res 39(8):1493–1500, 2015 26110815

Gowing L, Ali R, White JM: Opioid antagonists with minimal sedation for opioid withdrawal. Cochrane Database Syst Rev (4):CD002021, 2009 19821290

Gowing L, Ali R, White JM: Opioid antagonists under heavy sedation or anaesthesia for opioid withdrawal. Cochrane Database Syst Rev (1):CD002022, 2010 20091529

Grant BF, Stinson FS, Dawson DA, et al: Prevalence and co-occurrence of substance use disorders and independent mood and anxiety disorders: results from the National Epidemiologic Survey on Alcohol and Related Conditions. Arch Gen Psychiatry 61(8):807–816, 2004 15289279

Grant BF, Goldstein RB, Saha TD, et al: Epidemiology of DSM-5 alcohol use disorder: results from the National Epidemiologic Survey on Alcohol and Related Conditions III. JAMA Psychiatry 72(8):757–766, 2015 26039070

Grant BF, Saha TD, Ruan WJ, et al: Epidemiology of DSM-5 drug use disorder: results from the National Epidemiologic Survey on Alcohol and Related Conditions-III. JAMA Psychiatry 73(1):39–47, 2016 26580136

Greenfield SF, Pettinati HM, O'Malley S, et al: Gender differences in alcohol treatment: an analysis of outcome from the COMBINE study. Alcohol Clin Exp Res 34(10):1803–1812, 2010 20645934

Greenhalgh T, Robert G, Macfarlane F, et al: Diffusion of innovations in service organizations: systematic review and recommendations. Milbank Q 82(4):581–629, 2004 15595944

Gual A, Lehert P: Acamprosate during and after acute alcohol withdrawal: a double-blind placebo-controlled study in Spain. Alcohol Alcohol 36(5):413–418, 2001 11524307

Gual A, Balcells M, Torres M, et al: Sertraline for the prevention of relapse in detoxicated alcohol dependent patients with a comorbid depressive disorder: a randomized controlled trial. Alcohol Alcohol 38(6):619–625, 2003 14633652

Guardia J, Caso C, Arias F, et al: A double-blind, placebo-controlled study of naltrexone in the treatment of alcohol-dependence disorder: results from a multicenter clinical trial. Alcohol Clin Exp Res 26(9):1381–1387, 2002 12351933

Gueorguieva R, Wu R, Donovan D, et al: Baseline trajectories of drinking moderate acamprosate and naltrexone effects in the COMBINE study. Alcohol Clin Exp Res 35(3):523–531, 2011 21143249

Gueorguieva R, Wu R, O'Connor PG, et al: Predictors of abstinence from heavy drinking during treatment in COMBINE and external validation in PREDICT. Alcohol Clin Exp Res 38(10):2647–2656, 2014 25346505

Gupta KK, Gupta VK, Shirasaka T: An update on fetal alcohol syndrome—pathogenesis, risks, and treatment. Alcohol Clin Exp Res 40(8):1594–1602, 2016 27375266

Guyatt G, Gutterman D, Baumann MH, et al: Grading strength of recommendations and quality of evidence in clinical guidelines: report from an American College of Chest Physicians Task Force. Chest 129(1):174–181, 2006 16424429

Guyatt GH, Oxman AD, Kunz R, et al; GRADE Working Group: Going from evidence to recommendations. BMJ 336(7652):1049–1051, 2008 18467413

Guyatt G, Eikelboom JW, Akl EA, et al: A guide to GRADE guidelines for the readers of JTH. J Thromb Haemost 11(8):1603–1608, 2013 23773710

Hagedorn HJ, Brown R, Dawes M, et al: Enhancing access to alcohol use disorder pharmacotherapy and treatment in primary care settings: ADaPT-PC. Implement Sci 11:64, 2016 27164835

Harasymiw J, Bean P: The Early Detection of Alcohol Consumption (EDAC) test shows better performance than gamma-glutamyltransferase (GGT) to detect heavy drinking in a large population of males and females. Med Sci Monit 13(9):PI19–PI24, 2007 17767129

Harris AH, Ellerbe L, Reeder RN, et al: Pharmacotherapy for alcohol dependence: perceived treatment barriers and action strategies among Veterans Health Administration service providers. Psychol Serv 10(4):410–419, 2013 23356858

Harris AH, Bowe T, Hagedorn H, et al: Multifaceted academic detailing program to increase pharmacotherapy for alcohol use disorder: interrupted time series evaluation of effectiveness. Addict Sci Clin Pract 11(1):15, 2016 27633982

Harris BS, Bishop KC, Kemeny HR, et al: Risk factors for birth defects. Obstet Gynecol Surv 72(2):123–135, 2017 28218773

Hartung DM, McCarty D, Fu R, et al: Extended-release naltrexone for alcohol and opioid dependence: a meta-analysis of healthcare utilization studies. J Subst Abuse Treat 47(2):113–121, 2014 24854219

Hasin DS, Grant BF: The National Epidemiologic Survey on Alcohol and Related Conditions (NESARC) Waves 1 and 2: review and summary of findings. Soc Psychiatry Psychiatr Epidemiol 50(11):1609–1640, 2015 26210739

Hasin DS, Goodwin RD, Stinson FS, Grant BF: Epidemiology of major depressive disorder: results from the National Epidemiologic Survey on Alcoholism and Related Conditions. Arch Gen Psychiatry 62(10):1097–1106, 2005 16203955

Hasin DS, O'Brien CP, Auriacombe M, et al: DSM-5 criteria for substance use disorders: recommendations and rationale. Am J Psychiatry 170(8):834–851, 2013 23903334

Hauser P, Fuller B, Ho SB, et al: The safety and efficacy of baclofen to reduce alcohol use in veterans with chronic hepatitis C: a randomized controlled trial. Addiction 112(7):1173–1183, 2017 28192622

Hazlehurst JM, Armstrong MJ, Sherlock M, et al: A comparative quality assessment of evidence-based clinical guidelines in endocrinology. Clin Endocrinol (Oxf) 78(2):183–190, 2013 22624723

Heinälä P, Alho H, Kiianmaa K, et al: Targeted use of naltrexone without prior detoxification in the treatment of alcohol dependence: a factorial double-blind, placebo-controlled trial. J Clin Psychopharmacol 21(3):287–292, 2001 11386491

Helander A, Husa A, Jeppsson JO: Improved HPLC method for carbohydrate-deficient transferrin in serum. Clin Chem 49(11):1881–1890, 2003 14578320

Helander A, Olsson I, Dahl H: Postcollection synthesis of ethyl glucuronide by bacteria in urine may cause false identification of alcohol consumption. Clin Chem 53(10):1855–1857, 2007 17717128

Hepner KA, Watkins KE, Farmer CM, et al: Quality of care measures for the management of unhealthy alcohol use. J Subst Abuse Treat 76:11–17, 2017 28340902

Herbeck DM, Jeter KE, Cousins SJ, et al: Gender differences in treatment and clinical characteristics among patients receiving extended release naltrexone. J Addict Dis 35(4):305–314, 2016 27192330

Hien DA, Levin FR, Ruglass LM, et al: Combining seeking safety with sertraline for PTSD and alcohol use disorders: a randomized controlled trial. J Consult Clin Psychol 83(2):359–369, 2015 25622199

Hietala J, Koivisto H, Anttila P, Niemelä O: Comparison of the combined marker GGT-CDT and the conventional laboratory markers of alcohol abuse in heavy drinkers, moderate drinkers and abstainers. Alcohol Alcohol 41(5):528–533, 2006 16799164

Higgins ST, Budney AJ, Bickel WK, et al: Disulfiram therapy in patients abusing cocaine and alcohol. Am J Psychiatry 150(4):675–676, 1993 8465895

Higuchi S; Japanese Acamprosate Study Group: Efficacy of acamprosate for the treatment of alcohol dependence long after recovery from withdrawal syndrome: a randomized, double-blind, placebo-controlled study conducted in Japan (Sunrise Study). J Clin Psychiatry 76(2):181–188, 2015 25742205

Hock B, Schwarz M, Domke I, et al: Validity of carbohydrate-deficient transferrin (%CDT), gamma-glutamyl-transferase (gamma-GT) and mean corpuscular erythrocyte volume (MCV) as biomarkers for chronic alcohol abuse: a study in patients with alcohol dependence and liver disorders of non-alcoholic and alcoholic origin. Addiction 100(10):1477–1486, 2005 16185209

Horvitz-Lennon M, Donohue JM, Domino ME, Normand SL: Improving quality and diffusing best practices: the case of schizophrenia. Health Aff (Millwood) 28(3):701–712, 2009 19414878

Huang J, Zhu T, Qu Y, Mu D: Prenatal, perinatal and neonatal risk factors for intellectual disability: a systemic review and meta-analysis. PLoS One 11(4):e0153655, 2016 27110944

Huang MC, Chen CH, Yu JM, Chen CC: A double-blind, placebo-controlled study of naltrexone in the treatment of alcohol dependence in Taiwan. Addict Biol 10(3):289–292, 2005 16109592

Humeniuk R, Ali R, Babor TF, et al: Validation of the alcohol, smoking and substance involvement screening test (ASSIST). Addiction 103(6):1039–1047, 2008 18373724

Iheanacho T, Issa M, Marienfeld C, Rosenheck R: Use of naltrexone for alcohol use disorders in the Veterans' Health Administration: a national study. Drug Alcohol Depend 132(1-2):122–126, 2013 23434041

Institute of Medicine, Committee on Quality of Health Care in America: Crossing the Quality Chasm: A New Health System for the 21st Century. Washington, DC, National Academies Press, 2001. Available at: www.ncbi.nlm.nih.gov/books/NBK222274/. Accessed March 28, 2017.

Institute of Medicine: Clinical Practice Guidelines We Can Trust. Washington, DC, National Academies Press, 2011

Ipser JC, Wilson D, Akindipe TO, et al: Pharmacotherapy for anxiety and comorbid alcohol use disorders. Cochrane Database Syst Rev (1):CD007505, 2015 25601826

Isaksson A, Walther L, Hansson T, et al: Phosphatidylethanol in blood (B-PEth): a marker for alcohol use and abuse. Drug Test Anal 3(4):195–200, 2011 21438164

Iyer SP, Spaeth-Rublee B, Pincus HA: Challenges in the operationalization of mental health quality measures: an assessment of alternatives. Psychiatr Serv 67(10):1057–1059, 2016 27301768

Jatlow PI, Agro A, Wu R, et al: Ethyl glucuronide and ethyl sulfate assays in clinical trials, interpretation, and limitations: results of a dose ranging alcohol challenge study and 2 clinical trials. Alcohol Clin Exp Res 38(7):2056–2065, 2014 24773137

Jeppsson JO, Arndt T, Schellenberg F, et al; International Federation of Clinical Chemistry and Laboratory Medicine Working Group on Standardization of Carbohydrate-deficient Transferin (IFCC-WG-CDT): Toward standardization of carbohydrate-deficient transferrin (CDT) measurements: I. analyte definition and proposal of a candidate reference method. Clin Chem Lab Med 45(4):558–562, 2007 17439340

Johnson BA, Ait-Daoud N, Bowden CL, et al: Oral topiramate for treatment of alcohol dependence: a randomised controlled trial. Lancet 361(9370):1677–1685, 2003 12767733

Johnson BA, Ait-Daoud N, Akhtar FZ, Ma JZ: Oral topiramate reduces the consequences of drinking and improves the quality of life of alcohol-dependent individuals: a randomized controlled trial. Arch Gen Psychiatry 61(9):905–912, 2004a 15351769

Johnson BA, Ait-Daoud N, Aubin HJ, et al: A pilot evaluation of the safety and tolerability of repeat dose administration of long-acting injectable naltrexone (Vivitrex) in patients with alcohol dependence. Alcohol Clin Exp Res 28(9):1356–1361, 2004b 15365306

Johnson BA, Rosenthal N, Capece JA, et al; Topiramate for Alcoholism Advisory Board; Topiramate for Alcoholism Study Group: Topiramate for treating alcohol dependence: a randomized controlled trial. JAMA 298(14):1641–1651, 2007 17925516

Johnson BA, Rosenthal N, Capece JA, et al; Topiramate for Alcoholism Advisory Board; Topiramate for Alcoholism Study Group: Improvement of physical health and quality of life of alcohol-dependent individuals with topiramate treatment: US multisite randomized controlled trial. Arch Intern Med 168(11):1188–1199, 2008 18541827

Jonas DE, Garbutt JC, Amick HR, et al: Behavioral counseling after screening for alcohol misuse in primary care: a systematic review and meta-analysis for the U.S. Preventive Services Task Force. Ann Intern Med 157(9):645–654, 2012a 23007881

Jonas DE, Garbutt JC, Brown JM, et al: Screening, Behavioral Counseling, and Referral in Primary Care to Reduce Alcohol Misuse. AHQR Comparative Effectiveness Review No 64. (Prepared by the RTI International-University of North Carolina Evidence-Based Practice Center under Contract No 290-2007-10056-I.) AHRQ Publ No 12-EHC055-EF. Rockville, MD, Agency for Healthcare Research and Quality, July 2012b. Available at: www.effectivehealthcare.ahrq.gov/reports/final.cfm. Accessed March 28, 2017.

Jonas DE, Amick HR, Feltner C, et al: Pharmacotherapy for Adults With Alcohol-Use Disorders in Outpatient Settings. AHRQ Comparative Effectiveness Review No 134. Report No 14-EHC029-EF. Rockville, MD, Agency for Healthcare Research and Quality, May 2014. Available at: www.ncbi.nlm.nih.gov/books/NBK208590/. Accessed March 28, 2017.

Jones AW: Pharmacokinetics of ethanol—issues of forensic importance. Forensic Sci Rev 23(2):91–136, 2011 26231237

Jones CM, Paulozzi LJ, Mack KA; Centers for Disease Control and Prevention (CDC): Alcohol involvement in opioid pain reliever and benzodiazepine drug abuse-related emergency department visits and drug-related deaths—United States, 2010. MMWR Morb Mortal Wkly Rep 63(40):881–885, 2014 25299603

Jørgensen CH, Pedersen B, Tønnesen H: The efficacy of disulfiram for the treatment of alcohol use disorder. Alcohol Clin Exp Res 35(10):1749–1758, 2011 21615426

Kabel DI, Petty F: A placebo-controlled, double-blind study of fluoxetine in severe alcohol dependence: adjunctive pharmacotherapy during and after inpatient treatment. Alcohol Clin Exp Res 20(4):780–784, 1996 8800399

Kalk NJ, Lingford-Hughes AR: The clinical pharmacology of acamprosate. Br J Clin Pharmacol 77(2):315–323, 2014 23278595

Kampman K, Jarvis M: American Society of Addiction Medicine (ASAM) national practice guideline for the use of medications in the treatment of addiction involving opioid use. J Addict Med 9(5):358–367, 2015 26406300

Kampman KM, Pettinati HM, Lynch KG, et al: A double-blind, placebo-controlled trial of topiramate for the treatment of comorbid cocaine and alcohol dependence. Drug Alcohol Depend 133(1):94–99, 2013 23810644

Kaner E, Bland M, Cassidy P, et al: Effectiveness of screening and brief alcohol intervention in primary care (SIPS trial): pragmatic cluster randomised controlled trial. BMJ 346:e8501, 2013 23303891

Kaskutas LA: Alcoholics anonymous effectiveness: faith meets science. J Addict Dis 28(2):145–157, 2009 19340677

Kaskutas LA, Subbaraman MS, Witbrodt J, Zemore SE: Effectiveness of making Alcoholics Anonymous easier: a group format 12-step facilitation approach. J Subst Abuse Treat 37(3):228–239, 2009 19339148

Kaufmann CN, Chen LY, Crum RM, Mojtabai R: Treatment seeking and barriers to treatment for alcohol use in persons with alcohol use disorders and comorbid mood or anxiety disorders. Soc Psychiatry Psychiatr Epidemiol 49(9):1489–1499, 2014 23900549

Kelly AT, Mozayani A: An overview of alcohol testing and interpretation in the 21st century. J Pharm Pract 25(1):30–36, 2012 22215644

Kelly E, Darke S, Ross J: A review of drug use and driving: epidemiology, impairment, risk factors and risk perceptions. Drug Alcohol Rev 23(3):319–344, 2004 15370012

Kelty E, Hulse G: Examination of mortality rates in a retrospective cohort of patients treated with oral or implant naltrexone for problematic opiate use. Addiction 107(10):1817–1824, 2012 22487087

Kendler KS, Ohlsson H, Sundquist J, Sundquist K: Alcohol use disorder and mortality across the life-span: a longitudinal cohort and co-relative analysis. JAMA Psychiatry 73(6):575–581, 2016 27097014

Kenneson A, Funderburk JS, Maisto SA: Substance use disorders increase the odds of subsequent mood disorders. Drug Alcohol Depend 133(2):338–343, 2013 23906994

Kerr-Corrêa F, Igami TZ, Hiroce V, Tucci AM: Patterns of alcohol use between genders: a cross-cultural evaluation. J Affect Disord 102(1–3):265–275, 2007 17084906

Kidney Disease: Improving Global Outcomes (KDIGO) CKD Work Group: KDIGO 2012 Clinical Practice Guideline for the Evaluation and Management of Chronic Kidney Disease. Kidney Int Suppl 3(1):1–150, 2013

Kiefer F, Jahn H, Tarnaske T, et al: Comparing and combining naltrexone and acamprosate in relapse prevention of alcoholism: a double-blind, placebo-controlled study. Arch Gen Psychiatry 60(1):92–99, 2003 12511176

Kiefer F, Andersohn F, Otte C, et al: Long-term effects of pharmacotherapy on relapse prevention in alcohol dependence. Acta Neuropsychiatr 16(5):233–238, 2004 26984435

Kiefer F, Helwig H, Tarnaske T, et al: Pharmacological relapse prevention of alcoholism: clinical predictors of outcome. Eur Addict Res 11(2):83–91, 2005 15785069

Killeen TK, Brady KT, Gold PB, et al: Effectiveness of naltrexone in a community treatment program. Alcohol Clin Exp Res 28(11):1710–1717, 2004 15547458

King AC, Cao D, O'Malley SS, et al: Effects of naltrexone on smoking cessation outcomes and weight gain in nicotine-dependent men and women. J Clin Psychopharmacol 32(5):630–636, 2012 22926596

Kim SG, Kim CM, Choi SW, et al: A mu opioid receptor gene polymorphism (A118G) and naltrexone treatment response in adherent Korean alcohol-dependent patients. Psychopharmacology (Berl) 201(4):611–618, 2009 18795264

Kiritzé-Topor P, Huas D, Rosenzweig C, et al: A pragmatic trial of acamprosate in the treatment of alcohol dependence in primary care. Alcohol Alcohol 39(6):520–527, 2004 15304381

Knapp CM, Ciraulo DA, Sarid-Segal O, et al: Zonisamide, topiramate, and levetiracetam: efficacy and neuropsychological effects in alcohol use disorders. J Clin Psychopharmacol 35(1):34–42, 2015 25427171

Knight JR, Shrier LA, Bravender TD, et al: A new brief screen for adolescent substance abuse. Arch Pediatr Adolesc Med 153(6):591–596, 1999 10357299

Knopman DS, Hartman M: Cognitive effects of high-dose naltrexone in patients with probable Alzheimer's disease. J Neurol Neurosurg Psychiatry 49(11):1321–1322, 1986 3794740

Kollmann D, Rasoul-Rockenschaub S, Steiner I, et al: Good outcome after liver transplantation for ALD without a 6 months abstinence rule prior to transplantation including post-transplant CDT monitoring for alcohol relapse assessment—a retrospective study. Transpl Int 29(5):559–567, 2016 26865285

Korthuis PT, Lum PJ, Vergara-Rodriguez P, et al; CTN-0055 CHOICES Investigators: Feasibility and safety of extended-release naltrexone treatment of opioid and alcohol use disorder in HIV clinics: a pilot/feasibility randomized trial. Addiction 112(6):1036–1044, 2017 28061017

Kosten TR, Wu G, Huang W, et al: Pharmacogenetic randomized trial for cocaine abuse: disulfiram and dopamine beta-hydroxylase. Biol Psychiatry 73(3):219–224, 2013 22906516

Kowinski J, Baker S, Carroll KM: Twelve Step Facilitation Therapy Manual: A Clinical Research Guide for Therapists Treating Individuals With Alcohol Abuse and Dependence. NIAAA Project MATCH Monograph Series, Vol 1, DHHS Publ No (ADM) 92-1893. Rockville, MD, National Institute on Alcohol Abuse and Alcoholism, 1992. Available at: https://pubs.niaaa.nih.gov/publications/ProjectMatch/match01.pdf. Accessed March 28, 2017.

Krampe H, Ehrenreich H: Supervised disulfiram as adjunct to psychotherapy in alcoholism treatment. Curr Pharm Des 16(19):2076–2090, 2010 20482514

Kranzler HR, Burleson JA, Korner P, et al: Placebo-controlled trial of fluoxetine as an adjunct to relapse prevention in alcoholics. Am J Psychiatry 152(3):391–397, 1995 7864265

Kranzler HR, Burleson JA, Brown J, Babor TF: Fluoxetine treatment seems to reduce the beneficial effects of cognitive-behavioral therapy in type B alcoholics. Alcohol Clin Exp Res 20(9):1534-1541, 1996 8986200

Kranzler HR, Armeli S, Tennen H, et al: Targeted naltrexone for early problem drinkers. J Clin Psychopharmacol 23(3):294–304, 2003 12826991

Kranzler HR, Wesson DR, Billot L; DrugAbuse Sciences Naltrexone Depot Study Group: Naltrexone depot for treatment of alcohol dependence: a multicenter, randomized, placebo-controlled clinical trial. Alcohol Clin Exp Res 28(7):1051–1059, 2004 15252291

Kranzler HR, Tennen H, Armeli S, et al: Targeted naltrexone for problem drinkers. J Clin Psychopharmacol 29(4):350–357, 2009 19593174

Kranzler HR, Armeli S, Tennen H, et al: A double-blind, randomized trial of sertraline for alcohol dependence: moderation by age of onset [corrected] and 5-hydroxytryptamine transporter-linked promoter region genotype. J Clin Psychopharmacol 31(1):22–30, 2011 21192139

Kranzler HR, Feinn R, Armeli S, Tennen H: Comparison of alcoholism subtypes as moderators of the response to sertraline treatment. Alcohol Clin Exp Res 36(3):509–516, 2012a 21895712

Kranzler HR, Armeli S, Tennen H: Post-treatment outcomes in a double-blind, randomized trial of sertraline for alcohol dependence. Alcohol Clin Exp Res 36(4):739–744, 2012b 21981418

Kranzler HR, Armeli S, Covault J, et al: Variation in OPRM1 moderates the effect of desire to drink on subsequent drinking and its attenuation by naltrexone treatment. Addiction Biol 18(1):193–201, 2013 22784013

Kranzler HR, Covault J, Feinn R, et al: Topiramate treatment for heavy drinkers: moderation by a GRIK1 polymorphism. Am J Psychiatry 171(4):445–452, 2014a 24525690

Kranzler HR, Armeli S, Tennen H, Gelernter J, et al: GRIK1 genotype and daily expectations of alcohol's positive effects moderate the reduction of heavy drinking by topiramate. Exp Clin Psychopharmacol 22(6):494–501, 2014b 25436841

Kranzler HR, Wetherill R, Feinn R, et al: Posttreatment effects of topiramate treatment for heavy drinking. Alcohol Clin Exp Res 38(12):3017–3023, 2014c 25581656

Krupitsky E, Nunes EV, Ling W, et al: Injectable extended-release naltrexone for opioid dependence: a double-blind, placebo-controlled, multicentre randomised trial. Lancet 377(9776):1506–1513, 2011 21529928

Krupitsky E, Zvartau E, Blokhina E, et al: Randomized trial of long-acting sustained-release naltrexone implant vs oral naltrexone or placebo for preventing relapse to opioid dependence. Arch Gen Psychiatry 69(9):973–981, 2012 22945623

Krupitsky E, Nunes EV, Ling W, et al: Injectable extended-release naltrexone (XR-NTX) for opioid dependence: long-term safety and effectiveness. Addiction 108(9):1628–1637, 2013 23701526

Krystal JH, Cramer JA, Krol WF, et al; Veterans Affairs Naltrexone Cooperative Study 425 Group: Naltrexone in the treatment of alcohol dependence. N Engl J Med 345(24):1734–1739, 2001 11742047

Kulkarni RR, Bairy BK: Disulfiram-induced de novo convulsions without alcohol challenge: case series and review of literature. Indian J Psychol Med 37(3):345–348, 2015 26664087

Kwo PY, Cohen SM, Lim JK: ACG clinical guideline: evaluation of abnormal liver chemistries. Am J Gastroenterol 112(1):18–35, 2017 27995906

Laaksonen E, Koski-Jännes A, Salaspuro M, et al: A randomized, multicentre, open-label, comparative trial of disulfiram, naltrexone and acamprosate in the treatment of alcohol dependence. Alcohol Alcohol 43(1):53–61, 2008 17965444

Lai HM, Cleary M, Sitharthan T, Hunt GE: Prevalence of comorbid substance use, anxiety and mood disorders in epidemiological surveys, 1990–2014: A systematic review and meta-analysis. Drug Alcohol Depend 154:1–13, 2015 26072219

Laramée P, Leonard S, Buchanan-Hughes A, et al: Risk of all-cause mortality in alcohol-dependent individuals: a systematic literature review and meta-analysis. EBioMedicine 2(10):1394–1404, 2015 26629534

Larney S, Gowing L, Mattick RP, et al: A systematic review and meta-analysis of naltrexone implants for the treatment of opioid dependence. Drug Alcohol Rev 33(2):115–128, 2014 24299657

Larson EW, Olincy A, Rummans TA, Morse RM: Disulfiram treatment of patients with both alcohol dependence and other psychiatric disorders: a review. Alcohol Clin Exp Res 16(1):125–130, 1992 1558293

Latt NC, Jurd S, Houseman J, Wutzke SE: Naltrexone in alcohol dependence: a randomised controlled trial of effectiveness in a standard clinical setting. Med J Aust 176(11):530–534, 2002 12064984

Lee A, Tan S, Lim D, et al: Naltrexone in the treatment of male alcoholics—an effectiveness study in Singapore. Drug Alcohol Rev 20(2):193–199, 2001

Lee HS, Mericle AA, Ayalon L, Areán PA: Harm reduction among at-risk elderly drinkers: a site-specific analysis from the multi-site Primary Care Research in Substance Abuse and Mental Health for Elderly (PRISM-E) study. Int J Geriatr Psychiatry 24(1):54–60, 2009 18613283

Lee WM, Larson AM, Stravitz RT: AASLD position paper: The management of acute liver failure: update 2011. Available at: www.aasld.org/sites/default/files/guideline_documents/alfenhanced.pdf. Accessed March 31, 2017.

Lenz AS, Rosenbaum L, Sheperis D: Meta-analysis of randomized controlled trials of motivational enhancement therapy for reducing substance use. J Addict Offender Couns 37:66–86, 2016

Levounis P, Arnaout B, Marienfeld C (eds): Motivational Interviewing for Clinical Practice. Arlington, VA, American Psychiatric Association Publishing, 2017

Lhuintre JP, Daoust M, Moore ND, et al: Ability of calcium bis acetyl homotaurine, a GABA agonist, to prevent relapse in weaned alcoholics. Lancet 1(8436):1014–1016, 1985 2859465

Lhuintre JP, Moore N, Tran G, et al: Acamprosate appears to decrease alcohol intake in weaned alcoholics. Alcohol Alcohol 25(6):613–622, 1990 2085344

Liangpunsakul S, Qi R, Crabb DW, Witzmann F: Relationship between alcohol drinking and aspartate aminotransferase:alanine aminotransferase (AST:ALT) ratio, mean corpuscular volume (MCV), gamma-glutamyl transpeptidase (GGT), and apolipoprotein A1 and B in the U.S. population. J Stud Alcohol Drugs 71(2):249–252, 2010 20230722

Lieberman DZ, Cioletti A, Massey SH, et al: Treatment preferences among problem drinkers in primary care. Int J Psychiatry Med 47(3):231–240, 2014 25084819

Likhitsathian S, Uttawichai K, Booncharoen H, et al: Topiramate treatment for alcoholic outpatients recently receiving residential treatment programs: a 12-week, randomized, placebo-controlled trial. Drug Alcohol Depend 133(2):440–446, 2013 23906999

Ling W, Weiss DG, Charuvastra VC, O'Brien CP: Use of disulfiram for alcoholics in methadone maintenance programs: a Veterans Administration cooperative study. Arch Gen Psychiatry 40(8):851–854, 1983 6347118

Litten RZ, Bradley AM, Moss HB: Alcohol biomarkers in applied settings: recent advances and future research opportunities. Alcohol Clin Exp Res 34(6):955–967, 2010 20374219

Litten RZ, Ryan ML, Fertig JB, et al; NCIG (National Institute on Alcohol Abuse and Alcoholism Clinical Investigations Group) Study Group: A double-blind, placebo-controlled trial assessing the efficacy of varenicline tartrate for alcohol dependence. J Addict Med 7(4):277–286, 2013 23728065

Litten RZ, Falk D, Ryan M, Fertig J: Research opportunities for medications to treat alcohol dependence: addressing stakeholders' needs. Alcohol Clin Exp Res 38(1):27–32, 2014 23889161

Litten RZ, Wilford BB, Falk DE, et al: Potential medications for the treatment of alcohol use disorder: an evaluation of clinical efficacy and safety. Subst Abus 37(2):286–298, 2016 26928397

LoCastro JS, Youngblood M, Cisler RA, et al: Alcohol treatment effects on secondary nondrinking outcomes and quality of life: the COMBINE study. J Stud Alcohol Drugs 70(2):186–196, 2009 19261230

Longabaugh R, Wirtz PW, Gulliver SB, Davidson D: Extended naltrexone and broad spectrum treatment or motivational enhancement therapy. Psychopharmacology (Berl) 206(3):367–376, 2009 19639303

Lowe JM, McDonell MG, Leickly E, et al: Determining ethyl glucuronide cutoffs when detecting self-reported alcohol use in addiction treatment patients. Alcohol Clin Exp Res 39(5):905–910, 2015 25866234

Lucey MR, Silverman BL, Illeperuma A, O'Brien CP: Hepatic safety of once-monthly injectable extended-release naltrexone administered to actively drinking alcoholics. Alcohol Clin Exp Res 32(3):498–504, 2008 18241321

Ma JZ, Ait-Daoud N, Johnson BA: Topiramate reduces the harm of excessive drinking: implications for public health and primary care. Addiction 101(11):1561–1568, 2006 17034435

Maenhout TM, Poll A, Vermassen T, et al; ROAD Study Group: Usefulness of indirect alcohol biomarkers for predicting recidivism of drunk-driving among previously convicted drunk-driving offenders: results from the recidivism of alcohol-impaired driving (ROAD) study. Addiction 109(1):71–78, 2014 24438112

Maisel NC, Blodgett JC, Wilbourne PL, et al: Meta-analysis of naltrexone and acamprosate for treating alcohol use disorders: when are these medications most helpful? Addiction 108(2):275–293, 2013 23075288

Makoul G, Clayman ML: An integrative model of shared decision making in medical encounters. Patient Educ Couns 60(3):301–312, 2006 16051459

Malcolm R, O'Neil PM, Sexauer JD, et al: A controlled trial of naltrexone in obese humans. Int J Obes 9(5):347–353, 1985 3908352

Mann K, Lemenager T, Hoffmann S, et al; PREDICT Study Team: Results of a double-blind, placebo-controlled pharmacotherapy trial in alcoholism conducted in Germany and comparison with the US COMBINE study. Addict Biol 18(6):937–946, 2013 23231446

Mannelli P, Peindl K, Patkar AA, et al: Problem drinking and low-dose naltrexone-assisted opioid detoxification. J Stud Alcohol Drugs 72(3):507–513, 2011 21513688

Mannelli P, Peindl KS, Lee T, et al: Buprenorphine-mediated transition from opioid agonist to antagonist treatment: state of the art and new perspectives. Curr Drug Abuse Rev 5(1):52–63, 2012 22280332

Marienfeld C, Iheanacho T, Issa M, Rosenheck RA: Long-acting injectable depot naltrexone use in the Veterans' Health Administration: a national study. Addict Behav 39(2):434–438, 2014 23790742

Mark TL, Kassed CA, Vandivort-Warren R, et al: Alcohol and opioid dependence medications: prescription trends, overall and by physician specialty. Drug Alcohol Depend 99(1–3):345–349, 2009 18819759

Mark TL, Lubran R, McCance-Katz EF, et al: Medicaid coverage of medications to treat alcohol and opioid dependence. J Subst Abuse Treat 55:1–5, 2015 25921475

Marques P, Tippetts S, Allen J, et al: Estimating driver risk using alcohol biomarkers, interlock blood alcohol concentration tests and psychometric assessments: initial descriptives. Addiction 105(2):226–239, 2010 19922520

Martin GW, Rehm J: The effectiveness of psychosocial modalities in the treatment of alcohol problems in adults: a review of the evidence. Can J Psychiatry 57(6):350–358, 2012 22682572

Martinotti G, Di Nicola M, De Vita O, Hatzigiakoumis DS, et al: Low-dose topiramate in alcohol dependence: a single-blind, placebo-controlled study. J Clin Psychopharmacol 34(6)709–715, 2014 25275672

Martins SS, Gorelick DA: Conditional substance abuse and dependence by diagnosis of mood or anxiety disorder or schizophrenia in the U.S. population. Drug Alcohol Depend 119(1–2):28–36, 2011 21641123

Mason BJ, Kocsis JH, Ritvo EC, Cutler RB: A double-blind, placebo-controlled trial of desipramine for primary alcohol dependence stratified on the presence or absence of major depression. JAMA 275(10):761–767, 1996 8598592

Mason BJ, Goodman AM, Chabac S, Lehert P: Effect of oral acamprosate on abstinence in patients with alcohol dependence in a double-blind, placebo-controlled trial: the role of patient motivation. J Psychiatr Res 40(5):383–393, 2006 16546214

Mason BJ, Quello S, Goodell V, et al: Gabapentin treatment for alcohol dependence: a randomized clinical trial. JAMA Intern Med 174(1):70–77, 2014 24190578

Mattick RP, Breen C, Kimber J, Davoli M: Buprenorphine maintenance versus placebo or methadone maintenance for opioid dependence. Cochrane Database Syst Rev Feb 6;(2):CD002207, 2014

McCance-Katz EF, Gruber VA, Beatty G, et al: Interaction of disulfiram with antiretroviral medications: efavirenz increases while atazanavir decreases disulfiram effect on enzymes of alcohol metabolism. Am J Addict 23(2):137–144, 2014 24118434

McCaul ME, Wand GS, Eissenberg T, et al: Naltrexone alters subjective and psychomotor responses to alcohol in heavy drinking subjects. Neuropsychopharmacology 22(5):480–492, 2000a 10731623

McCaul ME, Wand GS, Rohde C, Lee SM: Serum 6-beta-naltrexol levels are related to alcohol responses in heavy drinkers. Alcohol Clin Exp Res 24(9):1385–1391, 2000b 11003204

McConchie RD, Panitz DR, Sauber SR, Shapiro S: Disulfiram-induced de novo seizures in the absence of ethanol challenge. J Stud Alcohol 44(4):739–743, 1983 6632888

McDonell MG, Skalisky J, Leickly E, et al: Using ethyl glucuronide in urine to detect light and heavy drinking in alcohol dependent outpatients. Drug Alcohol Depend 157:184–187, 2015 26475403

McDonell MG, Leickly E, McPherson S, et al: A randomized controlled trial of ethyl glucuronide-based contingency management for outpatients with co-occurring alcohol use disorders and serious mental illness. Am J Psychiatry 174(4):370–377, 2017 28135843

McGrath PJ, Nunes EV, Stewart JW, et al: Imipramine treatment of alcoholics with primary depression: a placebo-controlled clinical trial. Arch Gen Psychiatry 53(3):232–240, 1996 8611060

McLean CP, Su YJ, Foa EB: Posttraumatic stress disorder and alcohol dependence: does order of onset make a difference? J Anxiety Disord 28(8):894–901, 2014 25445079

Mersfelder TL, Nichols WH: Gabapentin: abuse, dependence, and withdrawal. Ann Pharmacother 50(3):229–233, 2016 26721643

Meyer A, Wapp M, Strik W, Moggi F: Association between drinking goal and alcohol use one year after residential treatment: a multicenter study. J Addict Dis 33(3):234–242, 2014 25115147

Micromedex: Acamprosate. Ann Arbor, MI, Truven Health Analytics, 2017a. Available at: www.micromedexsolutions.com/home/dispatch. Accessed February 7, 2017.

Micromedex: Gabapentin. Ann Arbor, MI, Truven Health Analytics, 2017b. Available at: www.micromedexsolutions.com/home/dispatch. Accessed February 7, 2017.

Micromedex: Naltrexone. Ann Arbor, MI, Truven Health Analytics, 2017c. Available at: www.micromedexsolutions.com/home/dispatch. Accessed February 7, 2017.

Micromedex: Topiramate. Ann Arbor, MI, Truven Health Analytics, 2017d. Available at: www.micromedexsolutions.com/home/dispatch. Accessed February 7, 2017.

Miller PM, Ornstein SM, Nietert PJ, Anton RF: Self-report and biomarker alcohol screening by primary care physicians: the need to translate research into guidelines and practice. Alcohol Alcohol 39(4):325–328, 2004 15208165

Miller PM, Thomas SE, Mallin R: Patient attitudes towards self-report and biomarker alcohol screening by primary care physicians. Alcohol Alcohol 41(3):306–310, 2006 16574672

Miller WR, Rollnick S: Motivational Interviewing: Helping People Change, 3rd Edition. New York, Guilford, 2013

Miller WR, Zweben A, DiClemente CC, Rychtarik RG: Motivational Enhancement Therapy Manual: A Clinical Research Guide for Therapists Treating Individuals With Alcohol Abuse and Dependence. Project MATCH Monograph Series, Vol 2. NIH Publ No 94-3723. Rockville, MD, National Institute on Alcohol Abuse and Alcoholism, 1994. Available at: https://pubs.niaaa.nih.gov/publications/ProjectMatch/match02.pdf. Accessed February 4, 2017.

Miller WR, Tonigan JS, Longabaugh R: The Drinker Inventory of Consequences (DrInC): An Instrument for Assessing Adverse Consequences of Alcohol Abuse: Test Manual. Project MATCH Monograph Series, Vol 4. NIH Publ No 95-3911. Rockville, MD, National Institute on Alcohol Abuse and Alcoholism, 1995

Minozzi S, Amato L, Vecchi S, et al: Oral naltrexone maintenance treatment for opioid dependence. Cochrane Database Syst Rev (4):CD001333, 2011 21491383

Mitchell AA, Gilboa SM, Werler MM, et al; National Birth Defects Prevention Study: Medication use during pregnancy, with particular focus on prescription drugs: 1976–2008. Am J Obstet Gynecol 205(1):51.e1–51.e8, 2011 21514558

Mitchell AJ, Meader N, Bird V, Rizzo M: Clinical recognition and recording of alcohol disorders by clinicians in primary and secondary care: meta-analysis. Br J Psychiatry 201:93–100, 2012 22859576

Mitchell JE, Morley JE, Levine AS, et al: High-dose naltrexone therapy and dietary counseling for obesity. Biol Psychiatry 22(1):35–42, 1987 3790639

Mitchell MC, Memisoglu A, Silverman BL: Hepatic safety of injectable extended-release naltrexone in patients with chronic hepatitis C and HIV infection. J Stud Alcohol Drugs 73(6):991–997, 2012 23036218

Moak DH, Anton RF, Latham PK, et al: Sertraline and cognitive behavioral therapy for depressed alcoholics: results of a placebo-controlled trial. J Clin Psychopharmacol 23(6):553–562, 2003 14624185

Monroe AK, Lau B, Mugavero MJ, et al: Heavy alcohol use is associated with worse retention in HIV care. J Acquir Immune Defic Syndr 73(4):419–425, 2016 27243904

Monterosso JR, Flannery BA, Pettinati HM, et al: Predicting treatment response to naltrexone: the influence of craving and family history. Am J Addict 10(3):258–268, 2001 11579624

Monti PM, Rohsenow DJ, Swift RM, et al: Naltrexone and cue exposure with coping and communication skills training for alcoholics: treatment process and 1-year outcomes. Alcohol Clin Exp Res 25(11):1634–1647, 2001 11707638

Moore AA, Giuli L, Gould R, et al: Alcohol use, comorbidity, and mortality. J Am Geriatr Soc 54(5):757–762, 2006 16696740

Moos RH, Moos BS: Rates and predictors of relapse after natural and treated remission from alcohol use disorders. Addiction 101(2):212–222, 2006 16445550

Morgenstern J, Kuerbis AN, Chen AC, et al: A randomized clinical trial of naltrexone and behavioral therapy for problem drinking men who have sex with men. J Consult Clin Psychol 80(5):863–875, 2012 22612306

Morley KC, Teesson M, Reid SC, et al: Naltrexone versus acamprosate in the treatment of alcohol dependence: a multi-centre, randomized, double-blind, placebo-controlled trial. Addiction 101(10):1451–1462, 2006 16968347

Morley KC, Teesson M, Sannibale C, et al: Clinical predictors of outcome from an Australian pharmacological relapse prevention trial. Alcohol Alcohol 45(6):520–526, 2010 20952764

Morris PL, Hopwood M, Whelan G, et al: Naltrexone for alcohol dependence: a randomized controlled trial. Addiction 96(11):1565–1573, 2001 11784454

Mowbray O, Krentzman AR, Bradley JC, et al: The effect of drinking goals at treatment entry on longitudinal alcohol use patterns among adults with alcohol dependence. Drug Alcohol Depend 132(1–2):182–188, 2013 23433899

Moyer VA; U.S. Preventive Services Task Force: Screening and behavioral counseling interventions in primary care to reduce alcohol misuse: U.S. preventive services task force recommendation statement. Ann Intern Med 159(3):210–218, 2013 23698791

Mundle G, Ackermann K, Mann K: Biological markers as indicators for relapse in alcohol-dependent patients. Addict Biol 4(2):209–214, 1999 20575788

Naranjo CA, Bremner KE, Lanctôt KL: Effects of citalopram and a brief psycho-social intervention on alcohol intake, dependence and problems. Addiction 90(1):87–99, 1995 7888983

Narayana PL, Gupta AK, Sharma PK: Use of anti-craving agents in soldiers with alcohol dependence syndrome. Med J Armed Forces India 64(4):320–324, 2008 27688567

National Collaborating Centre for Mental Health: National Institute for Health & Clinical Excellence. Alcohol Use Disorders: The NICE Guidelines on Diagnosis, Assessment and Management of Harmful Drinking and Alcohol Dependence. The British Psychological Society and The Royal College of Psychiatrists, 2011. Available at: www.nice.org.uk/guidance/cg115/evidence/full-guideline-136423405. Accessed April 3, 2017.

National Institute of Allergy and Infectious Disease: Hepatitis. Bethesda, MD, National Institute of Allergy and Infectious Disease, 2017. Available at: www.niaid.nih.gov/diseases-conditions/hepatitis. Accessed March 31, 2017.

National Library of Medicine: LiverTox: Clinical and Research Information on Drug Induced Liver Injury: Acamprosate. Bethesda, MD, National Library of Medicine, 2017a. Available at: https://livertox.nih.gov/Acamprosate.htm. Accessed March 24, 2017.

National Library of Medicine: LiverTox: Clinical and Research Information on Drug-Induced Liver Injury: Acute Hepatitis. Bethesda, MD, National Library of Medicine, 2017b. Available at: https://livertox.nih.gov/Phenotypes_acutehepatitis.html. Accessed March 31, 2017.

National Library of Medicine: LiverTox: Clinical and Research Information on Drug-Induced Liver Injury: Disulfiram. Bethesda, MD, National Library of Medicine, 2017c. Available at: https://livertox.nih.gov/Disulfiram.htm. Accessed March 23, 2017.

National Quality Measures Clearinghouse: Measure Summary: Preventive Care and Screening: Percentage of Patients Aged 18 Years and Older Who Were Screened for Unhealthy Alcohol Use Using a Systematic Screening Method at Least Once Within the Last 24 Months AND Who Received Brief Counseling If Identified as an Unhealthy Alcohol User. Rockville, MD, Agency for Healthcare Research and Quality, 2016. Available at: www.qualitymeasures.ahrq.gov/summaries/summary/50213/preventive-care-and-screening-percentage-of-patients-aged-18-years-and-older-who-were-screened-for-unhealthy-alcohol-use-using-a-systematic-screening-method-at-least-once-within-the-last-24-months-and-who-received-brief-counseling-if-identified-as-an-unhealthy?q=Measure+summary+preventive+care+and+screening+. Accessed April 1, 2017.

Nava F, Premi S, Manzato E, Lucchini A: Comparing treatments of alcoholism on craving and biochemical measures of alcohol consumptions. J Psychoactive Drugs 38(3):211–217, 2006 17165363

Nehlin C, Fredriksson A, Jansson L: Brief alcohol screening in a clinical psychiatric population: special attention needed. Drug Alcohol Rev 31(4):538–543, 2012 21726312

Niemelä O: Biomarker-based approaches for assessing alcohol use disorders. Int J Environ Res Public Health 13(2):166, 2016 26828506

Norström T, Rossow I: Alcohol consumption as a risk factor for suicidal behavior: a systematic review of associations at the individual and at the population level. Arch Suicide Res 20(4):489–506, 2016 26953621

O'Farrell TJ, Allen JP, Litten RZ: Disulfiram (Antabuse) contracts in treatment of alcoholism. NIDA Res Monogr 150:65–91, 1995 8742773

Okuda M, Olfson M, Wang S, et al: Correlates of intimate partner violence perpetration: results from a National Epidemiologic Survey. J Trauma Stress 28(1):49–56, 2015 25624189

Oliveto A, Poling J, Mancino MJ, et al: Randomized, double blind, placebo-controlled trial of disulfiram for the treatment of cocaine dependence in methadone-stabilized patients. Drug Alcohol Depend 113(2–3):184–191, 2011 20828943

O'Malley SS, O'Connor PG: Medications for unhealthy alcohol use: across the spectrum. Alcohol Res Health 33(4):300–312, 2011 23580015

O'Malley SS, Jaffe AJ, Chang G, et al: Naltrexone and coping skills therapy for alcohol dependence: a controlled study. Arch Gen Psychiatry 49(11):881–887, 1992 1444726

O'Malley SS, Jaffe AJ, Chang G, et al: Six-month follow-up of naltrexone and psychotherapy for alcohol dependence. Arch Gen Psychiatry 53(3):217–224, 1996 8611058

O'Malley SS, Rounsaville BJ, Farren C, et al: Initial and maintenance naltrexone treatment for alcohol dependence using primary care vs specialty care: a nested sequence of 3 randomized trials. Arch Intern Med 163(14):1695–1704, 2003 12885685

O'Malley SS, Sinha R, Grilo CM, et al: Naltrexone and cognitive behavioral coping skills therapy for the treatment of alcohol drinking and eating disorder features in alcohol-dependent women: a randomized controlled trial. Alcohol Clin Exp Res 31(4):625–634, 2007 17374042

O'Malley SS, Robin RW, Levenson AL, et al: Naltrexone alone and with sertraline for the treatment of alcohol dependence in Alaska natives and non-natives residing in rural settings: a randomized controlled trial. Alcohol Clin Exp Res 32(7):1271–1283, 2008 18482155

O'Shea RS, Dasarathy S, McCullough AJ; Practice Guideline Committee of the American Association for the Study of Liver Diseases; Practice Parameters Committee of the American College of Gastroenterology: Alcoholic liver disease. Hepatology 51(1):307–328, 2010 20034030

Oslin D, Liberto JG, O'Brien J, et al: Naltrexone as an adjunctive treatment for older patients with alcohol dependence. Am J Geriatr Psychiatry 5(4):324–332, 1997 9363289

Oslin DW, Berrettini W, Kranzler HR, et al: A functional polymorphism of the mu-opioid receptor gene is associated with naltrexone response in alcohol-dependent patients. Neuropsychopharmacology 28(8):1546–1552, 2003 12813472

Oslin DW, Lynch KG, Pettinati HM, et al: A placebo-controlled randomized clinical trial of naltrexone in the context of different levels of psychosocial intervention. Alcohol Clin Exp Res 32(7):1299–1308, 2008 18540910

Oslin DW, Leong SH, Lynch KG, et al: Naltrexone vs placebo for the treatment of alcohol dependence: a randomized clinical trial. JAMA Psychiatry 72(5):430–437, 2015 25760804

Paille FM, Guelfi JD, Perkins AC, et al: Double-blind randomized multicentre trial of acamprosate in maintaining abstinence from alcohol. Alcohol Alcohol 30(2):239–247, 1995 7662044

Pani PP, Trogu E, Vacca R, et al: Disulfiram for the treatment of cocaine dependence. Cochrane Database Syst Rev (1):CD007024, 2010 20091613

Patel MM, Brown JD, Croake S, et al: The current state of behavioral health quality measures: where are the gaps? Psychiatr Serv 66(8):865–871, 2015 26073415

Peer K, Rennert L, Lynch KG, et al: Prevalence of DSM-IV and DSM-5 alcohol, cocaine, opioid, and cannabis use disorders in a largely substance dependent sample. Drug Alcohol Depend 127(1–3):215–219, 2013 22884164

Pelc I, Le Bon O, Verbanck P, et al: Calcium-acetylhomotaurinate for maintaining abstinence in weaned alcoholic patients: a placebo-controlled double-blind multi-centre study, in Novel Pharmacological Interventions for Alcoholism. Edited by Naranjo CA, Sellers EM. New York, Springer-Verlag, 1992, pp 348–352

Pelc I, Le Bon O, Lehert P, et al: Acamprosate in the treatment of alcohol dependence: a 6-month postdetoxification study, in Acamprosate in Relapse Prevention of Alcoholism. Edited by Soyka M. Berlin, Springer, 1996, pp 133–142

Pelc I, Verbanck P, Le Bon O, et al: Efficacy and safety of acamprosate in the treatment of detoxified alcohol-dependent patients: a 90-day placebo-controlled dose-finding study. Br J Psychiatry 171:73–77, 1997 9328500

Petrakis IL, O'Malley S, Rounsaville B, et al; VA Naltrexone Study Collaboration Group: Naltrexone augmentation of neuroleptic treatment in alcohol abusing patients with schizophrenia. Psychopharmacology (Berl) 172(3):291–297, 2004 14634716

Petrakis IL, Poling J, Levinson C, et al; VA New England VISN I MIRECC Study Group: Naltrexone and disulfiram in patients with alcohol dependence and comorbid psychiatric disorders. Biol Psychiatry 57(10):1128–1137, 2005 15866552

Petrakis IL, Poling J, Levinson C, et al: Naltrexone and disulfiram in patients with alcohol dependence and comorbid post-traumatic stress disorder. Biol Psychiatry 60(7):777–783, 2006 17008146

Petrakis I, Ralevski E, Nich C, et al; VA VISN I MIRECC Study Group: Naltrexone and disulfiram in patients with alcohol dependence and current depression. J Clin Psychopharmacol 27(2):160–165, 2007 17414239

Petrakis IL, Ralevski E, Desai N, et al: Noradrenergic vs serotonergic antidepressant with or without naltrexone for veterans with PTSD and comorbid alcohol dependence. Neuropsychopharmacology 37(4):996–1004, 2012 22089316

Pettinati HM, Volpicelli JR, Kranzler HR et al.: Sertraline treatment for alcohol dependence: interactive effects of medication and alcoholic subtype. Alcohol Clin Exp Res 24(7):1041–1049, 2000 10924008

Pettinati HM, Volpicelli JR, Luck G, et al: Double-blind clinical trial of sertraline treatment for alcohol dependence. J Clin Psychopharmacol 21(2):143–153, 2001 11270910

Pettinati HM, Weiss RD, Miller WR, et al: Medical Management Treatment Manual: A Clinical Research Guide for Medically Trained Clinicians Providing Pharmacotherapy as Part of the Treatment for Alcohol Dependence. COMBINE Monograph Series, Vol 2. DHHS Publ No (NIH) 04-5289. Bethesda, MD, National Institute on Alcohol Abuse and Alcoholism, 2004

Pettinati HM, Kampman KM, Lynch KG, et al: A double blind, placebo-controlled trial that combines disulfiram and naltrexone for treating co-occurring cocaine and alcohol dependence. Addict Behav 33(5):651–667, 2008a 18079068

Pettinati HM, Kampman KM, Lynch KG, et al: Gender differences with high-dose naltrexone in patients with co-occurring cocaine and alcohol dependence. J Subst Abuse Treat 34(4):378–390, 2008b 17664051

Pettinati HM, Gastfriend DR, Dong Q, et al: Effect of extended-release naltrexone (XR-NTX) on quality of life in alcohol-dependent patients. Alcohol Clin Exp Res 33(2):350–356, 2009 19053979

Pettinati HM, Oslin DW, Kampman KM, et al: A double-blind, placebo-controlled trial combining sertraline and naltrexone for treating co-occurring depression and alcohol dependence. Am J Psychiatry 167(6):668–675, 2010 20231324

Pfohl DN, Allen JI, Atkinson RL, et al: Naltrexone hydrochloride (Trexan): a review of serum transaminase elevations at high dosage. NIDA Res Monogr 67:66–72, 1986 3092099

Piano S, Marchioro L, Gola E, et al: Assessment of alcohol consumption in liver transplant candidates and recipients: the best combination of the tools available. Liver Transpl 20(7):815–822, 2014 24692331

Pincus HA, Scholle SH, Spaeth-Rublee B, et al: Quality measures for mental health and substance use: gaps, opportunities, and challenges. Health Aff (Millwood) 35(6):1000–1008, 2016 27269015

Poldrugo F: Acamprosate treatment in a long-term community-based alcohol rehabilitation programme. Addiction 92(11):1537–1546, 1997 9519495

Ponizovsky AM, Rosca P, Aronovich E, et al: Baclofen as add-on to standard psychosocial treatment for alcohol dependence: a randomized, double-blind, placebo-controlled trial with 1 year follow-up. J Subst Abuse Treat 52:24–30, 2015 25572706

Project MATCH Research Group: Matching alcoholism treatments to client heterogeneity: Project MATCH posttreatment drinking outcomes. J Stud Alcohol 58:7–29, 1997

Project MATCH Research Group: Matching alcoholism treatments to client heterogeneity: Project MATCH three-year drinking outcomes. Alcohol Clin Exp Res 22(6):1300–1311, 1998a 9756046

Project MATCH Research Group: Matching alcoholism treatments to client heterogeneity: treatment main effects and matching effects on drinking during treatment. J Stud Alcohol 59(6):631–639, 1998b 9811084

Puukka K, Hietala J, Koivisto H, et al: Obesity and the clinical use of serum GGT activity as a marker of heavy drinking. Scand J Clin Lab Invest 67(5):480–488, 2007 17763184

Ralevski E, Balachandra K, Gueorguieva R, et al: Effects of naltrexone on cognition in a treatment study of patients with schizophrenia and comorbid alcohol dependence. J Dual Diagn 2(4):53–69, 2006

Ralevski E, Ball S, Nich C, et al: The impact of personality disorders on alcohol-use outcomes in a pharmacotherapy trial for alcohol dependence and comorbid Axis I disorders. Am J Addict 16(6):443–449, 2007 18058408

Ralevski E, O'Brien E, Jane JS, et al: Effects of acamprosate on cognition in a treatment study of patients with schizophrenia spectrum disorders and comorbid alcohol dependence. J Nerv Ment Dis 199(7):499–505, 2011a 21716064

Ralevski E, O'Brien E, Jane JS, et al: Treatment with acamprosate in patients with schizophrenia spectrum disorders and comorbid alcohol dependence. J Dual Diagn 7(1–2):64–73, 2011b 26954912

Rashad I, Kaestner R: Teenage sex, drugs and alcohol use: problems identifying the cause of risky behaviors. J Health Econ 23(3):493–503, 2004 15120467

Rehm J, Samokhvalov AV, Shield KD: Global burden of alcoholic liver diseases. J Hepatol 59(1):160–168, 2013 23511777

Rehm J, Gmel GE Sr, Gmel G, et al: The relationship between different dimensions of alcohol use and the burden of disease-an update. Addiction 112(6):968–1001, 2017 28220587

Riley EP, Infante MA, Warren KR: Fetal alcohol spectrum disorders: an overview. Neuropsychol Rev 21(2):73–80, 2011 21499711

Rising Pharmaceuticals Inc: Disulfiram. Allendale, NJ, Rising Pharmaceuticals, 2016. Available at: www.risingpharma.com/Files/Prescribing-Info/Package%20Insert-Disulfiram%20Tablets-250mg-500mg.pdf. Accessed February 7, 2017.

Roache JD, Kahn R, Newton TF, et al: A double-blind, placebo-controlled assessment of the safety of potential interactions between intravenous cocaine, ethanol, and oral disulfiram. Drug Alcohol Depend 119(1–2):37–45, 2011 21696894

Rogers E, Sherman S: Tobacco use screening and treatment by outpatient psychiatrists before and after release of the American Psychiatric Association treatment guidelines for nicotine dependence. Am J Public Health 104(1):90–95, 2014 24228666

Rogers WK, Benowitz NL, Wilson KM, Abbott JA: Effect of disulfiram on adrenergic function. Clin Pharmacol Ther 25(4):469–477, 1979 106999

Rohsenow DJ, Colby SM, Monti PM, et al: Predictors of compliance with naltrexone among alcoholics. Alcohol Clin Exp Res 24(10):1542–1549, 2000 11045863

Rohsenow DJ, Miranda R Jr, McGeary JE, Monti PM: Family history and antisocial traits moderate naltrexone's effects on heavy drinking in alcoholics. Exp Clin Psychopharmacol 15(3):272–281, 2007 17563214

Rolland B, Paille F, Gillet C, et al: Pharmacotherapy for alcohol dependence: the 2015 recommendations of the French Alcohol Society, issued in partnership with the European Federation of Addiction Societies. CNS Neurosci Ther 22(1):25–37, 2016 26768685

Rösner S, Hackl-Herrwerth A, Leucht S, et al: Opioid antagonists for alcohol dependence. Cochrane Database Syst Rev (12):CD001867, 2010

Rothstein E, Clancy DD: Toxicity of disulfiram combined with metronidazole. N Engl J Med 280(18):1006–1007, 1969 4888076

Rubinsky AD, Dawson DA, Williams EC, et al: AUDIT-C scores as a scaled marker of mean daily drinking, alcohol use disorder severity, and probability of alcohol dependence in a U.S. general population sample of drinkers. Alcohol Clin Exp Res 37(8):1380–1390, 2013 23906469

Rubio G, Jiménez-Arriero MA, Ponce G, Palomo T: Naltrexone versus acamprosate: one year follow-up of alcohol dependence treatment. Alcohol Alcohol 36(5):419–425, 2001 11524308

Rubio G, Ponce G, Jiménez-Arriero MA, et al: Polymorphism for mu-opioid receptor (+118) as a prognostic variable of naltrexone in alcohol dependence treatment: Preliminary results. Eur Neuropsychopharmacol 12:397, 2002

Rubio G, Martínez-Gras I, Manzanares J: Modulation of impulsivity by topiramate: implications for the treatment of alcohol dependence. J Clin Psychopharmacol 29(6):584–589, 2009 19910725

Sachs HC; Committee on Drugs: The transfer of drugs and therapeutics into human breast milk: an update on selected topics. Pediatrics 132(3):e796–e809, 2013 23979084

Saitz R, Palfai TP, Cheng DM, et al: Screening and brief intervention for drug use in primary care: the ASPIRE randomized clinical trial. JAMA 312(5):502–513, 2014 25096690

Sass H, Soyka M, Mann K, Zieglgänsberger W: Relapse prevention by acamprosate. Results from a placebo-controlled study on alcohol dependence. Arch Gen Psychiatry 53(8):673–680, 1996 8694680

Saunders JB, Aasland OG, Babor TF, et al: Development of the Alcohol Use Disorders Identification Test (AUDIT): WHO Collaborative Project on Early Detection of Persons with Harmful Alcohol Consumption—II. Addiction 88(6):791–804, 1993 8329970

Schellenberg F, Wielders J, Anton R, et al: IFCC approved HPLC reference measurement procedure for the alcohol consumption biomarker carbohydrate-deficient transferrin (CDT): its validation and use. Clin Chim Acta 465:91–100, 2017 28025028

Schmitz JM, Stotts AL, Sayre SL, et al: Treatment of cocaine-alcohol dependence with naltrexone and relapse prevention therapy. Am J Addict 13(4):333–341, 2004 15370932

Schmitz JM, Lindsay JA, Green CE, et al: High-dose naltrexone therapy for cocaine-alcohol dependence. Am J Addict 18(5):356–362, 2009 19874153

Seibert J, Fields S, Fullerton CA, et al: Use of quality measures for Medicaid behavioral health services by state agencies: implications for health care reform. Psychiatr Serv 66(6):585–591, 2015 25726975

Sennesael J: Acamprosate pharmacokinetic study after a single oral administration of 2 acamprosate tablets (2×333 mg) to subjects with normal or impaired renal function, Lipha, France, 1992 (AOTA-CIN IR1-AD 1003 H) (data on file): cited in Saivin S, Hulot T, Chabac S, et al: Clinical pharmacokinetics of acamprosate. Clin Pharmacokinet 35(5):331–345, 1998

Shield KD, Gmel G, Kehoe-Chan T, et al: Mortality and potential years of life lost attributable to alcohol consumption by race and sex in the United States in 2005. PLoS One 8(1):e51923, 2013 23300957

Silverman BL; Alkermes, Inc: ALK21-014: efficacy and safety of Medisorb® naltrexone (VIVITROL®) after enforced abstinence, 2011. Available at: https://clinicaltrials.gov/ct2/show/NCT00501631. Accessed March 28 2017.

Skinner MD, Lahmek P, Pham H, Aubin HJ: Disulfiram efficacy in the treatment of alcohol dependence: a meta-analysis. PLoS One 9(2):e87366, 2014 24520330

Slade T, Chapman C, Swift W, et al: Birth cohort trends in the global epidemiology of alcohol use and alcohol-related harms in men and women: systematic review and metaregression. BMJ Open 6(10):e011827, 2016a 27797998

Slade T, Chiu WT, Glantz M, et al: A cross-national examination of differences in classification of lifetime alcohol use disorder between DSM-IV and DSM-5: findings from the world mental health survey. Alcohol Clin Exp Res 40(8):1728–1736, 2016b 27426631

Smith PC, Schmidt SM, Allensworth-Davies D, Saitz R: Primary care validation of a single-question alcohol screening test. J Gen Intern Med 24(7):783–788, 2009 19247718

Staufer K, Andresen H, Vettorazzi E, et al: Urinary ethyl glucuronide as a novel screening tool in patients pre- and post-liver transplantation improves detection of alcohol consumption. Hepatology 54(5):1640–1649, 2011 21809364

Stewart SH, Koch DG, Willner IR, et al: Validation of blood phosphatidylethanol as an alcohol consumption biomarker in patients with chronic liver disease. Alcohol Clin Exp Res 38(6):1706–1711, 2014 24848614

Stoddard J, Zummo J: Oral and long-acting injectable naltrexone: removal of boxed warning for hepatotoxicity. J Clin Psychiatry 76(12):1695, 2015 26717532

Substance Abuse and Mental Health Services Administration: The Role of Biomarkers in the Treatment of Alcohol Use Disorders, 2012 Revision. SAMHSA Advisory, Vol 11, Issue 2, 2012. Available at: http://store.samhsa.gov/shin/content/SMA12-4686/SMA12-4686.pdf. Accessed January 30, 2017.

Substance Abuse and Mental Health Services Administration: Results From the 2013 National Survey on Drug Use and Health: Summary of National Findings. NSDUH Series H-48, DHHS Publ No (SMA) 14-4863. Rockville, MD, Substance Abuse and Mental Health Services Administration, 2014

Substance Abuse and Mental Health Services Administration and National Institute on Alcohol Abuse and Alcoholism: Medication for the Treatment of Alcohol Use Disorder: A Brief Guide. DHHS Publ No (SMA) 15-4907. Rockville, MD, Substance Abuse and Mental Health Services Administration, 2015. Available at: http://store.samhsa.gov/shin/content//SMA15-4907/SMA15-4907.pdf. Accessed March 10, 2017

Sudhinaraset M, Wigglesworth C, Takeuchi DT: Social and cultural contexts of alcohol use: influences in a social-ecological framework. Alcohol Res 38(1):35–45, 2016 27159810

Sullivan MA, Bisaga A, Glass A, et al: Opioid use and dropout in patients receiving oral naltrexone with or without single administration of injection naltrexone. Drug Alcohol Depend 147:122–129, 2015 25555621

Syed YY, Keating GM: Extended-release intramuscular naltrexone (VIVITROL®: a review of its use in the prevention of relapse to opioid dependence in detoxified patients. CNS Drugs 27(10):851–861, 2013 24018540

Sylvia LG, Gold AK, Stange JP, et al: A randomized, placebo-controlled proof-of-concept trial of adjunctive topiramate for alcohol use disorders in bipolar disorder. Am J Addict 25(2):94–98, 2016 26894822

Tempesta E, Janiri L, Bignamini A, et al: Acamprosate and relapse prevention in the treatment of alcohol dependence: a placebo-controlled study. Alcohol Alcohol 35(2):202–209, 2000 10787398

Tennis P, Chan KA, Curkendall SM, et al: Topiramate use during pregnancy and major congenital malformations in multiple populations. Birth Defects Res A Clin Mol Teratol 103(4):269–275, 2015 25776342

Tetrault JM, Tate JP, McGinnis KA, et al; Veterans Aging Cohort Study Team: Hepatic safety and antiretroviral effectiveness in HIV-infected patients receiving naltrexone. Alcohol Clin Exp Res 36(2):318–324, 2012 21797892

Thomas CP, Garnick DW, Horgan CM, et al: Establishing the feasibility of measuring performance in use of addiction pharmacotherapy. J Subst Abuse Treat 45(1):11–18, 2013 23490233

Thomas SE, Randall PK, Book SW, Randall CL: A complex relationship between co-occurring social anxiety and alcohol use disorders: what effect does treating social anxiety have on drinking? Alcohol Clin Exp Res 32(1):77–84, 2008 18028529

Tiet QQ, Mausbach B: Treatments for patients with dual diagnosis: a review. Alcohol Clin Exp Res 31(4):513–536, 2007 17374031

Tiihonen J, Ryynänen OP, Kauhanen J, et al: Citalopram in the treatment of alcoholism: a double-blind placebo-controlled study. Pharmacopsychiatry 29(1):27–29, 1996 8852531

Timko C, Debenedetti A, Moos BS, Moos RH: Predictors of 16-year mortality among individuals initiating help-seeking for an alcoholic use disorder. Alcohol Clin Exp Res 30(10):1711–1720, 2006 17010138

Timko C, Schultz NR, Cucciare MA, et al: Retention in medication-assisted treatment for opiate dependence: A systematic review. J Addict Dis 35(1):22–35, 2016 26467975

Tuithof M, ten Have M, van den Brink W, et al: Alcohol consumption and symptoms as predictors for relapse of DSM-5 alcohol use disorder. Drug Alcohol Depend 140:85–91, 2014 24793368

Turncliff RZ, Dunbar JL, Dong Q, et al: Pharmacokinetics of long-acting naltrexone in subjects with mild to moderate hepatic impairment. J Clin Pharmacol 45(11):1259–1267, 2005 16239359

U.S. Department of Health and Human Services, National Institutes of Health, National Institute on Alcohol Abuse and Alcoholism: Helping Patients Who Drink Too Much: A Clinician's Guide. NIH Publ No 07-3769. Bethesda, MD, National Institute on Alcohol Abuse and Alcoholism, 2007. Available at: https://pubs.niaaa.nih.gov/publications/Practitioner/CliniciansGuide2005/clinicians_guide.htm. Accessed March 17, 2017.

U.S. Department of Veterans Affairs, U.S. Department of Defense: VA/DoD Clinical Practice Guideline for the Management of Substance Use Disorders, Version 3.0. Washington, DC, U.S. Department of Veterans Affairs, 2015. Available at: www.healthquality.va.gov/guidelines/MH/sud/VADoDSUDCPG Revised22216.pdf. Accessed April 3, 2017.

U.S. Preventive Services Task Force: Counseling and interventions to prevent tobacco use and tobacco-caused disease in adults and pregnant women: U.S. Preventive Services Task Force reaffirmation recommendation statement. Ann Intern Med 150(8):551–555, 2009 19380855

U.S. Preventive Services Task Force: Final Recommendation Statement: Alcohol Misuse: Screening and Behavioral Counseling Interventions in Primary Care. Rockville, MD, U.S. Preventive Services Task Force, May 2013. Available at: www.uspreventiveservicestaskforce.org/Page/Document/RecommendationStatementFinal/alcohol-misuse-screening-and-behavioral-counseling-interventions-in-primary-care. Accessed April 3, 2017.

Vagenas P, Di Paola A, Herme M, et al: An evaluation of hepatic enzyme elevations among HIV-infected released prisoners enrolled in two randomized placebo-controlled trials of extended release naltrexone. J Subst Abuse Treat 47(1):35–40, 2014 24674234

Verebey KG, Mulé SJ: Naltrexone (Trexan): a review of hepatotoxicity issues. NIDA Res Monogr 67:73–81, 1986 3092100

Vickers AP, Jolly A: Naltrexone and problems in pain management. BMJ 332(7534):132–133, 2006 16424470

Viswanathan M, Ansari MT, Berkman ND, et al: Assessing the Risk of Bias of Individual Studies in Systematic Reviews of Health Care Interventions. AHRQ Methods Guide for Comparative Effectiveness Reviews. AHRQ Publ No 12-EHC047-EF. Rockville, MD, Agency for Healthcare Research and Quality, March 2012. Available at: https://effectivehealthcare.ahrq.gov/ehc/products/322/998/MethodsGuideforCERs_Viswanathan_IndividualStudies.pdf. Accessed April 3, 2017.

Volicer L, Nelson KL: Development of reversible hypertension during disulfiram therapy. Arch Intern Med 144(6):1294–1296, 1984 6732388

Volpicelli JR, Alterman AI, Hayashida M, O'Brien CP: Naltrexone in the treatment of alcohol dependence. Arch Gen Psychiatry 49(11):876–880, 1992 1345133

Volpicelli JR, Clay KL, Watson NT, O'Brien CP: Naltrexone in the treatment of alcoholism: predicting response to naltrexone. J Clin Psychiatry 56(Suppl 7):39–44, 1995 7673104

Volpicelli JR, Rhines KC, Rhines JS, et al: Naltrexone and alcohol dependence. Role of subject compliance. Arch Gen Psychiatry 54(8):737–742, 1997 9283509

Walsham NE, Sherwood RA: Ethyl glucuronide and ethyl sulfate. Adv Clin Chem 67:47–71, 2014 25735859

Walther L, de Bejczy A, Löf E, et al: Phosphatidylethanol is superior to carbohydrate-deficient transferrin and gamma-glutamyltransferase as an alcohol marker and is a reliable estimate of alcohol consumption level. Alcohol Clin Exp Res 39(11):2200–2208, 2015 26503066

Watkins K, Horvitz-Lennon M, Caldarone LB, et al: Developing medical record-based performance indicators to measure the quality of mental healthcare. J Healthc Qual 33(1):49–66, quiz 66–67, 2011 21199073

Watkins KE, Farmer CM, De Vries D, Hepner KA: The Affordable Care Act: an opportunity for improving care for substance use disorders? Psychiatr Serv 66(3):310–312, 2015 25727120

Watkins KE, Smith B, Akincigil A, et al: The quality of medication treatment for mental disorders in the Department of Veterans Affairs and in private-sector plans. Psychiatr Serv 67(4):391–396, 2016 26567931

Weston J, Bromley R, Jackson CF, et al: Monotherapy treatment of epilepsy in pregnancy: congenital malformation outcomes in the child. Cochrane Database Syst Rev 11:CD010224, 2016, 27819746

Wetterling T, Dibbelt L, Wetterling G, et al: Ethyl glucuronide (EtG): better than breathalyser or self-reports to detect covert short-term relapses into drinking. Alcohol Alcohol 49(1):51–54, 2014 24133131

Weykamp C, Wielders JP, Helander A, et al; IFCC Working Group on Standardization of Carbohydrate-Deficient Transferrin (WG-CDT): Toward standardization of carbohydrate-deficient transferrin (CDT) measurements: III. performance of native serum and serum spiked with disialotransferrin proves that harmonization of CDT assays is possible. Clin Chem Lab Med 51(5):991–996, 2013 23241602

White A, Castle IJ, Chen CM, et al: Converging patterns of alcohol use and related outcomes among females and males in the United States, 2002 to 2012. Alcohol Clin Exp Res 39(9):1712–1726, 2015 26331879

Whiteford HA, Degenhardt L, Rehm J, et al: Global burden of disease attributable to mental and substance use disorders: findings from the Global Burden of Disease Study 2010. Lancet 382(9904):1575–1586, 2013 23993280

Whitfield JB: Gamma glutamyl transferase. Crit Rev Clin Lab Sci 38(4):263–355, 2001 11563810

Whitworth AB, Fischer F, Lesch OM, et al: Comparison of acamprosate and placebo in long-term treatment of alcohol dependence. Lancet 347(9013):1438–1442, 1996 8676626

Williams EC, Rubinsky AD, Lapham GT, et al: Prevalence of clinically recognized alcohol and other substance use disorders among VA outpatients with unhealthy alcohol use identified by routine alcohol screening. Drug Alcohol Depend 135:95–103, 2014 24360928

Williams EC, Hahn JA, Saitz R, et al: Alcohol use and human immunodeficiency virus (HIV) infection: current knowledge, implications, and future directions. Alcohol Clin Exp Res 40(10):2056–2072, 2016 27696523

Williams J, Powell LM, Wechsler H: Does alcohol consumption reduce human capital accumulation? Evidence from the college alcohol study. Appl Econ 35:1227–1239, 2003

Wolaver AM: Effects of heavy drinking in college on study effort, grade point average, and major choice. Contemp Econ Policy 20:415–428, 2002

Wölwer W, Frommann N, Jänner M, et al: The effects of combined acamprosate and integrative behaviour therapy in the outpatient treatment of alcohol dependence: a randomized controlled trial. Drug Alcohol Depend 118(2–3):417–422, 2011 21621929

Wurst FM, Thon N, Yegles M, et al: Ethanol metabolites: their role in the assessment of alcohol intake. Alcohol Clin Exp Res 39(11):2060–2072, 2015 26344403

Yen MH, Ko HC, Tang FI, et al: Study of hepatotoxicity of naltrexone in the treatment of alcoholism. Alcohol 38(2):117–120, 2006 16839858

Yoshimura A, Kimura M, Nakayama H, et al: Efficacy of disulfiram for the treatment of alcohol dependence assessed with a multicenter randomized controlled trial. Alcohol Clin Exp Res 38(2):572–578, 2014 24117666

Zandberg LJ, Rosenfield D, McLean CP, et al: Concurrent treatment of posttraumatic stress disorder and alcohol dependence: predictors and moderators of outcome. J Consult Clin Psychol 84(1):43–56, 2016 26460570

Zarkin GA, Bray JW, Aldridge A, et al; COMBINE Cost-Effectiveness Research Group: Cost and cost-effectiveness of the COMBINE study in alcohol-dependent patients. Arch Gen Psychiatry 65(10):1214–1221, 2008 18838638

Zarkin GA, Bray JW, Aldridge A, et al: The effect of alcohol treatment on social costs of alcohol dependence: results from the COMBINE study. Med Care 48(5):396–401, 2010 20393362

Disclosures

The Guideline Writing Group and Systematic Review Group reported the following disclosures during development and approval of this guideline:

Dr. Reus is employed as a professor of psychiatry at the University of California, San Francisco School of Medicine. He is past Chairman of the Board of the Accreditation Council for Continuing Medical Education (ACCME). He receives travel funds from the ACCME and the American Board of Psychiatry and Neurology (ABPN) for board meetings and test development. He receives research grant support from the National Institute of Mental Health (NIMH) and National Institute on Drug Abuse and honoraria for NIMH grant review service. He reports no conflicts of interest with his work on this guideline.

Dr. Fochtmann is employed as a professor of psychiatry, pharmacological sciences, and biomedical informatics at Stony Brook University. She consults for the American Psychiatric Association on the development of practice guidelines and has received travel funds to attend meetings related to these duties. She reports no conflicts of interest with her work on this guideline.

Dr. Bukstein is employed by Boston Children's Hospital, where he is Vice Chair for the Department of Psychiatry. He is also a professor of psychiatry at Harvard Medical School. He has received royalties from Taylor Francis Press and Wolters Kluwer. He is co-chair of the Committee on Quality Issues of the American Academy of Child and Adolescent Psychiatry. He reports no conflicts of interest with his work on this guideline.

Dr. Eyler is employed as a professor of psychiatry and family medicine at the Robert Larner, MD, College of Medicine at the University of Vermont in Burlington, Vermont, and as an attending psychiatrist at the University of Vermont Medical Center and its affiliated hospitals. During the period of preparation of this guideline, he received honoraria from non-industry-sponsored academic and community presentations. He has provided clinical consultation on gender dysphoria to the Department of Corrections of the state of New Hampshire and general psychiatric consultation at The Health Center, a federally qualified health center in Plainfield, Vermont. He is a member of the advisory committee of the Samara Fund, a philanthropic group serving the LGBT communities in Vermont. He has received fees or royalties from Johns Hopkins University Press, Taylor & Francis, and Healthwise, Inc. Travel funds have been provided by the American Psychiatric Association, related to service on the Assembly Executive Committee. He reports no conflicts of interest with his work on this guideline.

Dr. Hilty is employed as a professor of psychiatry at the University of Southern California. He reports no conflicts of interest with his work on this guideline.

Dr. Horvitz-Lennon is employed as a physician scientist at the RAND Corporation, as a professor at the Pardee RAND Graduate School, and as an attending psychiatrist with Cambridge Health Alliance. She reports no conflicts of interest with her work on this guideline.

Dr. Mahoney is employed as a researcher and clinical nurse specialist at The Menninger Clinic in Houston, Texas. She is also an associate professor in the Department of Psychiatry and Behavioral Sciences at Baylor College of Medicine. She reports no conflicts of interest with her work on this guideline.

Dr. Pasic is employed as a professor of psychiatry at the University of Washington. She is a member of the board of the American Association of Emergency Psychiatry. She reports no conflicts of interest with her work on this guideline.

Dr. Weaver is employed as a professor of psychiatry and medical director of the Center for Neurobehavioral Research on Addiction at The University of Texas Health Science Center at Houston.

He receives research grant support from the National Institute on Drug Abuse. He is Chair of the Addiction Medicine Sub-board for the American Board of Preventive Medicine. He is a member of the Publications Council and the Annual Conference Committee for the American Society of Addiction Medicine. He is a member of the Behavioral Health Advisory Committee for the Texas Children's Health Plan. He receives travel funds from The Addiction Medicine Foundation for presentations and exam development and from The Joint Commission as a member of a technical advisory panel. He receives royalties from UpToDate as a content author. He occasionally provides medical expert witness consultation for legal cases. During the period of preparation of this guideline, he received honoraria from the U.S. Drug Enforcement Administration. He reports no conflict of interest with his work on this guideline.

Dr. Wills is employed as an assistant professor of psychiatry at University Hospitals, Case Medical Center. She also has a private practice in forensic psychiatry. She receives no royalties from any entity. She receives travel funds but no honoraria from the American Academy of Psychiatry and the Law. She provides medicolegal consultation and expert testimony to courts. She reports no conflicts of interest with her work on this guideline.

Dr. Kidd is employed as a fourth-year resident in psychiatry at New York Presbyterian (Columbia University), Columbia University Medical Center, and the New York State Psychiatric Institute. He is a member of the APA Council on Quality Care, the Area 2 Resident-Fellow Member Representative to the APA Assembly, and the Chair of the APA/APAF Leadership fellowship, for which he receives travel funds. He reports no conflicts of interest with his work on this guideline.

Dr. McIntyre is a clinical professor of psychiatry at the University of Rochester. He is in full-time private practice and is Medical Director of HCR, a home health care agency. Dr. McIntyre is the Chair of the Board of PCPI and Chair of the Quality Collaborative of Monroe County Medical Society. He serves on the boards of several other not-for-profit organizations. He reports no conflicts of interest with his work on this guideline.

Dr. Yager is employed as a professor of psychiatry at the University of Colorado. He reports no conflicts of interest with his work on this guideline.

Ms. Hong is employed as a research manager for the practice guidelines program at American Psychiatric Association. She reports no conflicts of interest with her work on this guideline.

Individuals and Organizations That Submitted Comments

Hannu Alho, M.D., Ph.D.

Raymond F. Anton Jr., M.D.

Henri-Jean Aubin, M.D., Ph.D.

Jonathan Avery, M.D.

Snehal Bhatt, M.D.

F. Michler Bishop, Ph.D.

Greg Briscoe, M.D.

Chris Bundy, M.D., M.P.H.

Ronald M. Burd, M.D.

Hilary S. Connery, M.D., Ph.D.

Lane M. Cook, M.D.

E. Jennifer Edelman, M.D., M.H.S.

Kenneth S. Fink, M.D., M.G.A., M.P.H.

Stuart Gitlow M.D., M.P.H., M.B.A.

Jeffrey Guina, M.D.

Andreas Heinz, M.D.

Steven K. Hoge, M.D.

Margaret Jarvis, M.D.

Bankole A. Johnson, D.Sc., M.D., MBChB, MPhil

David A. Kahn, M.D.

Lori D. Karan, M.D.

Victor M. Karpyak, M.D., Ph.D.

Thomas Kosten, M.D.

John H. Krystal, M.D.

Nathan E. Lavid, M.D., DFAPA

Petros Levounis, M.D., M.A.

Raye Z. Litten, Ph.D.

Velandy Manohar, M.D.

Barbara J. Mason, Ph.D.

Eileen McGee, M.D.

Kenneth Minkoff, M.D.

Christian A. Müller, M.D.

Wade C. Myers, M.D.

John Nurnberger, M.D., Ph.D.

Louis A. Parrott, M.D., Ph.D.

Smita Patel, M.D.

Richard Ries, M.D.

Shannon Robinson, M.D.

Andrew J. Saxon, M.D.

John P.D. Shemo, M.D.

Stephen F. Signer, M.D., C.M., M.B.A.

Richard F. Summers, M.D.

Bick Wanck, M.D.

Jill M Williams, M.D.

Jeffrey DeVido, M.D.

Kimberly A. Yonkers, M.D.

Bonnie Zima, M.D., M.P.H.

Paula Zimbrean, M.D.

APA Council on Addiction Psychiatry

AMDA—The Society for Post-Acute and Long-Term Care Medicine

American Academy of Addiction Psychiatry

American Academy of Family Physicians

American Association of Community Psychiatrists

American Psychoanalytic Association

American Psychological Association

American Society of Addiction Medicine

Association for Behavioral and Cognitive Therapies

Canadian Psychiatric Association

Mental Health America

National Council for Behavioral Health

New Jersey Psychiatric Association

APPENDICES:
REVIEW OF RESEARCH EVIDENCE

Appendix A.
Clinical Questions and Search Strategies

Clinical Questions

The evidence reviews for both the Agency for Healthcare Research and Quality (AHRQ) report on pharmacotherapy for alcohol use disorder (AUD) (Jonas et al. 2014) and this guideline were premised on the following clinical questions:

1A. Which medications are efficacious for improving consumption outcomes for adults with AUD in outpatient settings?

1B. How do medications for adults with AUD compare for improving consumption outcomes in outpatient settings?

2A. Which medications are efficacious for improving health outcomes for adults with AUD in outpatient settings?

2B. How do medications for adults with AUD compare for improving health outcomes in outpatient settings?

3A. What adverse effects are associated with medications for adults with AUD in outpatient settings?

3B. How do medications for adults with AUD compare for adverse effects in outpatient settings?

4. Are medications for treating adults with AUD effective in primary care settings?

5. Are any of the medications more or less effective than other medications for men or women, older adults, young adults, racial or ethnic minorities, smokers, or those with co-occurring disorders?

6. Are any of the medications more or less effective for adults with specific genotypes (e.g., related to polymorphisms of the μ-opioid receptor gene [OPRM1])?

Search Strategies

The AHRQ's systematic review, *Pharmacotherapy for Adults With Alcohol-Use Disorders in Outpatient Settings* (Jonas et al. 2014), served as the predominant source of information for this guideline. The search strategies used by the AHRQ can be found in the appendix of the AHRQ review (Jonas et al. 2014). Since the AHRQ searches were conducted from January 1, 1970 through October 11, 2013, the APA also conducted a search of the literature to supplement the AHRQ review, which ranged from September 1, 2013 to April 24, 2016 and used search strategies identical to those used in the AHRQ review. Databases that were searched for both the AHRQ and APA reviews are MEDLINE (PubMed), PsycINFO (EBSCO), CINAHL (EBSCO), EMBASE (Elsevier), and Cochrane (Wiley). Details on the search terms and numbers of the articles found in the updated search are provided in the following tables.

PubMed

Search	Query	Items found
#1	Search "Alcohol-Related Disorders" [MeSH]	101450
#2	Search "Alcoholism" [MeSH]	69036
#3	Search "Alcohol Drinking" [MeSH]	55907
#4	Search alcohol depend*	10367
#5	Search "alcohol misuse"	1872
#6	Search alcohol addiction*	1041
#7	Search "alcohol abuse"	14980
#8	Search problem drink*	2557
#9	Search alcohol problem*	3524
#10	Search "alcohol consumption"	32259
#11	Search harmful alcohol*	386
#12	Search harmful drink*	385
#13	Search ((((drinking[tiab] OR drinker[tiab] OR drinkers[tiab]) AND alcohol[tiab]))	32042
#14	Search (#1 or #2 or #3 or #4 or #5 or #6 or #7 or #8 or #9 or #10 or #11 or #12 or #13)	169531
#15	Search "Alcohol Deterrents"[MeSH]	1211
#16	Search (("Naltrexone"[Mesh] OR naltrexone))	8614
#17	Search ReVia	8616
#18	Search Vivitrol	29
#19	Search (("acamprosate" [Supplementary Concept] OR acamprosate))	735
#20	Search Campral	737
#21	Search (("Disulfiram"[Mesh] OR Disulfiram))	3960
#22	Search Antabuse	4005
#23	Search (("Amitriptyline"[Mesh] OR Amitriptyline))	8489
#24	Search (("aripiprazole" [Supplementary Concept] OR aripiprazole))	2982
#25	Search (("atomoxetine" [Supplementary Concept] OR atomoxetine))	1366
#26	Search (("Baclofen"[Mesh] OR Baclofen))	7067
#27	Search (("Buspirone"[Mesh] OR Buspirone))	2764
#28	Search (("Citalopram"[Mesh] OR citalopram))	5752
#29	Search (("Desipramine"[Mesh] OR Desipramine))	7634
#30	Search escitalopram	6211
#31	Search (("Fluoxetine"[Mesh] OR Fluoxetine))	11983
#32	Search (("Fluvoxamine"[Mesh] OR Fluvoxamine))	2712
#33	Search (("gabapentin" [Supplementary Concept] OR gabapentin))	5237
#34	Search (("Imipramine"[Mesh] OR Imipramine))	12756
#35	Search (("nalmefene" [Supplementary Concept] OR nalmefene))	339
#36	Search (("olanzapine" [Supplementary Concept] OR olanzapine))	7659
#37	Search (("Ondansetron"[Mesh] OR Ondansetron))	4157
#38	Search (("Paroxetine"[Mesh] OR paroxetine))	5642
#39	Search (("Prazosin"[Mesh] OR Prazosin))	13129
#40	Search (("quetiapine" [Supplementary Concept] OR quetiapine))	4056
#41	Search (("Sertraline"[Mesh] OR Sertraline))	4196
#42	Search (("topiramate"[Supplementary Concept] OR topiramate))	4003
#43	Search (((("Valproic Acid"[Mesh] OR Valproate))) OR "divalproex"	16643
#44	Search (("varenicline"[Supplementary Concept] OR varenicline))	1348
#45	Search (("Viloxazine"[Mesh] OR Viloxazine))	321

Search	Query	Items found
#46	Search ((#15 or #16 or #17 or #18 or #19 or #20 or #21 or #22 or #23 or #24 or #25 or #26 or #27 or #28 or #29 or #30 or #31 or #32 or #33 or #34 or #35 or #36 or #37 or #38 or #39 or #40 or #41 or #42 or #43 or #44 or #45))	120290
#47	Search ((#14 and #46))	4533
#48	Search (((#14 and #46))) AND "humans"[Filter]	3469
#49	Search (((#14 and #46)) AND "humans"[Filter]) AND "english"[Filter]	2867
#50	Search ((((#14 and #46)) AND "humans"[Filter]) AND "english"[Filter]) AND "adult"[Filter]	1273
#51	Search (#50) AND ("1970/01/01"[Date - Publication] : "3000"[Date - Publication])	1253
#52	Search ((comment[pt] OR editorial[pt] OR letter[pt] OR news[pt])))	1635136
#53	Search ((#51 NOT #52))	1185
#54	Search (((#51 NOT #52))) AND ("2013/09/01"[Date - Publication] : "3000"[Date - Publication])	124
#55	Search ((#47 AND ("retraction"[All Fields] OR "Retracted Publication"[pt]))	5
#56	Search #54 NOT #55	124

Search ID#	Search terms (using Boolean/phrase search mode)	Actions
S1	"Alcohol-Related Disorders"	280
S2	DE "Alcoholism"	26797
S3	(DE "Alcohol Drinking Attitudes" OR DE "Alcohol Drinking Patterns") OR (DE "Alcohol Intoxication")	22573
S4	alcohol depend*	18723
S5	"alcohol misuse"	1647
S6	alcohol addiction*	3846
S7	"alcohol abuse"	24544
S8	problem drink*	5810
S9	alcohol problem*	12102
S10	"alcohol consumption"	15177
S11	harmful alcohol*	724
S12	harmful drink*	498
S13	TI ((drinking OR drinker OR drinkers) AND alcohol) OR AB ((drinking OR drinker OR drinkers) AND alcohol)	24062
S14	S1 OR S2 OR S3 OR S4 OR S5 OR S6 OR S7 OR S8 OR S9 OR S10 OR S11 OR S12 OR S13	82937
S15	"Alcohol Deterrents"	2
S16	naltrexone	2986
S17	ReVia	18
S18	Vivitrol	23
S19	acamprosate	416
S20	Campral	14
S21	Disulfiram	654
S22	Antabuse	160
S23	Amitriptyline	2333
S24	aripiprazole	2049
S25	atomoxetine	787
S26	Baclofen	1221
S27	Buspirone	1400
S28	Citalopram	2365
S29	Desipramine	2090
S30	escitalopram	1185
S31	Fluoxetine	6074
S32	Fluvoxamine	1522
S33	gabapentin	1207
S34	Imipramine	4044
S35	nalmefene	114
S36	olanzapine	5556
S37	Ondansetron	446
S38	Paroxetine	3057
S39	Prazosin	594
S40	quetiapine	3074
S41	Sertraline	2469
S42	topiramate	1450
S43	"Valproic Acid" OR Valproate OR divalproex	4342

Search ID#	Search terms (using Boolean/phrase search mode)	Actions
S44	varenicline	562
S45	Viloxazine	109
S46	S15 OR S16 OR S17 OR S18 OR S19 OR S20 OR S21 OR S22 OR S23 OR S24 OR S25 OR S26 OR S27 OR S28 OR S29 OR S30 OR S31 OR S32 OR S33 OR S34 OR S35 OR S36 OR S37 OR S38 OR S39 OR S40 OR S41 OR S42 OR S43 OR S44 OR S45	40367
S47	S14 AND S46	2411
S48	S14 AND S46 Limiters - English; Age Groups: Adulthood (18 yrs & older); Population Group: Human	1197
S49	S14 AND S46 Limiters - Published Date: 20130901-20160531; English; Age Groups: Adulthood (18 yrs & older); Population Group: Human	181

Search ID#	Search terms (using Boolean/phrase search mode)	References retrieved
S1	MH "Alcohol-Related Disorders"	1275
S2	MH "Alcoholism"	12790
S3	MH "Alcohol Drinking"	19424
S4	alcohol depend*	4003
S5	"alcohol misuse"	855
S6	alcohol addiction*	507
S7	"alcohol abuse"	9104
S8	problem drink*	1694
S9	alcohol problem*	3696
S10	"alcohol consumption"	7140
S11	harmful alcohol*	368
S12	harmful drink*	238
S13	TI ((drinking OR drinker OR drinkers) AND alcohol) OR AB ((drinking OR drinker OR drinkers) AND alcohol)	8163
S14	S1 OR S2 OR S3 OR S4 OR S5 OR S6 OR S7 OR S8 OR S9 OR S10 OR S11 OR S12 OR S13	43236
S15	MH "Alcohol Deterrents"	253
S16	naltrexone	1506
S17	ReVia	11
S18	Vivitrol	50
S19	acamprosate	196
S20	Campral	7
S21	Disulfiram	271
S22	Antabuse	20
S23	Amitriptyline	865
S24	aripiprazole	920
S25	atomoxetine	517
S26	Baclofen	1005
S27	Buspirone	253
S28	Citalopram	1217
S29	Desipramine	177
S30	escitalopram	475
S31	Fluoxetine	1676
S32	Fluvoxamine	227
S33	gabapentin	1584
S34	Imipramine	343
S35	nalmefene	50
S36	olanzapine	1747
S37	Ondansetron	936
S38	Paroxetine	1120
S39	Prazosin	316
S40	quetiapine	1084
S41	Sertraline	1028
S42	topiramate	1165
S43	"Valproic Acid" OR Valproate OR divalproex	2193

Search ID#	Search terms (using Boolean/phrase search mode)	References retrieved
S44	varenicline	555
S45	Viloxazine	5
S46	S15 OR S16 OR S17 OR S18 OR S19 OR S20 OR S21 OR S22 OR S23 OR S24 OR S25 OR S26 OR S27 OR S28 OR S29 OR S30 OR S31 OR S32 OR S33 OR S34 OR S35 OR S36 OR S37 OR S38 OR S39 OR S40 OR S41 OR S42 OR S43 OR S44 OR S45	17496
S47	S14 AND S46	1201
S48	S14 AND S46 Limiters - English; Age Groups: Adulthood (18 yrs & older); Population Group: Human	1196
S49	S14 AND S46 Limiters - Published Date: 20130901-20160531; English; Age Groups: Adulthood (18 yrs & older); Population Group: Human	239

EMBASE

Search ID#	Search terms	References retrieved
#1	'alcohol-related disorders'/exp OR 'alcohol-related disorders'	109,688
#2	'alcoholism'/exp	109,506
#3	'drinking behavior'/exp	39,554
#4	'alcohol'/exp AND depend*	37,628
#5	'alcohol misuse'	2,372
#6	'alcohol'/exp AND addiction*	12,146
#7	'alcohol abuse'/exp	29,673
#8	problem AND drink*	9,845
#9	'alcohol'/exp AND problem*	14,123
#10	'alcohol consumption'/exp	90,443
#11	harmful AND alcohol*	3,691
#12	harmful AND drink*	2,250
#13	drinking:ti OR drinker:ti OR drinkers:ti AND alcohol:ti OR (drinking:ab OR drinker:ab OR drinkers:ab AND alcohol:ab)	40,816
#14	#1 OR #2 OR #3 OR #4 OR #5 OR #6 OR #7 OR #8 OR #9 OR #10 OR #11 OR #12 OR #13	258,040
#15	'alcohol deterrents'	15
#16	'naltrexone'/exp OR naltrexone	13,218
#17	'revia'/exp OR revia	12,211
#18	'vivitrol'/exp OR vivitrol	12,203
#19	'acamprosate'/exp OR acamprosate	2,082
#20	'campral'/exp OR campral	2,025
#21	'disulfiram'/exp OR disulfiram	8,453
#22	'antabuse'/exp OR antabuse	8,134
#23	'amitriptyline'/exp OR amitriptyline	36,056
#24	'aripiprazole'/exp OR aripiprazole	11,148
#25	'atomoxetine'/exp OR atomoxetine	4,233
#26	'baclofen'/exp OR baclofen	15,835
#27	'buspirone'/exp OR buspirone	8,567
#28	'citalopram'/exp OR citalopram	19,423
#29	'desipramine'/exp OR desipramine	21,591
#30	'escitalopram'/exp OR escitalopram	8,570
#31	'fluoxetine'/exp OR fluoxetine	41,023
#32	'fluvoxamine'/exp OR fluvoxamine	12,745
#33	'gabapentin'/exp OR gabapentin	23,826
#34	'imipramine'/exp OR imipramine	35,132
#35	'nalmefene'/exp OR nalmefene	1,087
#36	'olanzapine'/exp OR olanzapine	28,340
#37	'ondansetron'/exp OR ondansetron	14,436
#38	'paroxetine'/exp OR paroxetine	24,817
#39	'prazosin'/exp OR prazosin	23,785
#40	'quetiapine'/exp OR quetiapine	18,698
#41	'sertraline'/exp OR sertraline	21,836
#42	'topiramate'/exp OR topiramate	17,639
#43	'valproic acid'/exp OR 'valproic acid' OR 'valproate'/exp OR valproate OR divalproex	57,157

Search ID#	Search terms	References retrieved
#44	'varenicline'/exp OR varenicline	3,309
#45	'viloxazine'/exp OR viloxazine	1,451
#46	#15 OR #16 OR #17 OR #18 OR #19 OR #20 OR #21 OR #22 OR #23 OR #24 OR #25 OR #26 OR #27 OR #28 OR #29 OR #30 OR #31 OR #32 OR #33 OR #34 OR #35 OR #36 OR #37 OR #38 OR #39 OR #40 OR #41 OR #42 OR #43 OR #44 OR #45	289,719
#47	#14 AND #46	11,439
#48	#47 AND ([adult]/lim OR [aged]/lim) AND [humans]/lim AND [english]/lim AND [embase]/lim AND [1970-2016]/py	2,401
#49	editorial:it OR letter:it OR note:it AND [1970-2016]/py	2,041,776
#50	#48 NOT #49 AND [1970-2016]/py	2,161
#51	#48 NOT #49 AND [2013-2016]/py	545

ID	Search	Hits
#1	MeSH descriptor: [Alcohol-Related Disorders] explode all trees	3886
#2	MeSH descriptor: [Alcoholism] explode all trees	2638
#3	MeSH descriptor: [Alcohol Drinking] explode all trees	2804
#4	alcohol depend*	5822
#5	"alcohol misuse"	299
#6	alcohol addiction*	1893
#7	"alcohol abuse"	1452
#8	problem drink*	1027
#9	alcohol problem*	3480
#10	"alcohol consumption'	3355
#11	harmful alcohol*	710
#12	harmful drink*	310
#13	(drinking:ti or drinking:ab or drinker:ti or drinker:ab or drinkers:ti or drinkers:ab) and (alcohol:ti or alcohol:ab)	3324
#14	#1 or #2 or #3 or #4 or #5 or #6 or #7 or #8 or #9 or #10 or #11 or #12 or #13	13194
#15	MeSH descriptor: [Alcohol Deterrents] explode all trees	182
#16	[mh Naltrexone] or naltrexone	1559
#17	ReVia	13
#18	Vivitrol	16
#19	acamprosate	256
#20	Campral	8
#21	[mh Disulfiram] or Disulfiram	291
#22	Antabuse	26
#23	[mh Amitriptyline] or Amitriptyline	2536
#24	aripiprazole	917
#25	atomoxetine	407
#26	[mh Baclofen] or Baclofen	475
#27	[mh Buspirone] or Buspirone	569
#28	[mh Citalopram] or Citalopram	1797
#29	[mh Desipramine] or Desipramine	848
#30	escitalopram	1013
#31	[mh Fluoxetine] or Fluoxetine	3173
#32	[mh Fluvoxamine] or Fluvoxamine	963
#33	gabapentin	1402
#34	[mh Imipramine] or Imipramine	2264
#35	nalmefene	120
#36	olanzapine	2653
#37	[mh Ondansetron] or Ondansetron	2431
#38	[mh Paroxetine] or Paroxetine	2402
#39	[mh Prazosin] or Prazosin	1138
#40	quetiapine	1323
#41	[mh Sertraline] or Sertraline	2013
#42	topiramate	979
#43	[mh "Valproic Acid"] or Valproate or Divalproex	1674
#44	[mh Viloxazine] or Viloxazine	151

ID	Search	Hits
#45	varenicline	480
#46	#15 or #16 or #17 or #18 or #19 or #20 or #21 or #22 or #23 or #24 or #25 or #26 or #27 or #28 or #29 or #30 or #31 or #32 or #33 or #34 or #35 or #36 or #37 or #38 or #39 or #40 or #41 or #42 or #43 or #44 or #45	25834
#47	#14 and #46	1847
#48	comment:pt or editorial:pt or letter:pt or news:pt	7973
#49	#47 not #48	1838

Additional Target Searches

Search of MEDLINE (PubMed) on January 19, 2017
related to patient preferences and AUD pharmacotherapy

Search	Items found
("patient preference" OR "patient preferences" OR "patient choice" OR "patient choices" OR "shared decision making" OR "patient centered") AND ("alcohol use disorder" OR "alcohol use disorders" OR "alcohol abuse" OR "alcohol dependence" OR "alcoholism" OR "alcoholic")	88
Limited to "english"[Language] AND "humans"[Filter]	67

Articles were screened by one reviewer (L.J.F.) for relevance based on whether the patient population was primarily individuals with AUD and whether specific preferences for AUD treatments were discussed. Three articles were identified but were of limited relevance because one addressed only patients who were undomiciled, one was in a primary care setting, and one was based on a survey of the Swedish general population. None of the articles commented on preferences for specific pharmacotherapies.

Search of MEDLINE (PubMed) on January 22, 2017
related to use of quantitative measures to detect the presence and severity of alcohol misuse

Search	Items found
("audit" OR "promis" OR "rating scale" OR "rating scales" OR "quantitative measure" OR "quantitative measurement" OR "quantitative measurements" OR "quantitative measures" OR "measurement based") AND ("alcohol use disorder" OR "alcohol use disorders" OR "alcohol abuse" OR "alcohol dependence" OR "alcoholism" OR "alcoholic")	4376
Limited to ("english"[Filter] AND "humans"[Filter] AND ("2006"[Date - Publication] : "2016"[Date - Publication])) NOT ("comment"[Publication Type] OR "editorial"[Publication Type] OR "letter"[Publication Type])	1859

Articles were screened by one reviewer (L.J.F.) for relevance based on whether the quantitative measure was used to support a diagnosis of AUD and establish its severity. Articles were excluded if they focused on the use of quantitative measures for screening purposes in community samples or primary care settings. Three articles were identified, one of which was a systematic review of properties of the AUDIT.

Search of MEDLINE (PubMed) on January 22, 2017 related to use of laboratory biomarkers for alcohol use

Search	Items found
("biomarker" OR "biomarkers" OR "cdt" OR "carbohydrate deficient transferrin" OR "ast" OR "alt" OR "aspartate amino transferase" OR "alanine amino transferase" OR "ethylglucuronide" OR "ethyl glucuronide" OR "ethyl sulfate" OR "ethylsulfate" OR "ggt" OR "gamma glutamyl transferase" OR "gamma-glutamyltransferase" OR "mcv" OR "mean corpuscular volume" OR "phosphatidylethanol" OR "phosphatidyl ethanol" OR "peth") AND ("alcohol use disorder" OR "alcohol use disorders" OR "alcohol abuse" OR "alcohol dependence" OR "alcoholism" OR "alcoholic")	6175
Limited to ("english"[Filter] AND "humans"[Filter] AND ("2006"[Date - Publication] : "2016"[Date - Publication])) NOT ("comment"[Publication Type] OR "editorial"[Publication Type] OR "letter"[Publication Type])	2562

Articles were screened by one reviewer (L.J.F.) for relevance based on whether the laboratory biomarker was used as part of an initial evaluation of AUD or for ongoing monitoring of alcohol consumption patterns during treatment. Articles were included if they focused on the impact of quantitative measures on patient outcomes and used a randomized controlled design or a controlled or prospective cohort design with at least 50 individuals. Articles that were aimed primarily at establishing threshold values to optimize sensitivity and specificity or optimizing laboratory assay methodologies were excluded. Three articles were identified, of which one was a systematic review that included articles on use of phosphatidylethanol as a possible marker for chronic alcohol consumption or binge drinking. Two articles addressed the utility of biomarkers in identifying relapse of AUD in individuals who had received a liver transplant.

Search of MEDLINE (PubMed) on January 19, 2017 related to use of AUD medications in pregnancy and while breastfeeding

Search	Items found
("disulfiram" OR "acamprosate" OR "naltrexone" OR "topiramate" OR "ondansetron" OR "gabapentin") AND ("pregnant" OR "pregnancy" OR "breast feeding" OR "breastfeeding" OR "lactation" OR "lactating" OR "puerperal disorders" OR "puerperium" OR "perinatal" OR "prenatal")	646
Limited to "english"[Language] AND "humans"[Filter] AND ("2006"[Date - Publication] : "2016"[Date - Publication])	229

Articles were screened by one reviewer (L.J.F.) for relevance based on whether treatment using the medications listed above was at least 3 weeks in duration and not just at delivery or on an as-needed basis (e.g., for intermittent nausea). Included articles were randomized controlled trials, clinical trials of at least 50 women, or data from registries (e.g., MotherRisk). On the basis of these criteria, 11 articles were identified for full text review for possible citation in the discussion of evidence for guideline Statement 14.

Appendix B.
Review of Research Evidence Supporting Guideline Statements

Assessment and Determination of Treatment Goals

STATEMENT 1: Assessment of Substance Use

APA *recommends* **(1C)** that the initial psychiatric evaluation of a patient with suspected alcohol use disorder include assessment of current and past use of tobacco and alcohol as well as any misuse of other substances, including prescribed or over-the-counter medications or supplements.

Evidence for this statement comes from general principles of assessment and clinical care in psychiatric practice. Expert opinion suggests that conducting such assessments as part of the initial psychiatric evaluation improves the identification and diagnosis of substance use disorders. See APA *Practice Guidelines for the Psychiatric Evaluation of Adults* (American Psychiatric Association 2016) for additional details. A detailed systematic review to support this statement was outside the scope of this guideline; however, less comprehensive searches of the literature did not yield any studies that related to this recommendation in the context of AUD treatment. Consequently, the strength of research evidence is rated as low. Indirect evidence from outpatient primary care settings suggests that screening for use of tobacco, alcohol, and other substances can be beneficial if coupled with a brief intervention. Screening and intervention for tobacco use has been recommended by the U.S. Preventive Services Task Force (2009). Screening for at-risk drinking or AUD has also been recommended by the USPSTF (Moyer and U.S. Preventive Services Task Force 2013) as well as by professional organizations such as the American College of Obstetricians and Gynecologists (2011). Although several outpatient randomized controlled trials (RCTs) have not found a significant benefit of screening and brief intervention for alcohol (Kaner et al. 2013) or substance use (Saitz et al. 2014), screening may increase the likelihood that these disorders will be identified and documented in the clinical record (Mitchell et al. 2012; Williams et al. 2014), which would be expected to improve clinical decision making. Recognition of these disorders is particularly important given the high rates of comorbidity in individuals with AUD (S. P. Chou et al. 2016; Grant et al. 2016) and the frequent lack of treatment for these disorders (Centers for Disease Control and Prevention 2011; Hasin and Grant 2015).

STATEMENT 2: Use of Quantitative Behavioral Measures

APA *recommends* **(1C)** that the initial psychiatric evaluation of a patient with suspected alcohol use disorder include a quantitative behavioral measure to detect the presence of alcohol misuse and assess its severity.

Evidence for this statement is indirect and comes from studies of screening for alcohol use disorder (AUD) and studies of the properties of commonly used alcohol-related quantitative measures (Jonas et al. 2012a, 2012b). The strength of research evidence for this statement is rated as low. Findings from the Combined Pharmacotherapies and Behavioral Interventions for Alcohol Dependence (COMBINE) study suggest that in individuals receiving treatment for AUD, scores on the Alcohol Use Disorders Identification Test (AUDIT) reflect the severity of the disorder (Donovan et al. 2006). Severity of AUD is also reflected by AUDIT or AUDIT-C scores in other outpatient settings and community samples (Chavez et al. 2012; Dawson et al. 2012; Rubinsky et al. 2013; Williams et al. 2014). In primary care settings, the USPSTF (Moyer and U.S. Preventive Services Task Force 2013, p. 212) recommends screening for alcohol misuse and notes that "both the AUDIT and the abbreviated AUDIT-C have good sensitivity and specificity for detecting the full spectrum of alcohol misuse across multiple populations." Other scales that have been used for screening purposes in routine care (Cherpitel 2002; Dhalla and Kopec 2007; Humeniuk et al. 2008) have been less well studied as an indicator of AUD severity.

The USPSTF notes that their recommendations do not apply to individuals seeking treatment for alcohol misuse, but the ability to implement screening with these measures in primary care settings suggests that it would be feasible to use them in outpatient alcohol treatment. In addition to use for screening in hospital and emergency department settings, quantitative measures have been used for screening purposes in outpatient psychiatric settings, again suggesting the feasibility of implementation in AUD treatment (Nehlin et al. 2012). This recommendation is also consistent with Guideline VII on Quantitative Assessment as part of the APA *Practice Guidelines for the Psychiatric Evaluation of Adults* (American Psychiatric Association 2016).

STATEMENT 3: Use of Physiological Biomarkers

APA *suggests* (2C) that physiological biomarkers be used to identify persistently elevated levels of alcohol consumption as part of the initial evaluation of patients with alcohol use disorder or in the treatment of individuals who have an indication for ongoing monitoring of their alcohol use.

Evidence for this statement is indirect, and the strength of research evidence for this statement is rated as low. Evidence comes from information on the sensitivity and specificity of physiological biomarkers in detecting alcohol consumption (Alatalo et al. 2009; Bergström and Helander 2008a; Hietala et al. 2006; Hock et al. 2005; Lowe et al. 2015; Substance Abuse and Mental Health Services Administration 2012; Walther et al. 2015; Wurst et al. 2015). In addition, some (Harasymiw and Bean 2007; Wetterling et al. 2014) but not all (Bertholet et al. 2014; Liangpunsakul et al. 2010) studies suggest that physiological biomarkers can supplement patient self-report in identifying alcohol use in community samples, primary care, and other medical settings. Research also suggests that physiological biomarkers can be used to identify relapse to drinking (Mundle et al. 1999) and to promote abstinence (McDonell et al. 2017) or to demonstrate risk for alcohol-related behaviors such as driving while intoxicated (Maenhout et al. 2014; Marques et al. 2010) or health complications after liver transplant (Kollmann et al. 2016; Piano et al. 2014; Staufer et al. 2011). Additional information on the rationale for using physiological biomarkers in the management of individuals with AUD can be found in the advisory from the Substance Abuse and Mental Health Services Administration (2012).

STATEMENT 4: Assessment of Co-occurring Conditions

APA *recommends* (1C) that patients be assessed for co-occurring conditions (including substance use disorders, other psychiatric disorders, and other medical disorders) that may influence the selection of pharmacotherapy for alcohol use disorder.

Evidence for this statement comes from general principles of assessment and clinical care in psychiatric practice. Expert opinion suggests that conducting such assessments as part of the initial psychiatric evaluation improves diagnostic accuracy, appropriateness of treatment selection, and treatment safety. For additional details, see Guideline I, "Review of Psychiatric Symptoms, Trauma History, and Psychiatric Treatment History," and Guideline VI, "Assessment of Medical Health," in the APA *Practice Guidelines for the Psychiatric Evaluation of Adults* (American Psychiatric Association 2016). A detailed systematic review to support this statement was outside the scope of this guideline; however, less comprehensive searches of the literature did not yield any studies that related to this recommendation in the context of AUD treatment. Consequently, the strength of research evidence is rated as low.

STATEMENT 5: Determination of Initial Treatment Goals

APA *suggests* **(2C)** that the initial goals of treatment of alcohol use disorder (e.g., abstinence from alcohol use, reduction or moderation of alcohol use, other elements of harm reduction) be agreed on between the patient and clinician and that this agreement be documented in the medical record.

Evidence for this statement comes from general principles of assessment and clinical care in psychiatric practice. Also, in choosing pharmacotherapy for AUD and particularly before deciding to prescribe disulfiram, it is essential to know whether or not the patient has a goal of abstinence from alcohol use. More generally, expert opinion suggests that engaging patients in shared decision making improves the therapeutic alliance and adherence. For additional details, see Guideline VIII, "Involvement of the Patient in Treatment Decision Making," in the APA *Practice Guidelines for the Psychiatric Evaluation of Adults* (American Psychiatric Association 2016). There has also been increasing attention to shared decision making in treatment of AUD (Bradley and Kivlahan 2014) as well as in other areas of medicine (Durand et al. 2014; Makoul and Clayman 2006).

A detailed systematic review to support this statement was outside the scope of this guideline; however, a less comprehensive search of the literature did not yield any studies that were directly related to this recommendation. Consequently, the strength of research evidence is rated as low. However, secondary analyses of clinical trial data show that patient-stated goals of abstinence at study initiation are associated with more days abstinent and greater reductions in alcohol consumption than patient-stated goals of reduced alcohol use (Adamson et al. 2010; Al-Otaiba et al. 2008; Berger et al. 2016; Bujarski et al. 2013; Chang et al. 2006; Dunn and Strain 2013; Gueorguieva et al. 2014; Meyer et al. 2014; Mowbray et al. 2013). In addition, patient goals sometimes changed in the course of treatment. Several smaller studies also related to determining patient goals at the start of treatment. One small study examined the number and types of goals set in the course of treatment by individuals with AUD who were chronically homeless (Collins et al. 2015). Drinking-related goals were most frequent and typically included reducing drinking and reducing alcohol-related consequences, rather than abstinence-based goals. Quality-of-life goals and health-related goals were also reported throughout the course of treatment. In addition, a small study of at-risk elderly drinkers who were treated in primary care compared enhanced referral with integrated care, which included treatment goal setting among multiple other components (Lee et al. 2009). Individuals receiving integrated care were more likely to access care and had fewer drinks in the past week and fewer binge-drinking episodes in the past 3 months than those assigned to receive enhanced referral.

STATEMENT 6: Discussion of Legal Obligations

APA *suggests* **(2C)** that the initial goals of treatment of alcohol use disorder include discussion of the patient's legal obligations (e.g., abstinence from alcohol use, monitoring of abstinence) and that this discussion be documented in the medical record.

Evidence for this statement comes from general principles of assessment and clinical care in psychiatric practice. A detailed systematic review to support this statement was outside the scope of this guideline; however, on the basis of prior searches related to psychiatric assessment and treatment planning, we would not anticipate finding any studies with a direct bearing on this recommendation.

STATEMENT 7: Review of Risks to Self and Others

APA *suggests* **(2C)** that the initial goals of treatment of alcohol use disorder include discussion of risks to self (e.g., physical health, occupational functioning, legal involvement) and others (e.g., impaired driving) from continued use of alcohol and that this discussion be documented in the medical record.

Evidence for this statement comes from general principles of clinical care in psychiatric practice. A detailed systematic review to support this statement was outside the scope of this guideline; however, evidence does suggest that abstaining from or reducing alcohol consumption is associated with significant health benefits (Charlet and Heinz 2017). In addition, having the patient identify negative consequences of drinking for himself or herself is an element of motivational enhancement therapy (Miller and Rollnick 2013; Miller et al. 1994). Assessment of drinking consequences has been a part of many studies of treatment for AUD, including Matching Alcoholism Treatments to Client Heterogeneity (Project MATCH; Miller et al. 1995; Project MATCH Research Group 1997) and the COMBINE study (Anton et al. 2006), although the specific effect of this element on outcomes has not been separated from other elements of treatment.

STATEMENT 8: Evidence-Based Treatment Planning

APA *recommends* **(1C)** that patients with alcohol use disorder have a documented comprehensive and person-centered treatment plan that includes evidence-based nonpharmacological and pharmacological treatments.

Evidence for this statement comes from general principles of assessment and clinical care in psychiatric practice. A detailed systematic review to support this statement was outside the scope of this guideline; however, less comprehensive searches of the literature did not yield any studies that directly related to this recommendation. Consequently, the strength of research evidence is rated as low.

Expert opinion suggests that when using pharmacotherapy to treat AUD, it is beneficial for a treatment plan to incorporate nonpharmacological treatments and have a patient-centered focus. Furthermore, major clinical trials of alcohol pharmacotherapy, such as the COMBINE study, include some form of nonpharmacological treatment in all treatment arms. For example, medication management included elements of education, encouragement, approaches to enhancing medication adherence, and supportive interactions to promote abstinence.

In terms of person-centered care, one meta-analysis (Barrio and Gual 2016) assessed the role of patient-centered care in individuals with AUD. Of the 40 included studies, 5 involved use of pharmacological agents on an "as needed" basis, and 35 involved motivational interviewing, with more than one session occurring in 15 of the studies. Despite significant heterogeneity in the studies, a benefit of "as needed" medication was described with positive alcohol-related outcomes in some of the multiple-session motivational interviewing studies.

In terms of treatment preferences related to AUD, a study of 399 primary care patients included 65 individuals (68% male) with a score of greater than 8 on the AUDIT (Lieberman et al. 2014). When asked about potential treatments, 68% reported interest in "getting help from my doctor," 37% reported interest in an Internet program, and 23% reported interest in Alcoholics Anonymous (AA). In terms of pharmacotherapy, 55% reported interest in "taking a medication that would make it easier to avoid alcohol (but would not make me sick if I drank)," with 20% reporting interest in "taking a medication that would make me sick if I drank." Alcohol-related treatment preferences were also assessed in a large (N=9,005) population-based study in Sweden (Andréasson et al. 2013). Among respondents who reported the highest number of standard drinks per week (>28 for men and >18 for women), approximately 40% expressed a preference for AA or another support group, approximately 40% expressed a preference for psychotherapy, approximately 15% expressed a preference for pharmacotherapy, and approximately 5% expressed a preference for Internet-based intervention. Data from the COMBINE study demonstrate that patient views of treatment, including treatment cost-effectiveness, may differ from clinician views (Dunlap et al. 2010). In addition, the time that patients must invest in attending treatment sessions and traveling to treatment is often considerable (Dunlap et al. 2010).

Selection of a Pharmacotherapy

STATEMENT 9: Naltrexone or Acamprosate

APA *recommends* **(1B)** that naltrexone or acamprosate be offered to patients with moderate to severe alcohol use disorder who

- have a goal of reducing alcohol consumption or achieving abstinence,
- prefer pharmacotherapy or have not responded to nonpharmacological treatments alone, and
- have no contraindications to the use of these medications.

Evidence supporting the use of naltrexone and acamprosate comes from multiple double-blind RCTs. All trials described below were conducted in the outpatient setting, with subject recruitment typically occurring by print and other media advertising or by referrals (e.g., from inpatient detoxification programs or other outpatient clinicians). Most studies were conducted in Europe or the United States; the remaining studies were conducted in Asia, Australia, or South America. To be included in the systematic review of evidence, trials needed to be at least 12 weeks in length, with some extending to 26 weeks or more. Posttreatment follow-up was typically minimal, but some trials followed subjects up to a year after treatment discontinuation. The majority of the trials included psychotherapies or other psychosocial interventions (e.g., motivational therapies, cognitive-behavioral interventions, manual-based medication management approaches) for all treatment groups.

The vast majority of trials established eligibility for the trial on the basis of DSM-IV criteria or ICD-10 criteria for alcohol dependence as well as numerical descriptions of alcohol use (e.g., days of drinking in past week or month, threshold numbers for drinks per day or drinks per week), typically with lower thresholds for women than for men. In framing the guideline recommendation in terms of DSM-5 AUD, we relied on evidence that DSM-IV alcohol dependence corresponds to DSM-5 AUD of at least moderate severity (Compton et al. 2013; Hasin et al. 2013; Peer et al. 2013). In terms of exclusion criteria, other substance use disorders, besides nicotine and sometimes marijuana, typically precluded participation, as did use of psychotropic medications, and significant physical or psychiatric illnesses were also exclusion criteria for most trials. Other exclusion criteria related to ability to consent (e.g., language barriers, cognitive deficits) and to potential safety risks with the medication such as pregnancy or breastfeeding or need for opioid medication (with naltrexone). Study subjects were generally limited to adults, with a mean age of subjects in the mid-40s. The majority of trials had a preponderance of men. Other demographic characteristics were often unreported.

Most study outcomes were focused on abstinence-related outcomes such as any drinking, time to first drink, or time to relapse or alcohol consumption–related outcomes such as number of drinking days, number of heavy drinking days, drinks per drinking day, or drinks per week. Other important outcomes such as quality of life, accidents, injuries, and mortality were reported infrequently. In trials that included information about adverse events, the methods for identifying such events were frequently unclear. Numbers of serious events (including suicide or suicide attempts) were small, making it impossible to identify whether differences existed among treatment conditions. Some studies reported information only about adverse events that were statistically different from placebo, which could affect the meta-analyses on harms.

Benefits of Acamprosate

The AHRQ review (Jonas et al. 2014) found that acamprosate treatment at a dose of 666 mg and three times daily (range 1,000 mg to 3,000 mg per day in divided doses) was associated with a decreased likelihood of returning to alcohol use as compared with placebo (moderate strength of evidence; risk difference [RD] –0.09; 95% confidence interval [CI] –0.14 to –0.04; number needed to treat [NNT]=12) (Table B–1). Number of drinking days was also reduced with acamprosate treatment relative to placebo (moderate strength of evidence; weighted mean difference [WMD] –8.8; 95% CI –12.8 to –4.8; 13 trials). However, for both outcomes, the benefits of acamprosate were seen primarily in studies done outside of the United States. Return to heavy drinking (moderate strength of evidence) and number of heavy drinking days (insufficient strength of evidence) showed no effect of acamprosate. The available evidence also did not permit any conclusions about the effect of acamprosate on outcomes such as quality of life, functioning, accidents, injuries, or mortality. In studies that assessed response rates by sex, men and women did not differ on any measure of efficacy.

In the studies with long-term use of acamprosate (48–52 weeks), there was an 11% absolute reduction in return to any drinking (RD, –0.11; 95% CI, –0.16 to –0.06; 4 trials) and 12.2% fewer drinking days than for those treated with placebo over 48–52 weeks (WMD, –12.2; 95% CI, –16.4 to –8.0; I^2 0%).

A number of relevant studies that are not included in the AHRQ meta-analysis or in Table B–1 have shown mixed results for acamprosate. In a pragmatic trial in France, 422 patients treated by 149 practitioners were randomly assigned to standard care (typically outpatient detoxification followed by psychotherapy) or to acamprosate plus standard care (Kiritzé-Topor et al. 2004). The trial reported better outcomes for the acamprosate group on a number of alcohol-related measures, with an NNT of about 7. A 24-week study (total N=327) with low risk of bias that was conducted in Japan (Higuchi and Japanese Acamprosate Study Group 2015) showed greater rates of abstinence with acamprosate than placebo at 24 weeks (47.2% for acamprosate vs. 36.0% for placebo; p=0.039), but there was no significant effect of treatment on secondary endpoints (i.e., cumulative days of abstinence during 24 weeks of treatment, time to first relapse, and time to 3 or more days of consecutive drinking). Furthermore, the generalizability of this study to the United States may be limited because patients were enrolled on discharge from 2 months of inpatient detoxification/rehabilitation.

In two additional RCTs, effects of acamprosate did not differ from placebo. The German PREDICT study (Mann et al. 2013), modeled after the COMBINE study, recruited subjects (total N=426) at time of discharge from medical detoxification (average length of stay 18 days). The time to first

Outcome	Number of studies; number of subjects	Risk of bias; design	Consistency	Directness	Precision	Summary effect size (95% CI)	NNT[h]	Strength of evidence grade
Return to any drinking	16;[a] 4,847	Medium; RCTs	Consistent[b]	Direct	Precise	RD: –0.09 (–0.14 to –0.04)	12	Moderate
Return to heavy drinking	7; 2,496	Low; RCTs	Consistent	Direct	Precise	RD: –0.01 (–0.04 to 0.03)	NA	Moderate[c]
Drinking days	13;[d] 4,485	Medium; RCTs	Consistent	Direct	Precise	WMD: –8.8 (–12.8 to –4.8)	NA	Moderate
Heavy drinking days	1; 100	Medium; RCT	Unknown	Direct	Imprecise	WMD: –2.6 (–11.4 to 6.2)	NA	Insufficient
Drinks per drinking day	1;[d] 116	Low; RCT	Unknown	Direct	Imprecise	WMD: 0.40 (–1.81 to 2.61)	NA	Insufficient
Accidents	0;[e] 0	NA	NA	NA	NA	NA	NA	Insufficient
Injuries	0; 0	NA	NA	NA	NA	NA	NA	Insufficient
Quality of life or function	1; 612	Low; RCT	Unknown	Direct	Unknown	NSD[f]	NA	Insufficient
Mortality	8;[g] 2,677	Medium; RCTs	Unknown	Direct	Imprecise	7 (ACA) vs. 6 (PBO)	NA	Insufficient

[a]Two additional studies were rated high risk of bias; one additional study was rated as unclear risk of bias.
[b]Although there was considerable statistical heterogeneity, 14 of 15 studies reported point estimates that favored acamprosate; differences were in magnitude of benefit.
[c]The relatively small number of studies reporting this outcome raises concern for potential reporting bias, hence the rating of moderate rather than high.
[d]One additional study was rated high risk of bias.
[e]The single study that reported this outcome was rated as unclear risk of bias. It reported that one patient in the placebo group died by "accident." No other details on the cause or nature of the accident were provided.
[f]Results were not reported for each treatment group separately, but there were no clinically significant differences across treatment groups.
[g]One additional study reported a death but did not specify in which treatment group it occurred.
[h]Values for NNT were added from Jonas et al. (2014), Table 37. For values marked NA, NNT was not calculated because either the risk difference (95% CI) was not statistically significant or the effect measure was not one that allows direct calculation of NNT (e.g., WMD). Abbreviations: ACA=acamprosate; CI=confidence interval; NA=not applicable; NNT=number needed to treat; NSD=no statistically significant difference; PBO=placebo; RCT=randomized controlled trial; RD=risk difference; WMD=weighted mean difference.
Source. Jonas et al. 2014, Table D–1.

heavy drinking (primary outcome) did not differ among the treatment groups. Relapse-free survival at 90 days was 48.3% for acamprosate versus 51.8% for placebo. Another study (total $N=100$) with low risk of bias in a primary care setting (Berger et al. 2013) found no effect of acamprosate on percent days abstinent (primary outcome), percent heavy drinking days, or change in gamma-glutamyl transferase (GGT) levels. Nevertheless, both acamprosate and placebo groups showed improvement during the 12-week trial, particularly among individuals with a treatment goal of abstinence.

Grading of the Overall Supporting Body of Research Evidence for Efficacy of Acamprosate

- **Magnitude of effect:** *Weak*. When present, the magnitude of the effect is small.
- **Risk of bias:** *Medium*. Studies are RCTs of low to medium bias based on their described randomization and blinding procedures and descriptions of study dropouts.
- **Applicability:** The included trials all involve individuals with AUD, by either prior diagnostic criteria or other evidence of harmful levels of drinking. The studies include subjects from around the world, including North America. However, studies from the United States, including the COMBINE study, showed minimal or no response to acamprosate, whereas benefits of acamprosate were found in studies from Europe, where acamprosate was typically started in the hospital during a period of abstinence. The doses of acamprosate and characteristics of subjects in the studies appear to be representative of outpatient clinical practice.
- **Directness:** *Direct*. Studies measured abstinence and alcohol consumption.
- **Consistency:** *Inconsistent*. There was considerable heterogeneity, as evidenced by I^2 values of 70%–80% on return to any drinking and on percent drinking days.
- **Precision:** *Imprecise*. Confidence intervals for studies cross the threshold for clinically significant benefit of the intervention.
- **Dose-response relationship:** *Present*. Although not analyzed as part of the AHRQ meta-analysis, all three trials that examined several doses of acamprosate found at least a trend for improved response at higher doses.
- **Confounding factors (including likely direction of effect):** *Absent*. No known confounding factors are present that would be likely to reduce the effect of the intervention.
- **Publication bias:** *Not identified*. No publication bias was noted by the AHRQ review; however, they note that they were unable to assess for publication bias for early clinical trials (prior to the advent of https://clinicaltrials.gov).
- **Overall strength of research evidence:** *Moderate*. A large number of RCTs have been conducted, most of which have low to medium risk of bias. Many of the RCTs are funded by governmental agencies. Although the studies have good applicability and measure outcomes of interest directly, the imprecision and inconsistency of findings are limitations.

Harms of Acamprosate

The AHRQ review (Jonas et al. 2014) found statistically significant increases in diarrhea and vomiting as compared with placebo, although statistical heterogeneity was high, particularly for diarrhea (Table B–2). In studies published since the AHRQ report (Jonas et al. 2014) and not included in Table B–2, diarrhea was also common. In a study by Berger et al. (2013), diarrhea occurred in almost one-third of subjects, but there was no difference between acamprosate and placebo. In a study by Higuchi and Japanese Acamprosate Study Group (2015), diarrhea occurred more frequently with acamprosate than with placebo (12.9% vs. 4.9%, respectively). In a study by Mann et al. (2013), diarrhea was also noted to be greater with acamprosate than with placebo.

Anxiety was also noted to be greater with acamprosate than with placebo in the AHRQ review, but this finding was based on one study, and other studies have noted no difference from placebo (Micromedex 2017a) or less anxiety (Mann et al. 2013) or even somnolence (Forest Pharmaceuticals 2005) with acamprosate. In studies published since the AHRQ report (Jonas et al. 2014), other side effects occurred in less than 10% of individuals treated with acamprosate or placebo (Berger et al. 2013; Higuchi and Japanese Acamprosate Study Group 2015), without differences in overall side effects (Higuchi and Japanese Acamprosate Study Group 2015) or study attrition due to adverse events (Mann et al. 2013) between the two groups.

TABLE B–2.   Acamprosate compared with placebo

Outcome	Number of studies; number of subjects	Risk of bias; design	Consistency	Directness	Precision	Summary effect size (95% CI)	Strength of evidence grade
Withdrawals due to AEs	13;[a] 4,653	Medium; RCTs	Consistent	Direct	Imprecise	RD 0.006 (−0.003 to 0.015)	Low
Anorexia	0; 0	NA	NA	NA	NA	NA	Insufficient
Anxiety	1;[b] 601	Medium; RCT	Unknown	Direct	Imprecise	RD 0.164 (0.095 to 0.234)	Insufficient
Cognitive dysfunction	0; 0	NA	NA	NA	NA	NA	Insufficient
Diarrhea	12; 3,299	Medium; RCTs	Consistent	Direct	Precise	RD 0.099 (0.030 to 0.168)	Moderate
Dizziness	2; 151	Low to medium; RCTs	Inconsistent	Direct	Imprecise	RD 0.08 (−0.22 to 0.38)	Low
Headache	6;[b] 1,074	Medium; RCTs	Inconsistent	Direct	Imprecise	RD 0.001 (−0.052 to 0.05)	Low
Insomnia	3;[b] 251	Medium; RCTs	Inconsistent	Direct	Imprecise	RD 0.019 (−0.10 to 0.138)	Low
Nausea	7;[b] 1,758	Low to medium; RCTs	Consistent	Direct	Imprecise	RD 0.006 (−0.012 to 0.023)	Moderate
Numbness/ tingling/ paresthesias	1;[b] 262	Medium; RCT	Unknown	Direct	Imprecise	RD 0.008 (−0.013 to 0.029)	Insufficient
Rash	1;[b] 35	Low; RCT	Unknown	Direct	Imprecise	RD 0.111 (−0.069 to 0.291)	Insufficient
Suicide attempts or suicidal ideation	1;[c] 581	Medium; RCT	Unknown	Direct	Imprecise	RD 0.007 (−0.005, 0.019)	Insufficient
Taste abnormalities	0; 0	NA	NA	NA	NA	NA	Insufficient
Vision changes	0; 0	NA	NA	NA	NA	NA	Insufficient
Vomiting	4;[b] 1,817	Medium; RCTs	Consistent	Direct	Precise	RD 0.024 (0.007 to 0.042)	Moderate

[a]Three additional studies were rated high or unclear risk of bias.
[b]One additional study was rated high or unclear risk of bias.
[c]Two additional studies were rated high or unclear risk of bias.
Abbreviations: AE=adverse effect; CI=confidence interval; RCT=randomized controlled trial; RD=risk difference.
Source.   Jonas et al. 2014, Table D–33.

In the package insert for acamprosate (Forest Pharmaceuticals 2005), adverse events of a suicidal nature were described as somewhat more common with acamprosate as compared with placebo (1.4% vs. 0.5% in studies of 6 months or less; 2.4% vs. 0.8% in year-long studies), with suicide in 3 of 2,272 (0.13%) patients in the pooled acamprosate group and 2 of 1,962 patients (0.10%) in the pooled placebo group. However, the AHRQ report notes that evidence was not sufficient to make a determination about the risk of suicide-related events (Jonas et al. 2014). The package insert also notes that acamprosate is contraindicated with severe renal impairment (creatinine clearance [CrCl] 30 mL/min or less) and requires dose adjustments for moderate renal impairment (CrCl of 30–50 mL/min). Other information on harms of acamprosate comes from nonrandomized trials and drug information databases and is noted in Statement 9, Implementation.

Grading of the Overall Supporting Body of Research Evidence for Harms of Acamprosate

- **Magnitude of effect:** *Weak.* When present, the magnitude of effect is small.
- **Risk of bias:** *High.* Studies are RCTs of low to medium bias based on their described randomization and blinding procedures and descriptions of study dropouts. However, methods for determining harms are not well specified, and there is potential for selective reporting of results.
- **Applicability:** The included trials all involve individuals with AUD, by either prior diagnostic criteria or other evidence of harmful levels of drinking. The studies include subjects from around the world, including North America. The doses of acamprosate and characteristics of subjects in the studies appear to be representative of outpatient clinical practice.
- **Directness:** *Direct.* Studies measured common side effects and dropouts due to adverse events.
- **Consistency:** *Inconsistent.* There was considerable heterogeneity, particularly in reported rates of diarrhea.
- **Precision:** *Imprecise.* Confidence intervals for studies are wide in many studies and cross the threshold for clinically significant harms of the intervention.
- **Dose-response relationship:** *Unknown.* Dose-response information on side effects was not well described.
- **Confounding factors (including likely direction of effect):** *Absent.* No known confounding factors are present that would be likely to modify adverse events of the intervention. Although abnormalities in renal function could affect blood levels of drugs, individuals with significant renal impairment were excluded from the clinical trials.
- **Publication bias:** *Not identified.* No publication bias was noted by the AHRQ review; however, they note that they were unable to assess for publication bias for early clinical trials (prior to the advent of https://clinicaltrials.gov).
- **Overall strength of research evidence:** *Low.* A large number of RCTs have been conducted, but few have assessed adverse events in a systematic and predefined fashion. Many of the RCTs are funded by governmental agencies. Although the studies have good applicability and measure outcomes of interest directly, imprecision and inconsistency of findings are a limitation.

Data Abstraction: Acamprosate

Studies related to acamprosate are listed in Table B–3.

TABLE B–3. Studies related to acamprosate

Author and year; trial name	Study characteristics	Treatment administered, including study arm, dose (mg/day), sample size (N), and co-intervention	Rx duration, weeks (follow-up)	Sample characteristics, including diagnostic inclusions and major exclusions	Outcome measures, main results, and overall percent attrition	Risk of bias
Anton and COMBINE Study Research Group 2003	Design: DBRCT Setting: 11 academic outpatient sites Country: United States Funding: govt, meds	ACA 3,000+CBI+MM (9); ACA 3,000+MM (9); NTX 100+CBI+MM (9); NTX 100+MM (9); PBO+CBI+MM (9); PBO+MM (8) Other Tx: as randomized	16	DSM-IV alcohol dependence Mean age: 38–42 years 17%–22% Nonwhite 22%–33% Female Other Dx: NR	Drinking outcomes were not reported for this pilot feasibility study. ACA-NTX group adherence was equal to, or better than, adherence with PBO, ACA alone, or NTX alone. Adverse events were comparable in all groups. Attrition: 31%	Medium
Anton et al. 2006; Donovan et al. 2008; LoCastro et al. 2009; COMBINE	Design: DBRCT Setting: 11 academic outpatient sites Country: United States Funding: govt, meds	ACA 3,000+CBI+MM (151); ACA 3,000+MM (152); NTX 100+CBI+MM (155); NTX 100+MM (154); PBO+CBI+MM (156); PBO+MM (153) Other Tx: as randomized; community support group participation (e.g., AA) encouraged	16 (68)	DSM-IV alcohol dependence Mean age: 44 years 23% Nonwhite 31% Female Other Dx: NR	All groups showed substantial reductions in alcohol use, but ACA did not have a significant effect compared with PBO by itself or with any combination of NTX, CBI, or both. Differences between ACA and PBO were percent drinking days: −0.1 (95% CI −4.21, 4.01), return to any drinking: −0.02 (95% CI −0.08, 0.04), and return to heavy drinking: −0.04 (95% CI −0.11, 0.04). Mean treatment adherence for ACA was 84.2%, and 94% of those in the study provided drinking data for 16 weeks. Diarrhea was more frequent with ACA (65% vs. 35% with PBO), but the proportion of serious adverse effects and withdrawals due to adverse effects did not differ.	Low

TABLE B–3. Studies related to acamprosate *(continued)*

Author and year; trial name	Study characteristics	Treatment administered, including study arm, dose (mg/day), sample size (N), and co-intervention	Rx duration, weeks (follow-up)	Sample characteristics, including diagnostic inclusions and major exclusions	Outcome measures, main results, and overall percent attrition	Risk of bias
Baltieri and De Andrade 2004	Design: DBRCT Setting: outpatient Country: Brazil Funding: NR	ACA 1,998 (40); PBO (35) Other Tx: AA encouraged	12 (24)	ICD-10 alcohol dependence Mean age: 18–60 years % Nonwhite NR 0% Female Other Dx: 0%	Differences between ACA and PBO for return to any drinking: −0.22 (95% CI −0.45, 0). Kaplan-Meier survival curves (ITT analysis) showed lower relapse rates for ACA vs. PBO (p=0.02). Attrition: 23% at 12 weeks	Medium
Berger et al. 2013, 2016	Design: DBRCT Setting: 2 outpatient primary care sites Country: United States Funding: Forest	ACA 1,998 (51); PBO (49) Other Tx: brief structured behavioral intervention from primary care physician	12	DSM-IV alcohol dependence Mean age: 48 years 9% Nonwhite 38% Female Other Dx: tobacco use 44%	Differences between ACA and PBO were percent drinking days: 0.9 (95% CI −11.59, 13.39), percent heavy drinking days: −2.6 (95% CI −11.38, 6.18), and return to any drinking: 0.12 (95% CI 0, 0.25). Both treatment groups improved with greater response in those with a goal of abstinence. No deaths or serious adverse events Attrition: 19%	Medium
Besson et al. 1998	Design: DBRCT Setting: 3 outpatient psychiatric sites Country: Switzerland Funding: govt, Lipha	ACA 1,300–1,998 (55); PBO (55) Other Tx: routine counseling 100%; voluntary disulfiram 22%–24%	52 (108)	DSM-III chronic or episodic alcohol dependence Mean age: 42 years % Nonwhite NR 20% Female Other Dx: 0%	Differences between ACA and PBO were percent drinking days: −19 (95% CI −32.43, −5.57) and return to any drinking: −0.11 (95% CI −0.26, 0.04). Diarrhea occurred more often with ACA. Attrition: 65% at 360 days	Medium

TABLE B–3. Studies related to acamprosate *(continued)*

Author and year; trial name	Study characteristics	Treatment administered, including study arm, dose (mg/day), sample size (*N*), and co-intervention	Rx duration, weeks (follow-up)	Sample characteristics, including diagnostic inclusions and major exclusions	Outcome measures, main results, and overall percent attrition	Risk of bias
Chick et al. 2000b	Design: DBRCT Setting: 20 outpatient clinics Country: United Kingdom Funding: Lipha	ACA 1,998 (289); PBO (292) Other Tx: usual psychosocial; outpatient treatment program	24	DSM-III alcohol dependence Mean age: 43 years % Nonwhite NR 16% Female Other Dx: 0%	Differences between ACA and PBO were percent drinking days: 2 (95% CI –3.71, 7.71), return to any drinking: –0.01 (95% CI –0.06, 0.04), and return to heavy drinking: 0.02 (95% CI –0.04, 0.08). Overall rate of abstinence was 12%. Only 43% were taking 90% of tablets at 2 weeks, and adherence was 28% at 24 weeks. Attrition: 64%	Medium
De Sousa and De Sousa 2005	Design: OLRCT Setting: outpatient private psychiatric hospital Country: India Funding: NR	ACA 1,998 (50); DIS 250 (50) Other Tx: weekly supportive group psychotherapy offered	35	DSM-IV alcohol dependence Exclusions: previous disulfiram or acamprosate treatment Mean age: 42–43 years 100% Nonwhite 0% Female Other Dx: NR	DIS had a lower relapse rate than ACA (88% vs. 46%; *p*=0.0001) and a longer mean time to first relapse (123 days vs. 71 days; *p*=0.0001). ACA had lower craving scores than DIS. Attrition: 7%	High
Geerlings et al. 1997	Design: DBRCT Setting: 22 outpatient substance use treatment centers Country: Belgium, the Netherlands, and Luxembourg Funding: Lipha	ACA 1,332–1,998 (128); PBO (134) Other Tx: ACA: benzodiazepines 5%; PBO: benzodiazepines 6%	26 (52)	DSM-III alcohol dependence Mean age: 40–42 years % Nonwhite NR 24% Female Other Dx: NR	Differences between ACA and PBO were percent drinking days: –10 (95% CI –18.66, –1.34) and return to any drinking: –0.12 (95% CI –0.21, –0.02). Diarrhea was more frequent with ACA: 19.5% vs. PBO 11.5%. Attrition: 64%	Medium

TABLE B–3. Studies related to acamprosate *(continued)*

Author and year; trial name	Study characteristics	Treatment administered, including study arm, dose (mg/day), sample size (M), and co-intervention	Rx duration, weeks (follow-up)	Sample characteristics, including diagnostic inclusions and major exclusions	Outcome measures, main results, and overall percent attrition	Risk of bias
Greenfield et al. 2010; Fucito et al. 2012; COMBINE	Design: secondary data analysis Setting: 11 academic outpatient sites Country: United States Funding: govt, meds	ACA 3,000+CBI+MM (151); ACA 3,000+MM (152); NTX 100+CBI+MM (155); NTX 100+MM (154); PBO+CBI+MM (156); PBO+MM (153) Other Tx: as randomized; community support group participation (e.g., AA) encouraged	68	DSM-IV alcohol dependence Mean age: 44 years 23% Nonwhite 31% Female Other Dx: 0%	There was a significant NTX by CBI interaction for women on two primary outcomes (percent days abstinent and time to first heavy drinking day) and also secondary outcome measures (good clinical response, percent heavy drinking days, and craving). Only the NTX by CBI interaction was significant for percent days abstinent. The NTX by CBI interaction was significant for time to first heavy drinking day in men ($p=0.048$), with each treatment showing slower relapse times. A nonsignificant trend was present in women. NTX or CBI alone was superior to groups receiving neither in the percent of heavy drinking days.	Low

TABLE B–3. Studies related to acamprosate (continued)

Author and year; trial name	Study characteristics	Treatment administered, including study arm, dose (mg/day), sample size (N), and co-intervention	Rx duration, weeks (follow-up)	Sample characteristics, including diagnostic inclusions and major exclusions	Outcome measures, main results, and overall percent attrition	Risk of bias
Gual and Lehert 2001	Design: DBRCT Setting: outpatient, multicenter hospitals Country: Spain Funding: Lipha	ACA 1,998 (148); PBO (148) Other Tx: NR	26	DSM-III-R alcohol dependence Mean age: 41 years % Nonwhite NR 20%–21% Female Other Dx: NR	Differences between ACA and PBO were percent drinking days: –10.6 (95% CI –18.11, –3.09) and return to any drinking: –0.09 (95% CI –0.19, 0.02). Rates of complete abstinence as estimated by survival analysis were 35% and 26% for ACA vs. PBO. Overall adverse effects were comparable, but gastrointestinal effects were more frequent with ACA vs. PBO. Attrition: 35%	Medium
Higuchi and Japanese Acamprosate Study Group 2015	Design: DBRCT Setting: outpatient Country: Japan Funding: Nippon Shinyaku Company	ACA 1,998 (163); PBO (184)	24 (24)	ICD-10 alcohol dependence Mean age: 52.4 years % Nonwhite NR 12.5% Female Other Dx: NR	Abstinence rates with ACA vs. PBO were 47.2% vs. 36.0% with 11.3% (95% CI 0.6%, 21.9%) difference (P=0.039). Overall adverse events and diarrhea were common and more frequent with ACA. Attrition: 38%	Low

TABLE B–3. Studies related to acamprosate (*continued*)

Author and year; trial name	Study characteristics	Treatment administered, including study arm, dose (mg/day), sample size (*N*), and co-intervention	Rx duration, weeks (follow-up)	Sample characteristics, including diagnostic inclusions and major exclusions	Outcome measures, main results, and overall percent attrition	Risk of bias
Kiefer et al. 2003, 2004, 2005	Design: DBRCT Setting: 1 outpatient site Country: Germany Funding: univ; meds	ACA 1,998 (40); NTX 50 (40); PBO (40); ACA 1,998+NTX 50 (40) Other Tx: group therapy	12	DSM-IV alcohol dependence without any withdrawal symptoms Exclusions: homelessness Mean age: 46 years % Nonwhite NR 26% Female Other Dx: 0%	Differences between ACA and PBO were return to any drinking; –0.17 (95% CI –0.33, –0.02) and return to heavy drinking; –0.13 (95% CI –0.33, 0.08). ACA was superior to PBO on time to first relapse by survival analysis. At the end of active treatment, relapse rates with ACA+NTX did not differ from ACA alone. Attrition: 66%	Low

Author and year; trial name	Study characteristics	Treatment administered, including study arm, dose (mg/day), sample size (N), and co-intervention	Rx duration, weeks (follow-up)	Sample characteristics, including diagnostic inclusions and major exclusions	Outcome measures, main results, and overall percent attrition	Risk of bias
Laaksonen et al. 2008	Design: OLRCT Setting: 6 outpatient sites in 5 cities Country: Finland Funding: govt	ACA 1,998 or 1,333 (81); DIS 100–200 (81); NTX 50 (81) Other Tx: manual-based CBT	Up to 52 (119)	ICD-10 alcohol dependence Mean age: 43 years 0% Nonwhite 29% Female Other Dx: NR	During the continuous medication period (1–12 weeks), the DIS group did significantly better than the NTX and ACA groups in time to first heavy drinking day ($p=0.001$), days to first drinking ($p=0.002$), abstinence days, and average weekly alcohol intake. During the targeted medication period (13–52 weeks), there were no significant differences between the groups in time to first heavy drinking day and days to first drinking, whereas the DIS group reported significantly more frequent abstinence days than the ACA and NTX groups. During the whole study period (1–52 weeks), the DIS group did significantly better in the time to the first drink compared with the other groups. Attrition: 52%	High

TABLE B–3. Studies related to acamprosate *(continued)*

Author and year; trial name	Study characteristics	Treatment administered, including study arm, dose (mg/day), sample size (*N*), and co-intervention	Rx duration, weeks (follow-up)	Sample characteristics, including diagnostic inclusions and major exclusions	Outcome measures, main results, and overall percent attrition	Risk of bias
Lhuintre et al. 1985	Design: DBRCT Setting: outpatient methadone maintenance clinics Country: France Funding: meds	ACA 1,000–2,250 (42); PBO (43) Other Tx: meprobamate 100% for first month	13	Alcohol dependence indicated by morning withdrawal, >200 g/day daily alcohol intake, or at least two failed treatment attempts; GGT >30 IU/L; and red blood cell volume >96 fL Mean age: 40–43 years % Nonwhite NR 11% Female Other Dx: NR	Difference between ACA and PBO for return to any drinking: −0.2 (95% CI −0.4, 0) Abstinence rates for those who remained in the study: ACA 61% vs. PBO 32% Attrition: 18%	High
Lhuintre et al. 1990	Design: DBRCT Setting: outpatient substance use disorders clinic Country: France Funding: NR	ACA 1,332 (279); PBO (290) Other Tx: psychotherapy allowed	12 (12)	At least one sign of alcohol dependence, GGT >2× normal, or mean red blood cell corpuscular volume >98 fL Mean age: 42–43 years % Nonwhite NR 18% Female Other Dx: NR	Difference between ACA and PBO for return to any drinking: −0.1 (95% CI −0.16, −0.03) GGT as a marker of alcohol use was significantly lower with ACA vs. PBO at 12 weeks. Diarrhea was more common with ACA vs. PBO. Attrition: 37%	High

TABLE B–3. Studies related to acamprosate *(continued)*

Author and year; trial name	Study characteristics	Treatment administered, including study arm, dose (mg/day), sample size (*N*), and co-intervention	Rx duration, weeks (follow-up)	Sample characteristics, including diagnostic inclusions and major exclusions	Outcome measures, main results, and overall percent attrition	Risk of bias
Mann et al. 2013; PREDICT	Design: DBRCT Setting: NR Country: Germany Funding: govt, meds	ACA 1,998 (172); NTX 50 (169); PBO (86) Other Tx: MM	12	Alcohol dependence Mean age: 45 years % Nonwhite NR 23% Female Other Dx: NR	Difference between ACA and PBO for return to heavy drinking: 0.04 (95% CI –0.09, 0.16) Point estimates for heavy drinking relapse free survival from the Kaplan Meier curves were 48.3% for ACA, 49.1% for NTX, and 51.8% for PBO. Diarrhea was greater in ACA-treated patients. Attrition: 34%	Medium
Mason et al. 2006	Design: DBRCT Setting: 21 outpatient clinics Country: United States Funding: Lipha	ACA 2,000 (258); ACA 3,000 (83); PBO (260) Other Tx: brief abstinence-oriented protocol-specific counseling and self-help materials 100%	24 (32)	DSM-IV alcohol dependence Mean age: 44–45 years 14%–15% Nonwhite 29%–36% Female Other Dx: tobacco use 77%	Differences between ACA and PBO were percent drinking days: –5.9 (95% CI –11.51, –0.29), return to any drinking: 0.04 (95% CI 0, 0.08), and return to heavy drinking: –0.04 (95% CI –0.12, 0.04). A linear effect of dose was present in ITT analysis and a subgroup of motivated subjects. Attrition: 51%	Low

TABLE B–3. Studies related to acamprosate *(continued)*

Author and year; trial name	Study characteristics	Treatment administered, including study arm, dose (mg/day), sample size (*N*), and co-intervention	Rx duration, weeks (follow-up)	Sample characteristics, including diagnostic inclusions and major exclusions	Outcome measures, main results, and overall percent attrition	Risk of bias
Morley et al. 2006, 2010	Design: DBRCT Setting: 3 outpatient intensive substance use treatment sites Country: Australia Funding: govt	ACA 1,998 (55); NTX 50 (53); PBO (61) Other Tx: all offered 4–6 sessions of manualized compliance therapy; uptake/attendance NR	12	DSM-IV alcohol dependence or abuse and with alcohol abstinence for 3–21 days Mean age: 45 years % Nonwhite NR 30% Female Other Dx: substantial levels of emotional distress (anxiety, stress, and depression); 3% severe concurrent illness (psychiatric or other)	Differences between ACA and PBO were drinks per drinking days: 0.4 (95% CI –1.81, 2.61), return to any drinking: –0.02 (95% CI –0.16, 0.12), and return to heavy drinking: –0.02 (95% CI –0.14, 0.19). No differences in side effects were noted, except headache was more frequent with PBO. Attrition: 36%	Low
Narayana et al. 2008	Design: prospective cohort Setting: military, outpatient Country: India Funding: NR	ACA 1,332–1,998 (28); NTX 50 (26); TOP 100–125 (38) Other Tx: various psychotherapies were offered	52	ICD-10 alcohol dependence Mean age: 38 years 100% Nonwhite 0% Female Other Dx: NR	TOP (76.3%) was significantly more effective (*p*<0.01) in sustaining abstinence, although 57.7% NTX and 60.7% ACA maintained complete abstinence. 7 TOP subjects (18.4%) reported decreased relapses compared with 8 NTX (30.8%) and 9 ACA (32.1%) subjects. Attrition: 18%	High

TABLE B–3. Studies related to acamprosate (continued)

Author and year; trial name	Study characteristics	Treatment administered, including study arm, dose (mg/day), sample size (N), and co-intervention	Rx duration, weeks (follow-up)	Sample characteristics, including diagnostic inclusions and major exclusions	Outcome measures, main results, and overall percent attrition	Risk of bias
Paille et al. 1995	Design: DBRCT Setting: NR Country: France Funding: NR	ACA 1.3 g (188); ACA 2 g (173); PBO (177) Other Tx: supportive psychotherapy 100%; hypnotics 6%–7%; anxiolytics 8%–12%; antidepressants 8%–9%	52 (78)	DSM-III-R alcohol dependence Exclusions: three previous detoxification attempts Mean age: 43 years % Nonwhite NR 20% Female Other Dx: NR	Differences between ACA and PBO were percent drinking days: –10.2 (95% CI –16.53, –3.87) and return to any drinking: –0.07 (95% CI –0.13, –0.01). Mean days of continuous abstinence and cumulative abstinence were greater with the higher dose of ACA vs. PBO (p≤0.005). No overall difference in side effects among groups except for a dose-dependent increase in diarrhea with ACA Attrition: 56%	Medium
Pelc et al. 1992, 1996	Design: DBRCT Setting: outpatient, multicenter Country: Belgium Funding: NR	ACA 1,332–1,998 (55); PBO (47) Other Tx: supportive psychotherapy 100%	26	DSM-III alcohol dependence and GGT values above normal Mean age: 43 years % Nonwhite NR 31% Female Other Dx: NR	Difference between ACA and PBO for return to any drinking: –0.19 (95% CI –0.32, –0.07) Survival analysis indicated rates of abstinence throughout the trial of 24% ACA vs. 4% PBO. Attrition: 45% day 90; 65% day 180	High

TABLE B–3. Studies related to acamprosate *(continued)*

Author and year; trial name	Study characteristics	Treatment administered, including study arm, dose (mg/day), sample size (N), and co-intervention	Rx duration, weeks (follow-up)	Sample characteristics, including diagnostic inclusions and major exclusions	Outcome measures, main results, and overall percent attrition	Risk of bias
Pelc et al. 1997	Design: DBRCT Setting: outpatient, after inpatient detoxification Country: Belgium, France Funding: Lipha	ACA 1,332 (63); ACA 1,998 (63); PBO (62) Other Tx: counseling, social support when needed 100%	13	DSM-III-R alcohol dependence Mean age: NR % Nonwhite NR % Female NR Other Dx: NR	Differences between ACA and PBO were percent drinking days: –22.2 (95% CI –35.7, –8.7) and return to any drinking: –0.27 (95% CI –0.39, –0.14). Cumulative abstinence duration was greater in both ACA groups vs. PBO. Of those taking ACA, 41% were abstinent through 13 weeks vs. 15% for PBO. Attrition: 37%	Medium
Poldrugo 1997	Design: DBRCT Setting: inpatient for 1–2 weeks, then outpatient; multicenter community-based alcohol rehabilitation program Country: Italy Funding: Lipha	ACA 1,332–1,998 (122); PBO (124) Other Tx: community-based rehabilitation program with group sessions, alcohol education, community meetings 100%	26 (52)	DSM-III chronic or episodic alcohol dependence Mean age: 43–45 years % Nonwhite NR 23%–31% Female Other Dx: 0%	Differences between ACA and PBO were percent drinking days: –16 (95% CI –30.3, –1.7) and return to any drinking: –0.16 (95% CI –0.28, –0.04). Adverse effects did not differ between groups. Attrition: 54%	Medium

TABLE B–3. Studies related to acamprosate *(continued)*

Author and year; trial name	Study characteristics	Treatment administered, including study arm, dose (mg/day), sample size (*N*), and co-intervention	Rx duration, weeks (follow-up)	Sample characteristics, including diagnostic inclusions and major exclusions	Outcome measures, main results, and overall percent attrition	Risk of bias
Ralevski et al. 2011a, 2011b	Design: DBRCT Setting: outpatient univ and VA health centers Country: United States Funding: govt, Forest	ACA 1,998 (12); PBO (11) Other Tx: weekly skills training that incorporated cognitive-behavioral drug relapse prevention strategies 100%	12	DSM-IV alcohol dependence and DSM-IV schizophrenia, schizoaffective disorder, or psychotic disorder NOS Mean age: 51 years 65% Nonwhite 17% Female Other Dx: schizophrenia spectrum disorders 100%	Differences between ACA and PBO were drinks per drinking day: 1.8 (95% CI –3.53, 7.13), percent drinking days: 3.7 (95% CI –12.5, 19.9), and percent heavy drinking days:1.9 (95% CI –6.86, 10.66). Positive symptoms (via PANSS) decreased in both groups, but there was no effect of treatment. Adverse effects did not differ for ACA vs. PBO. Attrition: 35%	High
Sass et al. 1996	Design: DBRCT Setting: psychiatric outpatient Country: Germany Funding: Lipha	ACA 1,332–1,998 (136); PBO (136) Other Tx: counseling/ psychotherapy 100%	48 (96)	At least 5 DSM-III-R alcohol dependence criteria Mean age: 41–42 years % Nonwhite NR 22% Female Other Dx: NR	Differences between ACA and PBO were percent drinking days:–17.1 (95% CI –27.18, –7.02) and return to any drinking: –0.2 (95% CI –0.31, –0.09). Median time to first relapse was 131 days for ACA vs. 45 days for PBO. Of those completing treatment, 44.8% of ACA-treated subjects had continuous abstinence vs. 25.3% with PBO. Attrition: 51%	Medium

TABLE B–3. Studies related to acamprosate (*continued*)

Author and year; trial name	Study characteristics	Treatment administered, including study arm, dose (mg/day), sample size (N), and co-intervention	Rx duration, weeks (follow-up)	Sample characteristics, including diagnostic inclusions and major exclusions	Outcome measures, main results, and overall percent attrition	Risk of bias
Tempesta et al. 2000	Design: DBRCT Setting: outpatient Country: Italy Funding: Lipha	ACA 1,998 (164); PBO (166) Other Tx: medical and behavioral counseling	26 (39)	DSM-III-R alcohol dependence and GGT values >2× normal or mean corpuscular volume >95 fL Mean age: 46 years % Nonwhite NR 17% Female Other Dx: 0%	Differences between ACA and PBO were percent drinking days: −11.7 (95% CI −21.17, −2.23) and return to any drinking: −0.16 (95% CI −0.27, −0.06). Median time of abstinence was greater with ACA (135 days) vs. PBO (58 days). Continuous abstinence for 26 weeks occurred in 48% of ACA subjects vs. 33% with PBO ($p<0.01$). Rates of adverse effects did not differ between groups. Attrition: 25%	Medium
Whitworth et al. 1996	Design: DBRCT Setting: outpatient specialty clinic Country: Austria Funding: Lipha	ACA 1,332 or 1,998 (224); PBO (224) Other Tx: NR	52 (104)	DSM-III chronic or episodic alcohol dependence Mean age: 42 years % Nonwhite NR 21% Female Other Dx: NR	Differences between ACA and PBO were percent drinking days: −10 (95% CI −17.76, −2.24) and return to any drinking: −0.11 (95% CI −0.17, −0.05). At 48 weeks, 18.3% of ACA subjects were continuously abstinent vs. 7.1% with PBO. Adverse effects did not differ between groups, except diarrhea was more frequent with ACA (20.1%) vs. PBO (12.1%). Attrition: 60%	Medium

Author and year; trial name	Study characteristics	Treatment administered, including study arm, dose (mg/day), sample size (N), and co-intervention	Rx duration, weeks (follow-up)	Sample characteristics, including diagnostic inclusions and major exclusions	Outcome measures, main results, and overall percent attrition	Risk of bias
Wölwer et al. 2011	Design: DBRCT Setting: outpatient; 4 univ hospitals, 1 nonacademic clinic Country: Germany Funding: govt, meds	ACA 1,998+IBT (124); ACA 1,998+TAU (122); PBO+IBT (125) Other Tx: NR	24 (52)	DSM-IV alcohol dependence Mean age: 46 years % Nonwhite NR 29% Female Other Dx: NR	Difference between ACA and PBO for return to heavy drinking: 0 (95% CI –0.12, 0.13). Differences among all treatment groups were not significant at 24 weeks of active treatment or at 52 weeks. Attrition: 55%	Medium

Note. Unless noted elsewhere, subjects were excluded if they had contraindications for specific medications; were pregnant, breastfeeding, or unreliable in using contraception; were receiving psychotropic medications; or had another substance use disorder (except nicotine dependence), other psychiatric conditions, suicidal or homicidal ideas, or significant physical illness (including renal or hepatic disease). Studies comparing ACA with PBO or ACA with comparators other than NTX are included here. Studies comparing ACA with NTX are in Table B–13. Industry-sponsored studies list the name of the pharmaceutical company.

Abbreviations: AA=Alcoholics Anonymous; ACA=acamprosate; CBI=combined behavioral intervention; CBT=cognitive-behavioral therapy; CI=confidence interval; DBRCT=double-blind, randomized controlled trial; DIS=disulfiram; Dx=diagnosis; fL=femtoliters; GGT=gamma-glutamyl transferase; govt=governmental; IBT=integrative behavior therapy; ITT=intention to treat; meds=medications supplied by pharmaceutical company; MM=medical management; NOS=not otherwise specified; NR=not reported; NTX=naltrexone; OLRCT=open-label, randomized controlled trial; PANSS=Positive and Negative Syndrome Scale; PBO=placebo; TAU=treatment as usual; TOP=topiramate; Tx=treatment; univ=university; VA=U.S. Department of Veterans Affairs.

Benefits of Naltrexone

In the AHRQ review (Jonas et al. 2014) (Table B–4), studies of oral naltrexone typically used a dose of 50 mg/day (Table B–5), but a few trials used doses of 100–150 mg/day (Table B–6); trials of long-acting injectable naltrexone used doses of 150–400 mg/month (Table B–7). With naltrexone treatment, 4% fewer subjects returned to any drinking than with placebo (RD, –0.04; 95% CI, –0.07 to –0.01; 21 trials of low or medium bias), and 7% fewer subjects returned to heavy drinking than with placebo (RD, –0.07; 95% CI, –0.11 to –0.03; 23 trials of low or medium bias). For oral naltrexone at a dose of 50 mg/day, the NNT was 20 to prevent one person from returning to any drinking, with a NNT of 12 to prevent one person from returning to heavy drinking. For doses of oral naltrexone of 100 mg/day and for injectable naltrexone, effects were similar to those for oral naltrexone at 50 mg/day but were not statistically significant. As compared with placebo, subjects who received naltrexone also had 4.6% fewer drinking days (WMD, –4.6; 95% CI, –6.6 to –2.5; 19 trials), 3.8% fewer heavy drinking days (WMD, –3.8; 95% CI, –5.8 to –1.8; 11 trials), and 0.5% fewer drinks per drinking day (WMD, –0.54; 95% CI, –1.01 to –0.07; 11 trials). The single study of injectable naltrexone found a large effect size (WMD, –8.6) for fewer drinking days relative to placebo.

Only a limited number of studies assessed factors related to quality of life, and these studies used different measures, making comparison or meta-analysis impossible. In addition, quality of life measures were secondary outcomes, and studies were not adequately powered to assess these effects. One study found better overall mental health, but not physical health, with long-acting injectable naltrexone at 380 mg/month but no benefit on either measure at a dose of 190 mg/month. A placebo-controlled study of 50 mg/day of oral naltrexone found fewer alcohol-related consequences in the naltrexone group (76% vs. 45%, $p=0.02$). The other two studies assessing quality of life measures showed no statistical difference with naltrexone as compared with placebo.

One trial did not meet inclusion criteria for the comparative effectiveness review but was described in some detail in the AHRQ report. In this study (O'Malley et al. 2003), individuals all received oral naltrexone with random assignment to 10 weeks of either primary care management (PCM) or cognitive-behavioral therapy (CBT). Responders in each group (84.1% for PCM vs. 86.5% for CBT) continued with their assigned psychosocial treatment and were randomly assigned to continue naltrexone or switch to placebo. In the CBT group, the rates of abstinence decreased in those assigned to placebo but did not reach statistical significance, whereas in the PCM group, the placebo group had a greater reduction in abstinence rates than those who remained on naltrexone (80.8% vs. 51.9%, $p=0.03$).

Several studies of oral naltrexone published since the AHRQ review (not included in Tables B–4, B–5, or B–6) have shown minimal benefits. In the German PREDICT study (total $N=426$), modeled after the COMBINE study, there was no difference among naltrexone, acamprosate, and placebo groups on the time to first heavy drinking (Mann et al. 2013). In a 12-week, low-risk-of-bias trial, subjects ($N=221$) were randomly assigned to 50 mg/day oral naltrexone or placebo in blocks on the basis of their OPRM1 genotype (Oslin et al. 2015). There was no difference in the odds of heavy drinking with naltrexone as compared with placebo for either genotype, although significant reductions in heavy drinking occurred in all treatment groups. A four-arm study ($N=200$, medium risk of bias) of men who had sex with men investigated oral naltrexone 100 mg/day versus placebo and brief behavioral compliance treatment with and without modified behavioral self-control therapy (MBSCT) (Morgenstern et al. 2012). MBSCT was associated with a 28% decrease in drinks per week and a 35% decrease in heavy drinking days per week, whereas treatment with naltrexone did not have a statistically significant effect. However, naltrexone did increase the likelihood (odds ratio=3.3) of achieving nonhazardous levels of drinking, which was the stated goal of study subjects.

In the majority of studies of naltrexone, individuals met criteria for alcohol dependence by DSM-IV criteria; however, one controlled trial of 153 early problem drinkers randomly assigned subjects to naltrexone, targeted naltrexone before high-risk drinking situations, or placebo (Kranzler et al. 2003), and found a reduced likelihood of drinking in the naltrexone or targeted treatment groups

Outcome	Number of studies; number of subjects	Risk of bias; design	Consistency	Directness	Precision	Summary effect size (95% CI)	NNT[g]	Strength of evidence grade
Return to any drinking	21;[a] 4,233	Medium; RCTs	Consistent	Direct	Precise	RD: –0.04 (–0.07 to –0.01)	NC	Moderate
Return to heavy drinking	23;[a] 4,347	Medium; RCTs	Consistent	Direct	Precise	RD: –0.07 (–0.11 to –0.03)	NC	Moderate
Drinking days	19;[b] 3,329	Medium; RCTs	Consistent	Direct	Precise	WMD: –4.57 (–6.61 to –2.53)	NC	Moderate
Heavy drinking days	11;[c] 2,034	Medium; RCTs	Consistent	Direct	Precise	WMD: –3.81 (–5.85 to –1.78)	NC	Moderate
Drinks per drinking day	11;[d] 1,422	Medium; RCTs	Consistent	Direct	Imprecise	WMD: –0.54 (–1.01 to –0.07)	NC	Low
Accidents	0; 0	NA	NA	NA	NA	NA	NC	Insufficient
Injuries	0; 0	NA	NA	NA	NA	NA	NA	Insufficient
Quality of life	4; 1,513	Medium; RCTs	Inconsistent	Direct	Imprecise	Unable to pool data; some conflicting results[e]	NA	Insufficient
Mortality	6;[f] 1,738	Medium; RCTs	Unknown	Direct	Imprecise	1 (NTX) vs. 2 (PBO)	NA	Insufficient

[a]Two additional studies were rated high risk of bias; two additional studies were rated as unclear risk of bias.
[b]Three additional studies were rated high risk of bias.
[c]Two additional studies were rated high risk of bias.
[d]Five additional studies were rated high risk of bias.
[e]Two studies found no significant difference between naltrexone- and placebo-treated subjects. One study reported that patients receiving injectable naltrexone 380 mg/month had greater improvement on the mental health summary score than those receiving placebo at 24 weeks (8.2 vs. 6.2, $p=0.044$). One study measured alcohol-related consequences (with the DrInC) and reported that more subjects who received placebo ($N=34$) had ≥1 alcohol-related consequence than those who received naltrexone ($N=34$): 76% vs. 45%, $P=0.02$.
[f]One additional study reported a death but did not specify in which treatment group it occurred.
[g]Values for NNT were added from Jonas et al. (2014), Table 37. For values marked NA, NNT was not calculated either because the risk difference (95% CI) was not statistically significant or the effect measure was not one that allows direct calculation of NNT (e.g., WMD); NC indicates that the Agency for Healthcare Research and Quality review did not comment on a NNT for these outcomes.
Abbreviations: CI=confidence interval; NA=not applicable; DrInC=Drinker Inventory of Consequences; NNT=number needed to treat; NSD=no significant difference; NTX=naltrexone; PBO=placebo; RCT=randomized controlled trial; RD=risk difference; WMD=weighted mean difference.
Source. Jonas et al. 2014, Table D–3.

over an 8-week period. Although these findings require replication, they are consistent with possible benefit of naltrexone treatment in individuals with less severe AUD.

Although most trials of naltrexone excluded individuals with co-occurring physical or psychiatric illness, one study of naltrexone for smoking cessation conducted a subgroup analysis for individuals who also reported heavy drinking (Fridberg et al. 2014). The total sample included 315 smokers who were randomly assigned to placebo or naltrexone 50 mg/day for 12 weeks. In the sub-

Oral naltrexone (50 mg) compared with placebo

Outcome	Number of studies; number of subjects	Risk of bias; design	Consistency	Directness	Precision	Summary effect size (95% CI)	NNT	Strength of evidence grade
Return to any drinking	16; 2,347	Medium; RCTs	Consistent	Direct	Precise	RD: –0.05 (–0.10 to –0.00)	20	Moderate
Return to heavy drinking	19; 2,875	Medium; RCTs	Consistent	Direct	Precise	RD: –0.09 (–0.13 to –0.04)	12	Moderate
Drinking days	15; 1,992	Medium; RCTs	Consistent	Direct	Precise	WMD: –5.4 (–7.5 to –3.2)	NA	Moderate
Heavy drinking days	6; 521	Medium; RCTs	Consistent	Direct	Precise	WMD: –4.1 (–7.6 to –0.61)	NA	Moderate
Drinks per drinking day	9; 1,018	Medium; RCTs	Consistent	Direct	Imprecise	WMD: –0.49 (–0.92 to –0.06)	NA	Low

Abbreviations: CI=confidence interval; NA=not applicable; NNT=number needed to treat; NSD=no significant difference; NTX=naltrexone; PBO=placebo; RCT=randomized controlled trial; RD=risk difference; WMD=weighted mean difference.
Source. Jonas et al. 2014, Table D–4, with values for NNT added from Table 37.

TABLE B–6. **Oral naltrexone (100 mg) compared with placebo**

Outcome	Number of studies; number of subjects	Risk of bias; design	Consistency	Directness	Precision	Summary effect size (95% CI)	NNT	Strength of evidence grade
Return to any drinking	3; 946	Medium; RCTs	Consistent	Direct	Imprecise	RD: –0.03 (–0.08 to 0.02)	NA	Low
Return to heavy drinking	2; 858	Medium; RCTs	Consistent	Direct	Imprecise	RD: –0.05 (–0.11 to 0.01)	NA	Low
Drinking days	2; 858	Medium; RCTs	Consistent	Direct	Imprecise	WMD: –0.9 (–4.2 to 2.5)	NA	Low
Heavy drinking days	2; 423	Medium; RCTs	Consistent	Direct	Imprecise	WMD: –3.1 (–5.8 to –0.3)	NA	Low
Drinks per drinking day	1; 240	Medium; RCT	Unknown	Direct	Imprecise	WMD: 1.9 (–1.5 to 5.2)	NA	Insufficient

Abbreviations: CI=confidence interval; NA=not applicable; NNT=number needed to treat; RCT=randomized controlled trial; RD=risk difference; WMD=weighted mean difference.
Source. Jonas et al. 2014, Table D–5, with values for NNT added from Table 37.

Outcome	Number of studies; number of subjects	Risk of bias; design	Consistency	Directness	Precision	Summary effect size (95% CI)	NNT	Strength of evidence grade
Return to any drinking	2; 939	Medium; RCTs	Consistent	Direct	Imprecise	RD: –0.04 (–0.10 to 0.03)	NA	Low
Return to heavy drinking	2; 615	Medium; RCTs	Inconsistent	Direct	Imprecise	RD: –0.01 (–0.14 to 0.13)	NA	Low
Drinking days	1; 315	Medium; RCT	Unknown	Direct	Imprecise	WMD: –8.6 (–16.0 to –1.2)	NA	Insufficient
Heavy drinking days	2;[a] 926	Medium; RCTs	Consistent	Direct	Imprecise	WMD: –4.6 (–8.5 to –0.56)	NA	Low
Drinks per drinking day	0; 0	NA	NA	NA	NA	NA	NA	Insufficient

[a]Contains data from personal communication (B. Silverman, November 14, 2013).
Abbreviations: CI=confidence interval; NA=not applicable; NNT=number needed to treat; RCT=randomized controlled trial; RD=risk difference; WMD=weighted mean difference.
Source.   Jonas et al. 2014, Table D–6, with values for NNT added from Table 37.

group of 69 heavy drinkers (at least two heavy drinking episodes per month), weekly alcohol consumption was reduced with naltrexone treatment (incidence rate ratio [IRR] 0.71, 95% CI=0.51–1.0, p=0.049), as was smoking urge. Smoking quit rates with naltrexone as compared with placebo were also significantly better in the heavy drinking subgroup at the end of the study and at 12-month follow-up. Another medium-risk-of-bias study (Foa et al. 2013) was excluded from the AHRQ review because of its study design but is of relevance to clinical practice. Subjects met DSM-IV criteria for posttraumatic stress disorder (PTSD) and for alcohol dependence and were randomly assigned to receive naltrexone 100 mg/day plus prolonged exposure therapy (N=40), placebo plus prolonged exposure therapy (N=40), naltrexone 100 mg/day plus supportive therapy (N=42), or placebo plus supportive therapy (N=43). Although attrition was relatively high in all groups during the 24-week trial, alcohol craving and the percentage of days drinking alcohol were reduced in all groups, with a greater mean difference in groups that received naltrexone as compared with placebo groups (p=0.008). PTSD severity was reduced in all groups, with no significant effect of prolonged exposure over supportive therapy; however, those in the prolonged exposure plus naltrexone group were more likely to achieve a low level of PTSD symptoms.

The AHRQ review (Jonas et al. 2014) also examined studies that assessed whether μ opioid receptor gene polymorphism status was associated with a more robust response to naltrexone (Table B–8). The main single-nucleotide polymorphism (SNP) that was tested was an asparagine to aspartate substitution in exon 1 of the μ opioid receptor. (Because of changes in the National Center for Biotechnology Information Human Genome Reference Assembly, this SNP has been referred to by a number of designations, including A118G, Asn40Asp, rs1799971, A355G, and Asn102Asp.) The review found no significant difference between A-allele homozygotes and those with at least one G allele in terms of the outcomes return to any drinking (RD, 0.01; 95% CI, –0.2 to 0.2) and return to heavy drinking (RD, 0.14; 95% CI, –0.03 to 0.3) when all available studies were considered together. However, in its conclusions, the AHRQ report also noted that for return to heavy drinking,

TABLE B–8. Results of included studies that assessed the association between μ opioid receptor gene polymorphisms and naltrexone response

Author and year	Reported a significant positive association?	AA genotype, N	AA genotype, return to any drinking	AA genotype, return to heavy drinking— relapse	AG/GG genotypes, N	AG/GG genotypes, return to any drinking	AG/GG genotypes, return to heavy drinking— relapse
Anton et al. 2008b	Yes[a]	115[b]	NR	52	31[b]	NR	4
Coller et al. 2011	No	NR	NR	NR	NR	NR	NR
Gelernter et al. 2007	No	98	NR	35	33	NR	12
Kim et al. 2009	Mixed[c]	16	8	6	16	9	3
Kranzler et al. 2013	Yes	59	NR	NR	22	NR	NR
O'Malley et al. 2008	No[d]	25	16	16	3	2	2
Rubio et al. 2002	No	29	9	9	16	4	4

[a]Statistically significant difference between groups for return to heavy drinking.
[b]Data are for those who received naltrexone and medical management and do not include those who received naltrexone+medical management+CBI. The study found no gene by medication by time interactions for the latter group for percentage of days abstinent or heavy drinking days and did not report specific numbers by genotype for the outcomes.
[c]Yes for time to first relapse ($p=0.014$); no for abstinent rate ($p=0.656$) and relapse rate ($p=0.072$).
[d]Study authors restricted analyses to A-allele homozygotes because they had only 17 of 92 genotyped participants with at least one G allele. The results for the 75 A-allele homozygotes were similar to the results for the total sample, indicating that treatment efficacy was not dependent on the presence of the G allele.
Abbreviations: N=number; NR=not reported.
Source. Jonas et al. 2014, Table 36.

"it is possible that patients with at least one G allele of A118G polymorphism of OPRM1 might be more likely to respond to naltrexone" (Jonas et al. 2014, p. 94). The reasons behind this interpretation are severalfold. Of the seven studies, three studies, including the COMBINE study (Anton et al. 2008b), reported positive associations between OPRM1 polymorphisms and naltrexone response. In the COMBINE study, individuals who received medical management (MM) without cognitive-behavioral intervention were more likely to have a good clinical outcome if they had at least one Asp40 allele and received naltrexone (87.1%), as compared with Asn40 homozygotes treated with naltrexone (54.8%). About half of those treated with placebo also had a good outcome, regardless of genotype. This difference in outcomes would be clinically significant. One additional study did not meet a priori inclusion criteria for the systematic review, but it also included information on naltrexone response and OPRM1 genotype (Oslin et al. 2003). This study also found that naltrexone-treated subjects with at least one Asp40 allele as compared with Asn40 homozygotes had significantly lower rates of relapse ($p=0.044$) and a longer time to return to heavy drinking ($p=0.04$). When the results of this study were added to the meta-analysis in a sensitivity analysis, a positive association between genotype and response emerged (RD, 0.16; 95% CI, 0.02 to 0.29).

Since the AHRQ review, additional studies have not found a relationship between genotype and naltrexone response. As described above, one study randomly assigned subjects ($N=221$) to 50 mg/day oral naltrexone or to placebo with stratification on the basis of their OPRM1 genotype (Oslin et al. 2015). In this 12-week trial, there was no difference in the odds of heavy drinking with naltrexone as compared with placebo for either genotype. A secondary analysis of OPRM1 genotype has been conducted in a sample of veterans with alcohol dependence and other psychiatric conditions (Arias et al. 2014). Subjects in this 12-week, medium-risk-of-bias study were randomly assigned to placebo alone ($N=64$), naltrexone 50 mg/day ($N=59$), disulfiram 250 mg/day plus placebo ($N=66$), or naltrexone 50 mg/day and disulfiram 250 mg/day ($N=65$). OPRM1 genotyping was conducted for a subset of 107 European American subjects. No significant interactions were found between genotype and the response to naltrexone.

Taken together, the findings on OPRM1 genotype and naltrexone response did not seem to indicate a current role for OPRM1 genotype determination in clinical practice, and no guideline statement was made. However, use of genotype to identify predictors of response remains a promising avenue for research.

Grading of the Overall Supporting Body of Research Evidence for Efficacy of Naltrexone

- **Magnitude of effect:** *Weak.* When present for specific outcomes, the magnitude of the effect is small.
- **Risk of bias:** *Medium.* Studies are RCTs of low to medium bias based on their described randomization and blinding procedures and descriptions of study dropouts.
- **Applicability:** The included trials all involve individuals with AUD, by either prior diagnostic criteria or other evidence of harmful levels of drinking. The studies include subjects from around the world, including North America. The doses of naltrexone appear to be representative of outpatient clinical practice, but in some studies, the proportion of females in the trial was small.
- **Directness:** *Direct.* Studies measured abstinence and heavy drinking rates as well as measures of alcohol consumption.
- **Consistency:** *Inconsistent.* There was considerable heterogeneity as evidenced by I^2 values on drinking-related outcomes.
- **Precision:** *Imprecise.* Confidence intervals for studies cross the threshold for clinically significant benefit of the intervention.
- **Dose-response relationship:** *Unclear.* Studies typically used a single dose of naltrexone, and when comparisons were available, outcomes were at least as good and in some instances better for 50 mg/day of oral naltrexone as compared with 100 mg/day.
- **Confounding factors (including likely direction of effect):** *Unclear.* Some studies suggest a possible effect of genetic polymorphisms on treatment response, which could confound study interpretation.
- **Publication bias:** *Not identified.* No publication bias was noted by the AHRQ review; however, they note that they were unable to assess for publication bias for early clinical trials (prior to the release of https://clinicaltrials.gov).
- **Overall strength of research evidence:** *Moderate.* A large number of RCTs have been conducted, most of which have low to medium risk of bias. Many of the RCTs are funded by governmental agencies. Although the studies have good applicability and measure outcomes of interest directly, the imprecision and inconsistency of findings are a limitation. Another limitation is that the majority of trials use oral formulations at a dose of 50 mg/day; the strength of research evidence is less robust for other formulations (e.g., long-acting injections) and doses.

Grading of the Overall Supporting Body of Research Evidence for Predicting Efficacy of Naltrexone Through OPRM1 Genetic Polymorphism Testing

- **Magnitude of effect:** *Unclear*. However, if present, the magnitude of the effect is small.
- **Risk of bias:** *High*. Studies are RCTs of low to medium bias based on their described randomization and blinding procedures and descriptions of study dropouts. However, with one exception, all of the genotyping studies are based on secondary analyses, often with a subset of the original sample.
- **Applicability:** The included trials all involve individuals with AUD, by either prior diagnostic criteria or other evidence of harmful levels of drinking. The studies include subjects from around the world, including North America. The doses of naltrexone appear to be representative of outpatient clinical practice; however, many of the studies have few or no women. Some of the studies limit the analysis to white/European American subjects.
- **Directness:** *Direct*. Studies measured abstinence, heavy drinking, and measures of alcohol consumption.
- **Consistency:** *Inconsistent*. There was considerable heterogeneity as evidenced by I^2 values in the meta-analysis.
- **Precision:** *Imprecise*. Confidence intervals for studies cross the threshold for clinically significant benefit.
- **Dose-response relationship:** *Not assessed*.
- **Confounding factors (including likely direction of effect):** *Likely*. Given the known differences in genotype frequency among different races and ethnicities, the inclusion or exclusion of non-whites could influence the study conclusions and the overall meta-analysis.
- **Publication bias:** *Not identified*. No publication bias was noted by the AHRQ review; however, they note that they were unable to assess for publication bias for early clinical trials (prior to the release of https://clinicaltrials.gov).
- **Overall strength of research evidence:** *Low*. Although a large number of secondary analyses have been conducted on the basis of government-funded RCTs, the applicability, inconsistency, lack of precision, and potential for confounding factors are limitations.

Harms of Naltrexone

The AHRQ review (Jonas et al. 2014) found a statistically significant increased risk of withdrawal due to adverse events, dizziness, nausea, and vomiting in individuals treated with naltrexone as compared with placebo (Table B–9). Of studies that reported on mortality, no studies found more than one death in any one treatment group (Jonas et al. 2014). Effects of naltrexone on hepatic enzymes were viewed as intermediate outcomes and were not included in the AHRQ meta-analysis (D. Jonas, personal communication, July 2016). None of the literature identified in the updated literature search provided additional information on harms of naltrexone. Other information on harms of naltrexone comes from nonrandomized trials and drug information databases and is noted in Statement 9, Implementation.

Grading of the Overall Supporting Body of Research Evidence for Harms of Naltrexone

- **Magnitude of effect:** *Small*. When present, the magnitude of effect is small.
- **Risk of bias:** *High*. Studies are RCTs of low to medium bias based on their described randomization and blinding procedures and descriptions of study dropouts. However, methods for determining harms are not well specified, and there is potential for selective reporting of results.

Outcome	Number of studies; number of subjects	Risk of bias; design	Consistency	Directness	Precision	Summary effect size (95% CI)	Strength of evidence grade
Withdrawals due to AEs	17;[a] 2,743	Medium; RCTs	Consistent	Direct	Precise	RD 0.021 (0.009 to 0.034)	Moderate
Anorexia	1; 175	Medium; RCT	Unknown	Direct	Imprecise	RD 0.077 (0.014 to 0.140)	Insufficient
Anxiety	7;[b] 1,461	Medium; RCTs	Consistent	Direct	Imprecise	RD 0.007 (−0.022 to 0.036)	Low
Cognitive dysfunction	1; 123	Medium; RCT	Unknown	Direct	Imprecise	RD 0.190 (0.038 to 0.341)	Insufficient
Diarrhea	11;[c] 2,358	Medium; RCTs	Consistent	Direct	Imprecise	RD 0.013 (−0.011 to 0.038)	Moderate
Dizziness	13;[d] 2,675	Medium; RCTs	Consistent	Direct	Precise	RD 0.063 (0.036 to 0.089)	Moderate
Headache	17;[e] 3,347	Medium; RCTs	Inconsistent	Direct	Imprecise	RD 0.008 (−0.019 to 0.034)	Low
Insomnia	8;[d] 1,637	Medium; RCTs	Consistent	Direct	Imprecise	RD 0.027 (−0.002 to 0.057)	Low
Nausea	24;[f] 4,655	Medium; RCTs	Consistent	Direct	Precise	RD 0.112 (0.075 to 0.149)	Moderate
Numbness/ tingling/ paresthesias	1;[b] 123	Medium; RCT	Unknown	Direct	Imprecise	RD -0.008 (−0.185 to 0.168)	Insufficient
Rash	4;[c] 469	Medium; RCTs	Consistent	Direct	Imprecise	RD -0.010 (−0.060 to 0.040)	Low
Suicide	0; 0	NA	NA	NA	NA	NA	Insufficient
Taste abnormalities	1; 123	Medium; RCT	Unknown	Direct	Imprecise	RD −0.006 (−0.182 to 0.171)	Insufficient
Vision changes (blurred vision)	2; 133	Medium; RCTs	Inconsistent	Direct	Imprecise	RD 0.079 (−0.172 to 0.331)	Low
Vomiting	9;[b] 2,438	Medium; RCTs	Consistent	Direct	Precise	RD 0.043 (0.023 to 0.062)	Moderate

[a]Three additional studies were rated high or unclear risk of bias.
[b]Two additional studies were rated high or unclear risk of bias.
[c]One additional study was rated high or unclear risk of bias.
[d]Four additional studies were rated high or unclear risk of bias.
[e]Five additional studies were rated high or unclear risk of bias.
[f]Seven additional studies were rated as high or unclear risk of bias.
Abbreviations: AE=adverse effect; CI=confidence interval; RCT=randomized controlled trial; RD=risk difference.
Source.　Jonas et al. 2014, Table D–34.

- **Applicability:** The included trials all involve individuals with AUD, by either prior diagnostic criteria or other evidence of harmful levels of drinking. The studies include subjects from around the world, including North America. The doses of naltrexone appear to be representative of outpatient clinical practice.
- **Directness:** *Direct.* Studies measured common side effects and dropouts due to adverse events.
- **Consistency:** *Consistent.* For adverse events that showed a significant effect (e.g., withdrawal due to adverse events, dizziness, nausea, and vomiting), the findings were consistent across trials.
- **Precision:** *Imprecise.* Confidence intervals for studies are wide in many studies and cross the threshold for clinically significant harms of the intervention.
- **Dose-response relationship:** *Unknown.* Dose-response information on side effects was not well described.
- **Confounding factors (including likely direction of effect):** *Absent.* No known confounding factors are present that would be likely to modify adverse events of the intervention.
- **Publication bias:** *Not identified.* No publication bias was noted by the AHRQ review; however, they note that they were unable to assess for publication bias for early clinical trials (prior to the release of https://clinicaltrials.gov).
- **Overall strength of research evidence:** *Moderate.* A large number of RCTs have been conducted, but few have assessed adverse events in a systematic and predefined fashion. Many of the RCTs are funded by governmental agencies. Although imprecision is a limitation, the studies have good applicability, measure outcomes of interest directly, and are relatively consistent in finding naltrexone to have greater frequencies of withdrawal due to adverse events, dizziness, nausea, and vomiting as compared with placebo.

Data Abstraction: Naltrexone

Studies related to naltrexone are listed in Table B–10.

Benefits of Acamprosate Compared With Naltrexone

The AHRQ meta-analysis (Jonas et al. 2014) found no statistically significant difference between naltrexone and acamprosate on return to any drinking (RD, 0.02; 95% CI, –0.03 to 0.08; three trials), return to heavy drinking (RD, 0.01; 95% CI, –0.05 to 0.06; four trials), or drinking days (WMD, –2.98; 95% CI, –13.4 to 7.5) (Table B–11). Patient characteristics did not appear to be associated with a preferential response to either medication.

The COMBINE study (Anton et al. 2006, p. 2003) found that "patients receiving medical management with naltrexone, CBI, or both fared better on drinking outcomes than those who received placebo, but acamprosate showed no evidence of efficacy, with or without CBI." Analyses of alternative summary measures of drinking, including drinks per drinking day ($p=0.03$) and heavy drinking days per month ($p=0.006$), were consistent with those for the co-primary end points (percentage of days abstinent from alcohol and time to first heavy drinking day) in showing a significant naltrexone by CBI interaction. Although the CBI and naltrexone treatment combination showed a statistically significant difference in quality of life measures, the AHRQ review noted that this was unlikely to be clinically significant (Jonas et al. 2014). In a subsequent analysis that examined predictors of abstinence from heavy drinking, assignment to a specific treatment was not a major contributor to outcome, but individuals with more consecutive days of abstinence, with a drinking goal of abstinence, or with a lesser frequency of alcohol use prior to treatment were more likely to achieve abstinence from heavy drinking (Gueorguieva et al. 2011, 2014). By 3 years, median but not mean costs (treatment cost plus social costs of AUD such as health care, arrests, and motor vehicle accidents) were diminished in the COMBINE study by a number of treatment combinations that included pharmacotherapy (Zarkin et al. 2010). Treatment arms that were cost-effective, from a policy (Dunlap et al. 2010) and patient-centered (Zarkin et al. 2008) standpoint, were MM with placebo, MM plus naltrexone therapy, and MM plus combined naltrexone and acamprosate therapy.

TABLE B–10. Studies related to naltrexone

Author and year; trial name	Study characteristics	Treatment administered, including study arm, dose (mg/day), sample size (N), and co-intervention	Rx duration, weeks (follow-up)	Sample characteristics, including diagnostic inclusions and major exclusions	Outcome measures, main results, and overall percent attrition	Risk of bias
Ahmadi and Ahmadi 2002; Ahmadi et al. 2004	Design: DBRCT Setting: outpatient Country: Iran Funding: NR	NTX 50 (58); PBO (58) Other Tx: individual counseling 100%	12	DSM-IV alcohol dependence Mean age: 43 years % Nonwhite NR 0% Female Other Dx: NR	Differences between NTX and PBO were return to heavy drinking: –0.36 (95% CI –0.53, –0.2) and return to any drinking; –0.19 (95% CI –0.36, –0.02). NTX was associated with more nausea than PBO. Attrition: 39%	High
Anton and COMBINE Study Research Group 2003	Design: DBRCT Setting: 11 academic outpatient sites Country: United States Funding: govt, meds	ACA 3,000+CBI+MM (9); ACA 3,000+MM (9); NTX 100+ CBI+MM (9); NTX 100+MM (9); PBO+CBI+MM (9); PBO+MM (8) Other Tx: as randomized	16	DSM-IV alcohol dependence Mean age: 38–42 years 17%–22% Nonwhite 22%–33% Female Other Dx: NR	ACA-NTX group adherence was equal to, or better than, adherence with PBO, ACA alone, or NTX alone. Adverse events were comparable in all groups. Attrition: 31%	Medium

TABLE B–10. Studies related to naltrexone (*continued*)

Author and year; trial name	Study characteristics	Treatment administered, including study arm, dose (mg/day), sample size (*M*), and co-intervention	Rx duration, weeks (follow-up)	Sample characteristics, including diagnostic inclusions and major exclusions	Outcome measures, main results, and overall percent attrition	Risk of bias
Anton et al. 1999, 2001	Design: DBRCT Setting: outpatient academic site Country: United States Funding: govt, meds	NTX 50 (68); PBO (63) Other Tx: CBT 100%	12	DSM-III-R alcohol dependence, including loss of control over drinking Mean age: 41–44 years 11%–18% Nonwhite 27%–31% Female Other Dx: 0%	Differences between NTX and PBO were drinks per drinking day: –1.7 (95% CI –3.02, –0.38), percent drinking days: –8 (95% CI –15.22, –0.78), return to any drinking: –0.14 (95% CI –0.3, 0.03), and return to heavy drinking: –0.22 (95% CI –0.39, –0.05). Kaplan-Meier survival analysis showed a longer time to first relapse with NTX vs. PBO ($p < 0.02$). Adverse effects that were more frequent with NTX vs. PBO were nausea/vomiting, abdominal pain, daytime sleepiness, and nasal congestion. Attrition: 17%	Medium
Anton et al. 2005	Design: DBRCT Setting: outpatient Country: United States Funding: govt, meds	NTX 50+CBT (39); NTX 50+MET (41); PBO+CBT (41); PBO+MET (39) Other Tx: CBT and MET as randomized	12	DSM-IV alcohol dependence, including loss of control over drinking Exclusions: >2 prior detoxification admissions requiring medication Mean age: 43–45 years 8%–23% Nonwhite 21%–27% Female Other Dx: NR	Differences between NTX and PBO were drinks per drinking day: –0.7 (95% CI –2.06, 0.66), percent drinking days: –6.8 (95% CI –15.12, 1.52), and return to heavy drinking: –0.17 (95% CI –0.32, –0.02). Kaplan-Meier survival analysis showed a longer time to first relapse in the NTX groups. The NTX+CBT group had fewer relapses than the other groups. Attrition: 19%	Medium

TABLE B–10. Studies related to naltrexone *(continued)*

Author and year; trial name	Study characteristics	Treatment administered, including study arm, dose (mg/day), sample size (N), and co-intervention	Rx duration, weeks (follow-up)	Sample characteristics, including diagnostic inclusions and major exclusions	Outcome measures, main results, and overall percent attrition	Risk of bias
Anton et al. 2006; Donovan et al. 2008; LoCastro et al. 2009; COMBINE	Design: DBRCT Setting: 11 academic outpatient sites Country: United States Funding: govt, meds	ACA 3,000+CBI+MM (151); ACA 3,000+ MM (152); NTX 100+ CBI+MM (155); NTX 100+MM (154); PBO+CBI+MM (156); PBO+MM (153) Other Tx: as randomized; community support group participation (e.g., AA) encouraged	16 (68)	DSM-IV alcohol dependence Mean age: 44 years 23% Nonwhite 31% Female Other Dx: NR	All groups had a substantial reduction in drinking. Differences between NTX and PBO were percent drinking days: –1.1 (95% CI –5.2, 3), return to any drinking: –0.04 (95% CI –0.1, 0.02), and return to heavy drinking: –0.06 (95% CI –0.13, 0.01). Nausea and somnolence were more common with NTX vs. PBO. Complete within-treatment drinking data were provided by 94% of study subjects.	Low
Anton et al. 2008b	Design: DBRCT Setting: 11 outpatient sites Country: United States Funding: govt, meds	NTX 100 (301); PBO (303) Other Tx: MM 100%, CBI 49%, ACA % NR	16	DSM-IV alcohol dependence Mean age: 45–46 years 0% Nonwhite 30% Female Other Dx: NR	NTX was associated with fewer heavy drinking days and trend for more abstinent days over time in subjects with at least one copy of the Asp40 allele.	Medium
Anton et al. 2011	Design: DBRCT Setting: outpatient Country: United States Funding: govt	NTX 50 (50); PBO (50); NTX 50+6 weeks gabapentin, with 1,200 maximum dose (50) Other Tx: used COMBINE's manual (CBT+MM+12-step techniques) 100%	16	DSM-IV alcohol dependence Exclusion: >1 prior detoxification admission Mean age: 43–47 years 13% Nonwhite 18% Female Other Dx: NR	During the first 6 weeks, the NTX/gabapentin group took a longer time to relapse and had fewer heavy drinking days and fewer drinks per drinking day than the placebo and NTX alone groups. Time to relapse did not differ at the end of study. Complete within-treatment drinking data were provided by 82%–88% of subjects.	Medium

TABLE B–10. Studies related to naltrexone *(continued)*

Author and year; trial name	Study characteristics	Treatment administered, including study arm, dose (mg/day), sample size (*N*), and co-intervention	Rx duration, weeks (follow-up)	Sample characteristics, including diagnostic inclusions and major exclusions	Outcome measures, main results, and overall percent attrition	Risk of bias
Balldin et al. 2003	Design: DBRCT Setting: 10 outpatient sites Country: Sweden Funding: DuPont, Meda AB	NTX 50+CBT (25); NTX 50 +ST (31); PBO+CBT (30); PBO+ST (32) Other Tx: none	26	DSM-IV alcohol dependence Mean age: 48–51 years % Nonwhite NR 9%–23% Female Other Dx: 0%	Differences between NTX and PBO were drinks per drinking day: 0.2 (95% CI –1.47, 1.87), percent drinking days: –9.9 (95% CI –20.54, 0.74), percent heavy drinking days: –11 (95% CI –20.95, –1.05), return to any drinking: 0.03 (95% CI –0.03, 0.09), and return to heavy drinking: 0.01 (95% CI –0.07, 0.1). Decreased libido and abdominal pain were reported more often with NTX vs. PBO but did not require treatment cessation. Attrition: 23%	Low
Baltieri et al. 2008, 2009	Design: DBRCT Setting: outpatient Country: Brazil Funding: govt	TOP to 200–400 (52); NTX 50 (49); PBO (54) Other Tx: psychosocial 100%; AA recommended	12	ICD-10 alcohol dependence Mean age: 44–45 years 29% Nonwhite 0% Female Other Dx: tobacco use 66%	Differences between NTX and PBO were percent heavy drinking days: –7.5 (95% CI –23.48, 8.48), percent drinking days: –8.3 (95% CI –23.93, 7.33), and return to any drinking: –0.01 (95% CI –0.18, 0.17). Smokers relapsed more rapidly than nonsmokers. Attrition: 45%	High

TABLE B–10. Studies related to naltrexone (*continued*)

Author and year; trial name	Study characteristics	Treatment administered, including study arm, dose (mg/day), sample size (N), and co-intervention	Rx duration, weeks (follow-up)	Sample characteristics, including diagnostic inclusions and major exclusions	Outcome measures, main results, and overall percent attrition	Risk of bias
Brown et al. 2009	Design: DBRCT Setting: outpatient univ health center Country: United States Funding: govt	NTX 50 (20); PBO (23) Other Tx: CBT 100%	12	Alcohol dependence and bipolar I or II disorder, with current depressed or mixed mood state Exclusions: severe mood symptoms Mean age: 41 years 26% Nonwhite 49% Female Other Dx: bipolar (current depressed or mixed mood) 100%; cannabis abuse 21%; cocaine abuse 12%; amphetamine abuse 7%	Differences between NTX and PBO were drinks per drinking day: –1.8 (95% CI –3.67, 0.07) and return to heavy drinking: –0.28 (95% CI –0.55, –0.01). Rates of medication adherence and number of CBT sessions attended were comparable for the two groups, as were adverse effects. Attrition: 48%	High
Carroll et al. 1993	Design: OLRCT Setting: outpatient Country: United States Funding: govt	DIS 250 (9); NTX 50 (9) Other Tx: weekly individual psychotherapy 100%	12	DSM-III-R alcohol abuse/dependence and cocaine dependence Mean age: 32 years 39% Nonwhite 72% Female Other Dx: cocaine dependence 100%	Subjects taking DIS showed lower percentage of alcohol use days compared with those taking NTX (4.0% vs. 26.3%, t=3.73, p<0.01). Subjects taking DIS also reported fewer total days using alcohol (2.4. vs. 10.4 days, t=3.00, p<0.01), fewer total drinks (2.3 vs. 27.0, t= –2.00, p=0.06), and more total weeks of abstinence (mean 7.2 vs. 1.1 weeks, t=4.72, p<0.001) compared with those taking NTX. Attrition: 67%	High

TABLE B–10. Studies related to naltrexone *(continued)*

Author and year; trial name	Study characteristics	Treatment administered, including study arm, dose (mg/day), sample size (N), and co-intervention	Rx duration, weeks (follow-up)	Sample characteristics, including diagnostic inclusions and major exclusions	Outcome measures, main results, and overall percent attrition	Risk of bias
Chick et al. 2000a	Design: DBRCT Setting: 6 outpatient sites—5 alcohol treatment units and 1 academic hepatology department Country: United Kingdom Funding: DuPont	NTX 50 (90); PBO (85) Other Tx: usual psychosocial treatment program	12	DSM-III-R alcohol dependence or abuse Mean age: 43 years % Nonwhite NR 25% Female Other Dx: 0%	Differences between NTX and PBO were return to any drinking: 0.01 (95% CI –0.11, 0.13) and return to heavy drinking: 0 (95% CI –0.14, 0.14) In adherent subjects, greater reductions in craving noted with NTX vs. PBO ($p<0.05$) Attrition: 59% at 12 weeks, 19% lost to follow-up	Medium
Coller et al. 2011	Design: Open label Setting: outpatient Country: Australia Funding: govt	NTX 50 (100) Other Tx: CBI 100%	12	DSM-IV alcohol dependence Exclusions: NTX use in last 6 months Mean age: 43 years % Nonwhite NR 43% Female Other Dx: NR	Alcohol use decreased significantly, as did GGT and MCV values, with no differences among OPRM1 A118G genotype groups, A/A (65) or A/G and G/G (35)	Medium
De Sousa and De Sousa 2004	Design: OLRCT Setting: outpatient Country: India Funding: NR	DIS 250 (50); NTX 50 (50) Other Tx: supportive group psychotherapy 100%	52	DSM-IV alcohol dependence Exclusions: previous NTX and/or DIS treatment Mean age: 43–47 years % Nonwhite NR 0% Female Other Dx: NR	DIS was associated with greater reduction in relapse, greater survival time until the first relapse, and more days of abstinence than NTX: At study endpoint, relapse was 14% with DIS vs. 56% with NTX. NTX group reported lower composite craving scores than DIS group. Attrition: 3%	High

TABLE B–10. Studies related to naltrexone (*continued*)

Author and year; trial name	Study characteristics	Treatment administered, including study arm, dose (mg/day), sample size (N), and co-intervention	Rx duration, weeks (follow-up)	Sample characteristics, including diagnostic inclusions and major exclusions	Outcome measures, main results, and overall percent attrition	Risk of bias
Flórez et al. 2008	Design: OLRCT Setting: outpatient substance use disorders clinic Country: Spain Funding: NR	TOP to 200 (51); NTX 50 (51) Other Tx: therapy based on relapse prevention model 100%	26	ICD-10 alcohol dependence Mean age: 47 years 0% Nonwhite 15% Female Other Dx: personality disorders 27%	TOP and NTX were both effective but did not differ in efficacy as measured by a composite alcohol use metric. Adverse effects, particularly weight loss, were greater with TOP vs. NTX. Attrition: 10%	High
Flórez et al. 2011	Design: OLRCT Setting: outpatient substance use disorders clinic Country: Spain Funding: NR	TOP 200 (91); NTX 50 (91) Other Tx: BRENDA 100%; at least monthly meeting with psychiatrist 100%	26	ICD-10 alcohol dependence Mean age: 47–48 years % Nonwhite NR 15% Female Other Dx: personality disorders 23%	At 3 and 6 months, patients with TOP reported lower scores than those with NTX on craving and alcohol-related measures; those with TOP also scored less on disability-related measures at 6 months. TOP was associated with fewer drinks per drinking day and fewer heavy drinking days at 3 and 6 months compared with NTX. The percentage of days abstinent and total drinking days were comparable for TOP and NTX. A greater proportion of TOP subjects reported adverse effects at 3 months but not 6 months. Attrition: 10%	High

TABLE B–10. Studies related to naltrexone *(continued)*

Author and year; trial name	Study characteristics	Treatment administered, including study arm, dose (mg/day), sample size (N), and co-intervention	Rx duration, weeks (follow-up)	Sample characteristics, including diagnostic inclusions and major exclusions	Outcome measures, main results, and overall percent attrition	Risk of bias
Foa and Williams 2010; Foa et al. 2013; McLean et al. 2014; Zandberg et al. 2016	Design: DBRCT Setting: outpatient Country: United States Funding: govt	NTX 100+PE (40); NTX 100+SuppTx (42); PBO+PE (40); PBO+SuppTx (43) Other Tx: single-blind randomization to prolonged exposure therapy (12 weekly 90-min sessions, then 6 biweekly sessions) vs. supportive therapy; BRENDA provided to all subjects	24 (52)	DSM-IV alcohol dependence and PTSD Mean age: 42.7 years 70% Nonwhite 34.5% Female Other Dx: PTSD 100%	Percentages of days drinking alcohol and craving were reduced in all groups, with largest effect in groups that received NTX ($p=0.008$). PTSD severity was reduced in all groups, with no significant effect of prolonged exposure versus supportive therapy. Low PTSD symptoms were more likely with prolonged exposure plus NTX. Attrition: 44%	Medium
Fogaça et al. 2011	Design: DBRCT Setting: outpatient Country: Brazil Funding: govt	NTX 50 (20); PBO (20); NTX 50+PUFA (20); PUFA (20) Other Tx: none	12	DSM-IV alcohol dependence; male; age 30–50 years Mean age: NR % Non-white NR 0% Female Other Dx: NR	All groups showed improvement at 3 months ($p<0.001$) on drinking days, alcohol dependence severity, and craving scores, with no difference in treatment groups. Attrition: 46%	High

TABLE B–10. Studies related to naltrexone *(continued)*

Author and year; trial name	Study characteristics	Treatment administered, including study arm, dose (mg/day), sample size (N), and co-intervention	Rx duration, weeks (follow-up)	Sample characteristics, including diagnostic inclusions and major exclusions	Outcome measures, main results, and overall percent attrition	Risk of bias
Garbutt et al. 2010; Lucey et al. 2008; Pettinati et al. 2009	Design: DBRCT Setting: inpatient and outpatient public hospitals, private and VA clinics, and tertiary care medical centers Country: United States Funding: Alkermes	NTX inj 380 every 4 weeks (208); NTX inj 190 every 4 weeks (210); PBO (209) Other Tx: BRENDA standardized supportive therapy 100%	26	DSM-IV alcohol dependence with goal of reduced drinking or abstinence Mean age: 45 years 17% Nonwhite 32% Female Other Dx: NR	Differences between NTX and PBO were percent heavy drinking days: –5.14 (95% CI –10.04, –0.23) and return to any drinking: –0.01 (95% CI –0.05, 0.03) Decreased appetite was greater with NTX vs. PBO and was related to dose; nausea, fatigue, and dizziness were also greater for NTX groups taken together vs. PBO. Attrition: 39%	Medium
Gastpar et al. 2002	Design: DBRCT Setting: 7 outpatient sites Country: Germany Funding: DuPont	NTX 50 (84); PBO (87) Other Tx: psychosocial treatment	12	DSM-III-R alcohol dependence or abuse Mean age: 43 years 0% Nonwhite 28% Female Other Dx: 0%	Differences between NTX and PBO were return to any drinking: –0.03 (95% CI –0.18, 0.12) and return to heavy drinking: –0.01 (95% CI –0.16, 0.14) Kaplan-Meier survival analysis showed no NTX vs. PBO difference in time to heavy drinking. Adverse effects did not differ between groups. Attrition: 36%	Medium

TABLE B–10. Studies related to naltrexone *(continued)*

Author and year; trial name	Study characteristics	Treatment administered, including study arm, dose (mg/day), sample size (N), and co-intervention	Rx duration, weeks (follow-up)	Sample characteristics, including diagnostic inclusions and major exclusions	Outcome measures, main results, and overall percent attrition	Risk of bias
Gelernter et al. 2007	Design: DBRCT Setting: multisite VAMCs Country: United States Funding: VA	NTX 50 (149); PBO (64) Other Tx: NR	13	DSM-IV alcohol dependence Mean age: 50 years 26% Nonwhite 0% Female Other Dx: cannabis and cocaine 27%; major depression 13.9%; social phobia 7.7%; generalized anxiety disorder 5.1%; PTSD 13.6%; antisocial personality disorder 8.1%; tobacco use 71.8%	Treatment condition, age, and number of drinks per drinking day at baseline were significant ($p < 0.05$) predictors of relapse rate and time to relapse. No significant interactions were found between individual SNP and NTX treatment response. In the subsample of patients with genotype information for OPRM1 Asn40Asp, OPRK1, or OPRD1 rs678849, NTX treatment significantly reduced the odds of relapse. Subjects in the PBO group were about twice as likely to relapse as subjects in the NTX group. Attrition: 65%	High

TABLE B–10. Studies related to naltrexone (continued)

Author and year; trial name	Study characteristics	Treatment administered, including study arm, dose (mg/day), sample size (N), and co-intervention	Rx duration, weeks (follow-up)	Sample characteristics, including diagnostic inclusions and major exclusions	Outcome measures, main results, and overall percent attrition	Risk of bias
Greenfield et al. 2010; Fucito et al. 2012; COMBINE	Design: secondary data analysis Setting: 11 academic outpatient sites Country: United States Funding: govt, meds	ACA 3,000+CBI+MM (151); ACA 3,000+ MM (152); NTX 100+CBI+MM (155); NTX 100+MM (154); PBO+CBI+MM (156); PBO+MM (153) Other Tx: as randomized; community support group participation (e.g., AA) encouraged	68	DSM-IV alcohol dependence Mean age: 44 years 23% Nonwhite 31% Female Other Dx: 0%	There was a significant NTX by CBI interaction for women on two primary outcomes (percent days abstinent and time to first heavy drinking day) and also secondary outcome measures (good clinical response, percent heavy drinking days, and craving). Only the NTX by CBI interaction was significant for percent days abstinent. The NTX by CBI interaction was significant for time to first heavy drinking day in men (p=0.048), with each treatment showing slower relapse times; a nonsignificant trend was present in women. NTX or CBI alone was superior to groups receiving neither in the percent of heavy drinking days. Complete within-treatment drinking data were provided by 94% of study subjects.	Low
Guardia et al. 2002	Design: DBRCT Setting: 7 outpatient sites Country: Spain Funding: Pharmazam/ Zambon	NTX 50 (101); PBO (101) Other Tx: psychosocial	12	DSM-IV alcohol dependence Mean age: NR % Nonwhite NR 25% Female Other Dx: NR	Differences between NTX and PBO were drinks per drinking day: −0.51 (95% CI −1.03, 0.01), percent drinking days: −2.3 (95% CI −9.31, 4.71), return to any drinking: −0.01 (95% CI −0.15, 0.13), and return to heavy drinking: −0.11 (95% CI −0.2, −0.02) Kaplan-Meier survival analysis showed greater time to first relapse with NTX vs. PBO (p<0.05). Rates of nausea and headache were greater with NTX vs. PBO. Attrition: 41%	Medium

TABLE B–10. Studies related to naltrexone (continued)

Author and year; trial name	Study characteristics	Treatment administered, including study arm, dose (mg/day), sample size (N), and co-intervention	Rx duration, weeks (follow-up)	Sample characteristics, including diagnostic inclusions and major exclusions	Outcome measures, main results, and overall percent attrition	Risk of bias
Heinälä et al. 2001	Design: DBRCT Setting: outpatient Country: Finland Funding: govt	NTX 50 daily for 12 weeks, then targeted+CS (34); PBO+CS (33); NTX 50 daily for 12 weeks, then targeted+ST (29); PBO+ST (25) Other Tx: none	32	DSM-IV alcohol dependence Mean age: 46 years % Nonwhite NR 29% Female Other Dx: 0%	There was a significant treatment effect on relapse rate to heavy drinking, and there was an interaction between the medication and the type of therapy, with best response for the coping/NTX group. Among patients never relapsed to heavy drinking, NTX showed a significantly better response than PBO in the coping groups ($p=0.08$). Among patients who relapsed to heavy drinking, 19.1% of the coping/NTX group relapsed only once, compared with 3.2% of the coping/PBO group. Coping/NTX had better outcomes on reported alcohol consumption (mean±SD g/week) than the other three groups (231 ± 40 for coping/NTX, 354 ± 62 for coping/PBO, 357 ± 81 for supportive/NTX, and 326 ± 80 for supportive/PBO). Attrition: 32%	High
Huang et al. 2005	Design: DBRCT Setting: 1 week alcohol treatment inpatient unit, then outpatient site Country: Taiwan Funding: NR	NTX 50 (20); PBO (20) Other Tx: weekly individual psychotherapy sessions 100%	14	Subjects admitted for alcohol detoxification and meeting DSM-III-R alcohol dependence Mean age: 38–43 years 100% Nonwhite 0% Female Other Dx: NR	Difference between NTX and PBO for return to heavy drinking: 0.05 (95% CI −0.18, 0.28). Craving was less with NTX vs. PBO, although relapse rates did not differ. Attrition: 40%	High

TABLE B–10. Studies related to naltrexone *(continued)*

Author and year; trial name	Study characteristics	Treatment administered, including study arm, dose (mg/day), sample size (N), and co-intervention	Rx duration, weeks (follow-up)	Sample characteristics, including diagnostic inclusions and major exclusions	Outcome measures, main results, and overall percent attrition	Risk of bias
Johnson et al. 2004b	Design: DBRCT Setting: 4 outpatient sites Country: United States, France, the Netherlands Funding: univ, meds	NTX inj 400 every 28 days (25); PBO inj (5) Other Tx: psychosocial support 100%	17	DSM-IV alcohol dependence Mean age: 43 years 37% Nonwhite 27% Female Other Dx: NR	Differences between NTX and PBO were drinks per drinking day: –2.2 (95% CI –3.19, –1.21), percent heavy drinking days: –13 (95% CI –44.48, 18.48), and percent drinking days: –6.8 (95% CI –53.75, 40.15). Injection site induration and angioedema led to NTX discontinuation in 2 of the 25 NTX subjects. Attrition: 30%	High
Kiefer et al. 2003, 2004, 2005	Design: DBRCT Setting: 1 outpatient site Country: Germany Funding: univ, meds	ACA 1,998 (40); NTX 50 (40); PBO (40); ACA 1,998+NTX 50 (40) Other Tx: group therapy	12	DSM-IV alcohol dependence without any withdrawal symptoms Exclusions: homelessness Mean age: 46 years % Nonwhite NR 26% Female Other Dx: 0%	Differences between NTX and PBO were return to any drinking: –0.28 (95% CI –0.44, –0.11) and return to heavy drinking: –0.25 (95% CI –0.45, –0.05) Kaplan-Meier survival analysis showed significantly longer time to relapse and to first alcohol use for NTX or NTX+ACA vs. PBO. At the end of active treatment, relapse rates with ACA+NTX did not differ from ACA alone. Adverse effects were minor, and differences between groups were not clinically significant. Attrition: 53%	Low

TABLE B–10. Studies related to naltrexone (continued)

Author and year; trial name	Study characteristics	Treatment administered, including study arm, dose (mg/day), sample size (N), and co-intervention	Rx duration, weeks (follow-up)	Sample characteristics, including diagnostic inclusions and major exclusions	Outcome measures, main results, and overall percent attrition	Risk of bias
Killeen et al. 2004	Design: DBRCT Setting: outpatient community substance use treatment center Country: United States Funding: govt	NTX 50+TAU (54); PBO+TAU(43); TAU alone (48) Other Tx: several types and intensities	12	Current alcohol use disorder Exclusions: >10 days outpatient treatment past 3 months Mean age: 37 years 24% Nonwhite 37% Female Other Dx: comorbid psychiatric disorder 51%; other substance use disorder 35%	Differences between NTX and PBO were drinks per drinking day: 1.6 (95% CI −0.55, 3.75), percent drinking days: −1.2 (95% CI −9.31, 7.33), percent heavy drinking days: −2.9 (95% CI −9.94, 4.14), return to any drinking: 0 (95% CI −0.21, 0.22), and return to heavy drinking: 0.08 (95% CI −0.13, 0.28). Daytime sleepiness, fatigue, and dizziness were more common with NTX vs. PBO. Attrition: 28%	Medium
King et al. 2012; Fridberg et al. 2014	Design: DBRCT Setting: outpatient Country: United States Funding: govt	NTX 50 (34); PBO (35) Other Tx: behavioral therapy and open-label nicotine patch	12 (52)	Healthy smokers with heavy drinking Mean age: 35.5 years 37% Nonwhite 38% Female Other Dx: nicotine dependence 100%	Weekly alcohol consumption was reduced with NTX (IRR 0.71; 95% CI 0.51, 1.0; p=0.049). Smoking quit rates were 23% NTX vs. 15% PBO at 12-month follow-up. Attrition: 25%	Medium

TABLE B–10. Studies related to naltrexone *(continued)*

Author and year; trial name	Study characteristics	Treatment administered, including study arm, dose (mg/day), sample size (N), and co-intervention	Rx duration, weeks (follow-up)	Sample characteristics, including diagnostic inclusions and major exclusions	Outcome measures, main results, and overall percent attrition	Risk of bias
Kranzler et al. 2004	Design: DBRCT Setting: outpatient Country: United States Funding: DrugAbuse Sciences	NTX inj once a month 150 (185); PBO inj (157) Other Tx: MET 100%	12	DSM-IV alcohol dependence Mean age: 44 years 17%–18% Nonwhite 33%–37% Female Other Dx: NR	Differences between NTX and PBO were percent drinking days: –8.6 (95% CI –16.01, –1.19), percent heavy drinking days: –3.4 (95% CI –10.24, 3.44), return to any drinking: –0.08 (95% CI –0.15, 0), return to heavy drinking: –0.07 (95% CI –0.16, 0.02). Difficulties giving the injection occurred in 21% of injections, with 4% withdrawing because of injection site reactions, but rates in NTX and PBO groups did not differ. Adverse effects did not differ between the groups. Attrition: 22%	Medium

TABLE B–10. Studies related to naltrexone (*continued*)

Author and year; trial name	Study characteristics	Treatment administered, including study arm, dose (mg/day), sample size (*N*), and co-intervention	Rx duration, weeks (follow-up)	Sample characteristics, including diagnostic inclusions and major exclusions	Outcome measures, main results, and overall percent attrition	Risk of bias
Kranzler et al. 2009	Design: DBRCT Setting: outpatient Country: United States Funding: govt	NTX 50 targeted (38); NTX 50 once daily (45); PBO targeted (39); PBO once daily (41) Other Tx: brief coping skills training 100%	12	Average weekly alcohol consumption of ≥24 standard drinks for men and ≥18 standard drinks for women Exclusions: recent unsuccessful attempt to reduce drinking or past/current significant alcohol withdrawal symptoms Mean age: 49 years 3% Nonwhite 42% Female Other Dx: substance use disorder <1%; social phobia 3%; antisocial personality disorder 3%; dysthymic disorder <1%; agoraphobia without panic disorder <1%; OCD <1%; GAD <1%	The difference between the targeted NTX group and the mean of the other three groups was not significant (*p*=0.038), but the targeted NTX group drank 16.5% less per day than the other groups. Heavier drinkers reported greater decreases in drinks per day during the study period (*b*=−0.004, SE=0.002, *p*=0.038). Men in the targeted NTX group had fewer drinks per drinking day than the daily NTX group (*p*=0.014). The targeted NTX group drank 19% less on drinking days than the other groups. Nausea and dizziness were more frequent with NTX vs. PBO. Attrition: 15%	Medium

TABLE B–10. Studies related to naltrexone (continued)

Author and year; trial name	Study characteristics	Treatment administered, including study arm, dose (mg/day), sample size (N), and co-intervention	Rx duration, weeks (follow-up)	Sample characteristics, including diagnostic inclusions and major exclusions	Outcome measures, main results, and overall percent attrition	Risk of bias
Krystal et al. 2001; VACS425	Design: DBRCT Setting: multisite outpatient Country: United States Funding: VA, meds	NTX 50 for 12 months (209); NTX 50 for 3 months, then PBO (209); PBO (209) Other Tx: 12-step facilitation	12 or 52	DSM-IV alcohol dependence Exclusions: homelessness; alcohol-related disability pension Mean age: 49 years 37% Nonwhite 3% Female Other Dx: 0%	Differences between NTX and PBO were percent drinking days: −2.7 (95% CI −6.62, 1.22), return to any drinking: −0.06 (95% CI −0.14, 0.02), return to heavy drinking: −0.06 (95% CI −0.15, 0.02), and drinks per drinking day: 0.2 (95% CI −1.38, 1.78) Median time to relapse was 135 days, with no differences by group. Adverse effects did not differ among groups. Attrition: 27%	Medium
Laaksonen et al. 2008	Design: OLRCT Setting: 6 outpatient sites in 5 cities Country: Finland Funding: govt	ACA 1,998 or 1,333 (81); DIS 100–200 (81); NTX 50 (81) Other Tx: manual-based CBT	Up to 52 (119)	ICD-10 alcohol dependence Mean age: 43 years 0% Nonwhite 29% Female Other Dx: NR	During the continuous medication period (1–12 weeks), the DIS group did significantly better than the NTX and ACA groups in time to first heavy drinking day (p=0.001), days to first drinking (p=0.002), abstinence days, and average weekly alcohol intake. During the targeted medication period (13–52 weeks), there were no significant differences between the groups in time to first heavy drinking day and days to first drinking, whereas the DIS group reported significantly more frequent abstinence days than the ACA and NTX groups. During the whole study period (1–52 weeks), the DIS group did significantly better in time to the first drink compared with the other groups. Attrition: 52%	High

TABLE B–10. Studies related to naltrexone *(continued)*

Author and year; trial name	Study characteristics	Treatment administered, including study arm, dose (mg/day), sample size (N), and co-intervention	Rx duration, weeks (follow-up)	Sample characteristics, including diagnostic inclusions and major exclusions	Outcome measures, main results, and overall percent attrition	Risk of bias
Latt et al. 2002	Design: DBRCT Setting: 4 hospital-based outpatient sites Country: Australia Funding: govt	NTX 50 (56); PBO (51) Other Tx: no extensive psychosocial interventions	12 (26)	DSM-IV alcohol dependence Mean age: 45 years % Nonwhite NR 30% Female Other Dx: 0%	Differences between NTX and PBO were percent drinking days: −0.9 (95% CI −26.7, 24.9) and return to heavy drinking: −0.19 (95% CI −0.37, −0.01). Kaplan-Meier survival analysis showed longer time to relapse for NTX (median 90 days) vs. PBO (median 42 days), with relapse in 33.9% with NTX vs. 52.9% with PBO. Headache was more common with PBO vs. NTX; other adverse effects did not differ. Attrition: 31%	Medium
Lee et al. 2001	Design: DBRCT Setting: inpatient for 1 month, then outpatient Country: Singapore Funding: meds	NTX 50 (35); PBO (18) Other Tx: intensive inpatient rehabilitation program; postdischarge therapy encouraged 100%	12	DSM-IV alcohol dependence Mean age: 45 years ≥88% Nonwhite 0% Female Other Dx: NR	Difference between NTX and PBO for return to any drinking: −0.07 (95% CI −0.35, 0.21) Decrease in craving was more frequent with NTX vs. PBO. Adverse effects were minor and did not differ with NTX vs. PBO. Attrition: 66% at 12 weeks; 26% with missing data	High

TABLE B–10. Studies related to naltrexone *(continued)*

Author and year; trial name	Study characteristics	Treatment administered, including study arm, dose (mg/day), sample size (N), and co-intervention	Rx duration, weeks (follow-up)	Sample characteristics, including diagnostic inclusions and major exclusions	Outcome measures, main results, and overall percent attrition	Risk of bias
Longabaugh et al. 2009	Design: DBRCT Setting: outpatient Country: United States Funding: govt	NTX 50 for 24 weeks+BST (36); NTX 50 for 12 weeks, then PBO for 12 weeks+BST (35); NTX 50 for 24 weeks+MET (33); NTX 50 for 12 weeks, then PBO for 12 weeks+MET (38) Other Tx: none	12–24 (72)	DSM-IV alcohol dependence Mean age: 44–46 years 6%–14% Nonwhite 33%–43% Female Other Dx: NR	With 12 additional weeks of NTX, the median time to first heavy drinking day was longer for those in the BST group than for those in the other three groups (61 days vs. between 11 and 20 days, Wilcoxon chi-square=5.05, $p<0.03$). With 12 additional weeks of NTX, the median time to first drink was longer for those in the BST group than for the other three groups (27.5 days vs. between 2 and 10 days, Wilcoxon chi-square=6.12, $p<0.02$). Neither percentage of abstinent days nor percentage of heavy drinking days was significantly greater for the BST/NTX condition than any other condition. Attrition: 18%	Medium
Mann et al. 2013; PREDICT	Design: DBRCT Setting: NR Country: Germany Funding: govt, meds	ACA 1,998 (172); NTX 50 (169); PBO (86) Other Tx: MM	12	Alcohol dependence Mean age: 45 years % Nonwhite NR 23% Female Other Dx: NR	Difference between NTX and PBO for return to heavy drinking: 0.03 (95% CI −0.1, 0.16) Point estimates for heavy drinking relapse–free survival from the Kaplan-Meier curves were 48.3% for ACA, 49.1% for NTX, and 51.8% for PBO. No adverse effects were greater with NTX than other groups. Attrition: 34%	Medium

TABLE B–10. Studies related to naltrexone (*continued*)

Author and year; trial name	Study characteristics	Treatment administered, including study arm, dose (mg/day), sample size (*N*), and co-intervention	Rx duration, weeks (follow-up)	Sample characteristics, including diagnostic inclusions and major exclusions	Outcome measures, main results, and overall percent attrition	Risk of bias
Monterosso et al. 2001	Design: DBRCT Setting: outpatient Country: United States Funding: govt	NTX 100 (121); PBO (62) Other Tx: BRENDA	12	DSM-III-R alcohol dependence Mean age: 46 years 27% Nonwhite 27% Female Other Dx: NR	Difference between NTX and PBO for percent heavy drinking days: –3.9 (95% CI –7.58, –0.22) NTX was most efficacious in those with higher craving (*p*=0.02). Attrition: 18%	Medium
Monti et al. 2001; Rohsenow et al. 2000, 2007	Design: DBRCT Setting: 2 weeks partial hospital (premedication), 52 weeks out-patient Country: United States Funding: govt	NTX 50 (64); PBO (64) Other Tx: brief physician outpatient contacts (intensive therapy occurred prior to medication portion of trial)	12 (52)	DSM-IV alcohol abuse or dependence Mean age: 39 years 3% Nonwhite 24% Female Other Dx: cocaine use 23%; sedative use 8%; opiate use 4%	Differences between NTX and PBO were return to heavy drinking: –0.05 (95% CI –0.2, 0.11) and drinks per drinking day: –3.83 (95% CI –5.55, –2.11). Survival analysis showed no difference in time to relapse between groups. Data were available for 91% of the sample at 3 months and 87% at 12 months, with no difference between groups.	Medium
Morgenstern et al. 2012; Chenet al. 2014	Design: DBRCT Setting: NR Country: United States Funding: govt	NTX 100+MBSCT (51); NTX 100 (51); PBO+MBSCT (50); PBO (48) Other Tx: brief behavioral medication compliance enhancement therapy 100%	12	Average weekly consumption of at least 24 standard drinks per week over the previous 90 days and being sexually active with other men; 90% with DSM-IV alcohol dependence Mean age: 40 years 26% Nonwhite 0% Female Other Dx: HIV 15%; any drug use 67%	Among those receiving usual care only, those receiving NTX were significantly more likely to have nonhazardous drinking during the treatment period than those receiving PBO (OR=3.33, 95% CI 2.14, 17.42). Among those receiving MBSCT, NTX had no significant effect (OR=0.53, 95% CI 0.26, 1.07). Adverse effects did not differ between groups at study endpoint. Attrition: 16%	Medium

TABLE B–10. Studies related to naltrexone (continued)

Author and year; trial name	Study characteristics	Treatment administered, including study arm, dose (mg/day), sample size (N), and co-intervention	Rx duration, weeks (follow-up)	Sample characteristics, including diagnostic inclusions and major exclusions	Outcome measures, main results, and overall percent attrition	Risk of bias
Morley et al. 2006, 2010	Design: DBRCT Setting: 3 outpatient intensive substance use treatment sites Country: Australia Funding: govt	ACA 1,998 (55); NTX 50 (53); PBO (61) Other Tx: all offered 4–6 sessions of manualized compliance therapy; uptake/attendance NR	12	DSM-IV alcohol dependence or abuse and with alcohol abstinence for 3–21 days Mean age: 45 years % Nonwhite NR 30% Female Other Dx: substantial levels of emotional distress (anxiety, stress, and depression); 3% severe concurrent illness (psychiatric or other)	Differences between NTX and PBO were drinks per drinking days: =–1.2 (95% CI –3.43, 1.03), percent drinking days: –1.3 (95% CI –14.56, 11.96), return to any drinking: –0.01 (95% CI –0.13, 0.15), and return to heavy drinking: 0.03 (95% CI –0.13, 0.20) No significant adverse effects were noted. Attrition: 35%	Low
Morris et al. 2001	Design: DBRCT Setting: outpatient Country: Australia Funding: govt, meds	NTX 50 (55); PBO (56) Other Tx: group psychoeducation and social support	12	DSM-III-R alcohol dependence Mean age: 47 years % Nonwhite NR 0% Female Other Dx: PTSD 23%; GAD 32%; panic disorder 4%; MDD 6%; BPD 1%	Differences between NTX and PBO were percent drinking days: –11 (95% CI –26.34, 4.34), return to any drinking: –0.09 (95% CI –0.23, 0.05), and return to heavy drinking: –0.26 (95% CI –0.43, –0.09) Survival analyses showed longer time to first relapse with NTX (6.7 weeks) vs. PBO (4.2 weeks) but no difference in time to first drink. Attrition: 36%	Medium

TABLE B–10. Studies related to naltrexone *(continued)*

Author and year; trial name	Study characteristics	Treatment administered, including study arm, dose (mg/day), sample size (N), and co-intervention	Rx duration, weeks (follow-up)	Sample characteristics, including diagnostic inclusions and major exclusions	Outcome measures, main results, and overall percent attrition	Risk of bias
Narayana et al. 2008	Design: prospective cohort Setting: military, outpatient Country: India Funding: NR	ACA 1,332–1,998 (28); NTX 50 (26); TOP 100–125 (38) Other Tx: various psychotherapies were offered	52	ICD-10 alcohol dependence Mean age: 38 years 100% Nonwhite 0% Female Other Dx: NR	TOP (76.3%) was significantly more effective ($p < 0.01$) in sustaining abstinence, although 57.7% NTX and 60.7% ACA maintained complete abstinence. 7 TOP subjects (18.4%) reported decreased relapses compared with 8 NTX (30.8%) and 9 ACA (32.1%) subjects. Attrition: 22%	High
Nava et al. 2006	Design: OLRCT Setting: outpatient Country: Italy Funding: govt	GHB 50 (28); NTX 50 (24); DIS 200 (28) Other Tx: CBT	52	DSM-IV-TR alcohol dependence Exclusions: any withdrawal syndrome, HIV antibodies, homelessness Mean age: 38.5–42.7 years % Nonwhite NR 15% Female Other Dx: 0%	At the end of the study, no statistical difference was found among groups in terms of the number of withdrawn, abstinent, nonabstinent, and relapsed patients. A significant reduction in alcohol intake, craving, and laboratory markers of alcohol abuse was found in all groups. The GHB group showed greater decreases in alcohol craving and in laboratory markers of alcohol abuse compared with the NTX and DIS groups. Attrition: 31%	High

Author and year; trial name	Study characteristics	Treatment administered, including study arm, dose (mg/day), sample size (N), and co-intervention	Rx duration, weeks (follow-up)	Sample characteristics, including diagnostic inclusions and major exclusions	Outcome measures, main results, and overall percent attrition	Risk of bias
O'Malley et al. 1992, 1996	Design: DBRCT Setting: outpatient univ alcohol treatment unit Country: United States Funding: govt, meds	NTX 50+CS (29); NTX 50+ST (23); PBO+CS (25); PBO+ST (27)	12 (38)	DSM-III-R alcohol dependence Mean age: 41 years 7% Nonwhite 26% Female Other Dx: NR	Differences between NTX and PBO were drinks per drinking day: –1.75 (95% CI –4.07, 0.57), percent drinking days: –5.6 (95% CI –11.07, –0.13), return to any drinking: –0.2 (95% CI –0.38, –0.02), and return to heavy drinking: –0.19 (95% CI –0.38, –0.01). Subjects treated with NTX were less likely to meet AUD criteria at treatment endpoint than with PBO treatment. Benefits of treatment lasted through only 1 month of follow-up. Attrition: 18%	Medium
O'Malley et al. 2007	Design: DBRCT stratified by eating disorder Setting: univ mental health center Country: United States Funding: govt	NTX 50 (57); PBO (50) Other Tx: cognitive-behavioral coping skills therapy 100%, based on manualized approach used in Project MATCH	12	DSM-IV alcohol dependence Exclusions: >30 days abstinence, obesity or significant underweight Mean age: 40 years 11% Nonwhite 100% Female Other Dx: eating disorder 28%	Differences between NTX and PBO were return to any drinking: 0.1 (95% CI –0.05, 0.25) and return to heavy drinking: 0.04 (95% CI –0.14, 0.22). Survival analysis showed no difference between NTX and PBO for time to first day of drinking or time to first day of heavy drinking. Decreased appetite, depression, dizziness, and overall reports of adverse effects were more common with NTX vs. PBO. Attrition: 43%	Medium

TABLE B–10. Studies related to naltrexone *(continued)*

Author and year; trial name	Study characteristics	Treatment administered, including study arm, dose (mg/day), sample size (*N*), and co-intervention	Rx duration, weeks (follow-up)	Sample characteristics, including diagnostic inclusions and major exclusions	Outcome measures, main results, and overall percent attrition	Risk of bias
O'Malley et al. 2008	Design: DBRCT Setting: Alaskan outpatient site Country: United States Funding: govt, meds	NTX 50 (34); PBO (34); NTX 50+SERT 100 (33) Other Tx: MM 100%	16	DSM-IV alcohol dependence Mean age: 40 years 70% Nonwhite 34% Female Other Dx: NR	Differences between NTX and PBO were drinks per drinking day: –0.3 (95% CI –0.7, 0.1), percent drinking days: –9.1 (95% CI –10.55, –7.65), percent heavy drinking days: –7.5 (95% CI –8.91, –6.09), return to any drinking: –0.24 (95% CI –0.43, –0.04), and return to heavy drinking: –0.18 (95% CI –0.38, 0.03). There was a statistically significant advantage of NTX over PBO but no additional benefit from the addition of SERT to NTX on total abstinence (NTX vs. PBO, *p*=0.04; NTX vs. NTX+SERT, *p*=0.56) or the percentage who reported a drinking-related problem during treatment (NTX vs. PBO, *p*=0.04; NTX vs. NTX+SERT, *p*=0.85). Time to first heavy drinking day was longer but not significantly greater for the NTX-only group compared with PBO (NTX vs. PBO, *p*=0.14; NTX vs. NTX+SERT, *p*=0.84). Treatment efficacy was not dependent on the presence of an Asn40 allele. Nausea, sleepiness, and dizziness were greater with NTX vs. PBO, with even greater rates with NTX+SERT. Attrition: 33%	Medium

TABLE B–10. Studies related to naltrexone (continued)

Author and year; trial name	Study characteristics	Treatment administered, including study arm, dose (mg/day), sample size (N), and co-intervention	Rx duration, weeks (follow-up)	Sample characteristics, including diagnostic inclusions and major exclusions	Outcome measures, main results, and overall percent attrition	Risk of bias
Oslin et al. 1997	Design: DBRCT Setting: outpatient substance use disorders clinic and VAMC Country: United States Funding: DuPont Merck	NTX 100 on Monday and Wednesday, 150 on Friday (21); PBO (23) Other Tx: group therapy and case manager 100%	12	DSM-III-R alcohol dependence Mean age: 58 years 64% Nonwhite % Female NR Other Dx: 0%	Differences between NTX and PBO were percent drinking days: –4.6 (95% CI –12.76, 3.56), return to any drinking: –0.06 (95% CI –0.34, 0.21), and return to heavy drinking: –0.2 (95% CI –0.45, 0.04). Adverse effects did not differ for NTX vs. PBO. Attrition: 39%	Medium
Oslin et al. 2008	Design: DBRCT Setting: outpatient psychiatry clinic Country: United States Funding: govt	NTX 100+CBT (40); NTX 100+BRENDA (39); NTX 100+doctor only (41); PBO+CBT (40); PBO+BRENDA (40); PBO+doctor only (40) Other Tx: none	24	DSM-IV alcohol dependence Mean age: 41 years 27% Nonwhite 27% Female Other Dx: NR	Differences between NTX and PBO were drinks per drinking day: 1.86 (95% CI –1.47, 5.19), percent drinking days: –0.4 (95% CI –6.14, 5.34), percent heavy drinking days: –2 (95% CI –6.2, 2.2), return to any drinking: –0.01 (95% CI –0.11, 0.09), and return to heavy drinking: –0.03 (95% CI –0.15, 0.1). There was no overall effect of NTX, but psychosocial treatment had a modest main effect favoring CBT. Insomnia was more frequent with NTX vs. PBO, but other adverse effects did not differ. Subjects attended 31.3% of psychosocial intervention sessions, and 50.4% of subjects adhered to medication. Attrition: 23%	Medium

TABLE B–10. Studies related to naltrexone (*continued*)

Author and year; trial name	Study characteristics	Treatment administered, including study arm, dose (mg/day), sample size (N), and co-intervention	Rx duration, weeks (follow-up)	Sample characteristics, including diagnostic inclusions and major exclusions	Outcome measures, main results, and overall percent attrition	Risk of bias
Oslin et al. 2015	Design: DBRCT, block randomized by Asn40 allele genotype Setting: outpatient Country: United States Funding: govt	NTX 50 (111); PBO (110) Other Tx: MM	12	DSM-IV alcohol dependence, European or Asian descent Mean age: 48.5 years 1.8% Nonwhite 14.1% Female Other Dx: NR	Time-dependent decrease in heavy drinking for all groups (GEE score test χ^2_1=12.18, P=0.001), with no significant group×time interactions. No moderating effect of OPRM1 gene status was found. Attrition: 31%	Low
Petrakis et al. 2004; Ralevski et al. 2006	Design: DBRCT Setting: New England Mental Illness and Research Education Clinical Center outpatient sites Country: United States Funding: VA	NTX 50 (16); PBO (15) Other Tx: CBT+psychiatric treatment as usual; neuroleptics 52%; benzodiazepines 16%; thymoleptics 39%	12	DSM-IV alcohol dependence or abuse and schizophrenia or schizoaffective disorder Mean age: 46 years 19% Nonwhite 0% Female Other Dx: schizophrenia or schizoaffective disorder 100%	Differences between NTX and PBO were drinks per drinking day: 2.98 (95% CI –4.63, 10.59), percent drinking days: –8.7 (95% CI –19.16, 1.76), and percent heavy drinking days: –1.5 (95% CI –4.49, 1.49). Adverse effects were similar for NTX and PBO, and psychotic symptoms (via the PANSS) and AIMS scores did not differ between groups. Attrition: 24%	Medium

Author and year; trial name	Study characteristics	Treatment administered, including study arm, dose (mg/day), sample size (N), and co-intervention	Rx duration, weeks (follow-up)	Sample characteristics, including diagnostic inclusions and major exclusions	Outcome measures, main results, and overall percent attrition	Risk of bias
Petrakis et al. 2005, 2006, 2007; Ralevski et al. 2007; VAMIRECC	Design: DBRCT Setting: outpatient VA Country: United States Funding: govt	DIS 250 (66); NTX 50 (59); PBO (64); NTX 50+DIS 250 (65) Other Tx: psychiatric treatment as usual 100%	12	DSM-IV alcohol dependence and other Axis I disorder Exclusions: psychosis Mean age: 47 years 26% Nonwhite 3% Female Other Dx: Axis I disorder 100%	Differences between NTX and PBO were percent drinking days: –1.9 (95% CI –6.46, 2.66), percent heavy drinking days: –2 (95% CI –6.25, 2.25), and return to any drinking: 0.01 (95% CI –0.16, 0.18). Those in both NTX and DIS groups had significantly fewer drinking days per week ($F_{1,246}=5.71$, $p=0.02$) and more consecutive days of abstinence ($F_{1,246}=4.49$, $p=0.04$) than those assigned to PBO. No significant differences were found between groups in terms of the percent days of abstinence, percent of heavy drinking days, and the number of subjects with total abstinence. DIS showed greater reductions over time of GGT ($F_{1,454}=5.85$, $p<0.02$) compared with NTX. DIS-treated subjects reported a significantly greater change over time in craving compared with the NTX-treated subjects ($z=3.98$, $p<0.01$). Adverse effects were most frequent in subjects treated with NTX+DIS. Attrition: 35%	High

TABLE B–10. Studies related to naltrexone *(continued)*

Author and year; trial name	Study characteristics	Treatment administered, including study arm, dose (mg/day), sample size (N), and co-intervention	Rx duration, weeks (follow-up)	Sample characteristics, including diagnostic inclusions and major exclusions	Outcome measures, main results, and overall percent attrition	Risk of bias
Petrakis et al. 2012	Design: DBRCT Setting: outpatient; multiple psychiatric centers, primarily VA Country: United States Funding: VA	DMI 200+PBO (24); paroxetine 40+PBO (20); DMI 200+NTX 50 (22); paroxetine 40+NTX 50 (22) Other Tx: clinical management; compliance enhancement therapy 100%	12	DSM-IV alcohol dependence and PTSD Exclusions: psychosis Mean age: 47 years 25% Nonwhite 9% Female Other Dx: PTSD 100%	Compared with paroxetine, DMI significantly reduced the percentage of heavy drinking days ($F_{1,84}=7.22$, $p=0.009$) and drinks per drinking days ($F_{1,84}=5.04$, $p=0.027$). There was a significant interaction for time by DMI/paroxetine treatment on drinks per week ($ATS_{6,82}=2.46$, $p=0.018$): DMI subjects had a greater reduction in their drinking over time compared with paroxetine subjects. NTX, compared with PBO, significantly decreased craving ($F_{1582,0}=6.39$, $p=0.012$); NTX=19.88 (SD=12.89) and PBO=21.1 (SD=12.89) at baseline vs. NTX=6.7 (SD=14.07) and PBO=8.3 (SD=13.38) at endpoint). GGT declined more in the DMI-treated participants ($F_{1229,5}=5.08$, $p=0.02$; DMI baseline=55.2, paroxetine baseline=86.4; DMI week 4=48.7, paroxetine week 4=46.1; DMI week 8=41.7, paroxetine week 8=47.1; DMI week 12=37.5, paroxetine week 12=57.1). Attrition: 44.3%	High

Author and year; trial name	Study characteristics	Treatment administered, including study arm, dose (mg/day), sample size (N), and co-intervention	Rx duration, weeks (follow-up)	Sample characteristics, including diagnostic inclusions and major exclusions	Outcome measures, main results, and overall percent attrition	Risk of bias
Pettinati et al. 2008b	Design: DBRCT Setting: univ-affiliated outpatient substance use disorder treatment research facility Country: United States Funding: govt, meds	NTX 150 (82); PBO (82); subjects also randomly assigned to either CBT or BRENDA (2×2 design) Other Tx: NR	12	DSM-IV alcohol dependence and cocaine dependence Mean age: 39 years 76% Nonwhite 29% Female Other Dx: cocaine dependence 100%	Differences between NTX and PBO were drinks per drinking day: –1.7 (95% CI –3.29, –0.11), percent drinking days: –2.3 (95% CI –6.85, 2.25), and percent heavy drinking days: –2.72 (95% CI –6.16, 0.72). Type of psychosocial treatment did not affect outcomes. Nausea was more frequent with NTX vs. PBO. Attrition: 36%	Medium
Pettinati et al. 2010	Design: DBRCT Setting: outpatient Country: United States Funding: govt, meds	SERT 200 (40); NTX 100 (49); PBO (39); SERT 200+NTX 100 (42) Other Tx: CBT 100%	14	DSM-IV alcohol dependence and major depression Mean age: 43 years 35% Nonwhite 38% Female Other Dx: depression 100%	Difference between NTX and PBO for return to any drinking: 0.03 (95% CI –0.15, 0.2) SERT+NTX was associated with a higher rate of abstinence and longer time to heavy drinking relapse than PBO or either drug alone. Rates of adverse effects were not significantly different among groups. Attrition: 43%	Medium
Schmitz et al. 2004	Design: DBRCT Setting: outpatient Country: United States Funding: govt	NTX 50+RPT (20); NTX 50+DC (20); PBO+RPT (20); PBO+DC (20) Other Tx: RPT or DC as randomized	12	DSM-IV alcohol dependence and cocaine dependence Mean age: 36 years 71% Nonwhite 16% Female Other Dx: cocaine dependence 100%	Differences between NTX and PBO were drinks per drinking day: 2 (95% CI –1.14, 5.14) and percent drinking days: –0.4 (95% CI –6.91, 6.11). Cocaine use was not affected by NTX vs. PBO. Adverse effects did not differ among groups. Attrition: 69%	High

TABLE B–10. Studies related to naltrexone *(continued)*

Author and year; trial name	Study characteristics	Treatment administered, including study arm, dose (mg/day), sample size (N), and co-intervention	Rx duration, weeks (follow-up)	Sample characteristics, including diagnostic inclusions and major exclusions	Outcome measures, main results, and overall percent attrition	Risk of bias
Schmitz et al. 2009	Design: DBRCT Setting: outpatient substance use disorders clinic Country: United States Funding: govt	NTX 100+CBT (20); NTX 100+CBT and CM (25); PBO+CBT (27); PBO+CBT and CM (14) Other Tx: CBT 100%	12	DSM-IV alcohol dependence and cocaine dependence Mean age: 34 years 84%–93% Nonwhite 13% Female Other Dx: cocaine use disorder 100%	The probability of drinking days (any drinking) showed an effect for time, $F_{1,365}=5.27$, $p\leq0.02$: for each successive week in treatment, the odds of drinking decreased by a factor of 0.94 (95% CI 0.89, 0.99). Mean percent drinking days: 40% for NTX with CBT, 33% for NTX with CBT+CM, 23% for PBO with CBT, and 33% for PBO with CBT+CM. In the CBT group, the odds of heavy drinking decreased by a factor of 0.81 over time in treatment (95% CI 0.74, 0.88), whereas for participants in the CBT+CM group, the odds of heavy drinking remained stable over time (OR=0.99; 95% CI 0.92, 1.06). For participants receiving NTX, the odds of a heavy drinking day decreased over time by a factor of 0.83 (95% CI 0.78, 0.88). For participants receiving PBO, the odds of heavy drinking did not change over time (OR=0.96; 95% CI 0.87, 1.07). Attrition: 76%	High
Silverman et al. 2011	Design: DBRCT Setting: outpatient Country: Germany, Austria Funding: Alkermes	NTX inj 380 every 4 weeks (152); PBO (148) Other Tx: NR	12	Dx NR Mean age: 46 years % Nonwhite NR 20% Female Other Dx: NR	Difference between NTX and PBO for return to heavy drinking: 0.07 (95% CI −0.05, 0.18) Attrition: 37%	Medium
Volpicelli et al. 1992, 1995	Design: DBRCT Setting: substance use disorder treatment unit of a VAMC Country: United States Funding: govt, meds	NTX 50 (54); PBO (45) Other Tx: outpatient treatment program and group therapy 100%	12	Score >5 on the Michigan Alcohol Screening Test (MAST) Mean age: NR ≥78% Nonwhite 0% Female Other Dx: NR	Differences between NTX and PBO were return to heavy drinking: −0.19 (95% CI −0.37, −0.02) and return to any drinking: −0.08 (95% CI −0.27, 0.12). Kaplan-Meier survival analysis found a longer time to relapse with NTX vs. PBO. Rates of craving were less with NTX than PBO. Adverse effects did not differ between groups. Attrition: NR	Medium

TABLE B–10. Studies related to naltrexone (continued)

Author and year; trial name	Study characteristics	Treatment administered, including study arm, dose (mg/day), sample size (N), and co-intervention	Rx duration, weeks (follow-up)	Sample characteristics, including diagnostic inclusions and major exclusions	Outcome measures, main results, and overall percent attrition	Risk of bias
Volpicelli et al. 1997	Design: DBRCT Setting: outpatient substance use disorders clinic; univ/VA treatment research center Country: United States Funding: govt, meds	NTX 50 (48); PBO (49) Other Tx: counseling 100%	12	DSM-III-R alcohol dependence and completed medical detoxification for alcohol withdrawal Exclusions: alcohol abstinence >21 days Mean age: 38–39 years 60%–65% Nonwhite 18%–26% Female Other Dx: NR	Differences between NTX and PBO were percent drinking days: –4.6 (95% CI –10.1, 0.9), return to any drinking: –0.09 (95% CI –0.28, 0.1), and return to heavy drinking: –0.18 (95% CI –0.37, 0.02). Of those who completed treatment, fewer relapses were seen with NTX (26%) vs. PBO (53%), with even greater effects in those who were adherent to medication. Adverse effects did not differ between groups. Attrition: 27%	Medium

Note. Unless noted elsewhere, subjects were excluded if they had contraindications for specific medications; were pregnant, breastfeeding, or unreliable in using contraception; were receiving psychotropic medications; or had another substance use disorder (except nicotine dependence), other psychiatric conditions, suicidal or homicidal ideas, or significant physical illness (including renal or hepatic disease). Studies comparing NTX with PBO or NTX with comparators other than ACA are included here. Studies comparing NTX with ACA are in Table B–13. Industry-sponsored studies list the name of the pharmaceutical company.

Abbreviations: AA=alcoholics anonymous; ACA=acamprosate; AIMS=Abnormal Involuntary Movement Scale; ATS=ANOVA-type statistic; AUD=alcohol use disorder; BPD=borderline personality disorder; BRENDA=Biopsychosocial evaluation, Report of findings to patient, Empathetic understanding of patient's situation, Needs to be addressed, Direct advice to patient on how to meet those needs, and Assessing reaction/behaviors of patient to advice and adjusting treatment plan as necessary for best care; BST=broad-spectrum treatment; CBI=combined behavioral intervention; CBT=cognitive-behavioral therapy; CI=confidence interval; CM=contingency management; COMBINE= Combined Pharmacotherapies and Behavioral Interventions for Alcohol Dependence; CS=coping skills; DBRCT=double-blind, randomized controlled trial; DC=drug counseling; DIS=disulfiram; DMI=desipramine; Dx=diagnosis; GAD=generalized anxiety disorder; GEE=generalized estimating equation; GGT=gamma-glutamyl transferase; GHB=gamma-hydroxybutyrate; govt=governmental; inj=injection; IRR=Incidence Rate Ratio; MATCH=Matching Alcoholism Treatments to Client Heterogeneity; MBSCT=modified behavioral self-control therapy; MCV=mean corpuscular volume; meds=medications supplied by pharmaceutical company; MET=motivational enhancement therapy; MM=medical management; NOS=not otherwise specified; NR=not reported; NTX=naltrexone; OCD=obsessive-compulsive disorder; OLRCT=open label, randomized controlled trial; OR=odds ratio; PANSS=Positive and Negative Syndrome Scale; PBO=placebo; PE=prolonged exposure therapy; PTSD=posttraumatic stress disorder; PUFA=polyunsaturated fatty acids; RPT=relapse prevention therapy; SD=standard deviation; SE=significant effect; SERT=sertraline; SNP=single nucleotide polymorphism; ST=supportive therapy; SuppTx=supportive counseling; TAU=treatment as usual; TOP=topiramate; Tx=treatment; univ=university; VA=U.S. Department of Veterans Affairs; VAMC=U.S. Veterans Affairs Medical Center; VAMIRECC=Veterans Affairs Mental Illness Research Education Clinical Centers.

TABLE B–11. Acamprosate compared with naltrexone

Outcome	Number of studies; number of subjects	Risk of bias; design	Consistency	Directness	Precision	Summary effect size (95% CI)	Strength of evidence grade
Return to any drinking	3; 800	Low; RCTs	Consistent	Direct	Imprecise	RD 0.02 (–0.03 to 0.08)[a]	Moderate
Return to heavy drinking	4; 1,141	Low; RCTs	Consistent	Direct	Imprecise	RD 0.01 (–0.05 to 0.06)[a]	Moderate
Drinking days	2; 720	Low; RCTs	Inconsistent	Direct	Imprecise	WMD –2.98 (–13.42 to 7.45)[a]	Low
Heavy drinking days	1; 612	Low; RCT	Unknown	Direct	Unknown	Significant NTX by CBI interaction, $P=0.006$	Insufficient
Drinks per drinking day	2; 720	Low; RCTs	Inconsistent	Direct	Unknown	Unable to pool data[b]	Insufficient
Accidents	0; 0	NA	NA	NA	NA	NA	Insufficient
Injuries	0; 0	NA	NA	NA	NA	NA	Insufficient
Quality of life or function	1;[c] 612	Low; RCT	Unknown	Direct	Imprecise	NSD for all measures except SF-12v2® physical health, which favored NTX+CBI	Insufficient
Mortality	0;[d] 0	NA	NA	NA	NA	NA	Insufficient

[a]Positive value indicates that naltrexone is favored.

[b]Two trials reported some information about drinks per drinking day, but there were not enough data for us to conduct a quantitative synthesis. One trial conducted in Australia reported no statistically significant difference between ACA and NTX (mean, SD: 7.5, 6.1 vs. 5.9, 6.1; P not reported)., The COMBINE study reported that analyses of alternative summary measures of drinking, including drinks per drinking day ($P=0.03$), were consistent with those for the co-primary endpoints (percent days abstinent from alcohol and time to first heavy drinking day), all showing a significant naltrexone by CBI interaction.

[c]One additional study was rated high risk of bias. It found that quality of life improved for both groups over the 52-week follow-up compared with baseline but found no difference between the ACA and NTX groups.

[d]One study that reported this outcome was rated high risk of bias; another reported one death but did not specify in which treatment group it occurred.

Abbreviations: ACA=acamprosate; CBI=combined behavioral intervention; CI=confidence interval; COMBINE= Combined Pharmacotherapies and Behavioral Interventions for Alcohol Dependence; NA=not applicable; NTX=naltrexone; NSD=no significant difference; RCT=randomized controlled trial; RD=risk difference; SD=standard deviation; WMD=weighted mean difference.

Source. Jonas et al. 2014, Table D–8.

The medium-risk-of-bias German PREDICT study (total $N=426$) is the only study identified in the updated literature search that included a head-to-head comparison of acamprosate and naltrexone (Mann et al. 2013) and is not included in Table B–11. This trial was modeled after the COMBINE study and found no difference among naltrexone, acamprosate, and placebo groups on the time to first heavy drinking. Point estimates for heavy drinking relapse free survival from the Kaplan-Meier curves were 48.3% for acamprosate, 49.1% for naltrexone, and 51.8% for placebo. A secondary analysis of adherent patients also showed no significant differences among the treatment groups.

Grading of the Overall Supporting Body of Research Evidence for Head-to-Head Comparison of Acamprosate and Naltrexone Benefits

- **Magnitude of effect:** *None.*
- **Risk of bias:** *Low.* Studies are RCTs that are generally of low bias based on their described randomization and blinding procedures and descriptions of study dropouts.
- **Applicability:** The included trials all involve individuals with AUD, by either prior diagnostic criteria or other evidence of harmful levels of drinking. The studies include subjects from around the world, including North America. The doses of acamprosate and naltrexone appear to be representative of outpatient clinical practice.
- **Directness:** *Direct.* Studies measured abstinence and heavy drinking rates as well as measures of alcohol consumption.
- **Consistency:** *Consistent.* There was some heterogeneity as evidenced by increased I^2 values on one drinking-related outcome, but confidence intervals are overlapping.
- **Precision:** *Imprecise.* Confidence intervals for studies cross the threshold for clinically significant benefit of the intervention.
- **Dose-response relationship:** *Unclear.* Studies used a single dose of naltrexone and acamprosate.
- **Confounding factors (including likely direction of effect):** *Unclear.* Some studies suggest a possible effect of genetic polymorphisms on treatment response, which could confound study interpretation.
- **Publication bias:** *Not identified.* No publication bias was noted by the AHRQ review; however, they note that they were unable to assess for publication bias for early clinical trials (prior to the release of https://clinicaltrials.gov).
- **Overall strength of research evidence:** *Moderate.* A number of RCTs have been conducted, most of which are governmentally funded and have a low risk of bias. Although the studies have good applicability, imprecision is a limitation. Another limitation is that the trials use oral formulations of naltrexone without considering the long-acting injectable formulation.

Harms of Acamprosate Compared With Naltrexone

In terms of adverse events, the risks of headache, nausea, and vomiting were noted to be slightly higher for individuals treated with naltrexone as compared with acamprosate in the AHRQ review (Jonas et al. 2014) (Table B–12). The number of deaths in head-to-head studies of naltrexone and acamprosate was extremely small, and no statistical comparison was possible (Jonas et al. 2014). In the PREDICT trial (not included in Table B–12), diarrhea was significantly greater with acamprosate, and nervousness/anxiety was greater in placebo subjects. Serious adverse events (9.9% of patients during active treatment and 17.4% during follow-up) and related dropouts (6.3%) did not differ among the treatment groups.

Grading of the Overall Supporting Body of Research Evidence for Head-to-Head Comparison of Acamprosate and Naltrexone Harms

- **Magnitude of effect:** *Very small.* When present, the magnitude of effect is very small.
- **Risk of bias:** *Medium.* Studies are RCTs of low bias based on their described randomization and blinding procedures and descriptions of study dropouts. However, methods for determining harms are not always well specified, and there is potential for selective reporting of results.
- **Applicability:** The included trials all involve individuals with AUD, by either prior diagnostic criteria or other evidence of harmful levels of drinking. The studies include subjects from around the world, including North America. The doses of acamprosate and naltrexone appear to be representative of outpatient clinical practice.

TABLE B–12. Acamprosate compared with naltrexone

Outcome	Number of studies; number of subjects	Risk of bias; design	Consistency	Directness	Precision	Summary effect size (95% CI)[a]	Strength of evidence grade
Withdrawals due to AEs	2;[b] 953	Medium; RCTs	Consistent	Direct	Imprecise	RD 0.015 (–0.04 to 0.07)	Low
Anorexia	0; 0	NA	NA	NA	NA	NA	Insufficient
Anxiety	0; 0	NA	NA	NA	NA	NA	Insufficient
Cognitive dysfunction	0; 0	NA	NA	NA	NA	NA	Insufficient
Diarrhea	4;[b] 836	Low to medium; RCTs	Consistent	Direct	Imprecise	RD 0.18 (–0.02 to 0.37)	Moderate
Dizziness	2;[b] 144	Low to medium; RCTs	Inconsistent	Direct	Imprecise	RD 0.08 (–0.23 to 0.39)	Low
Headache	3;[b] 301	Medium; RCTs	Inconsistent	Direct	Imprecise	RD –0.056 (–0.120 to 0.008)	Low[d]
Insomnia	2; 144	Low to medium; RCTs	Inconsistent	Direct	Imprecise	RD 0.07 (–0.20 to 0.34)	Low
Nausea	4;[c] 836	Low to medium; RCTs	Consistent	Direct	Imprecise	RD –0.08 (–0.18 to 0.02)	Low[e]
Numbness/ tingling/ paresthesias	0; 0	NA	NA	NA	NA	NA	Insufficient
Rash	0; 0	NA	NA	NA	NA	NA	Insufficient
Suicide	0; 0	NA	NA	NA	NA	NA	Insufficient
Taste abnormalities	0; 0	NA	NA	NA	NA	NA	Insufficient
Vision changes	0; 0	NA	NA	NA	NA	NA	Insufficient
Vomiting	2; 648	Low; RCTs	Consistent	Direct	Precise	RD –0.06 (–0.11 to –0.01)	Moderate

[a]In this column, a positive value favors naltrexone.
[b]One additional study was rated high or unclear risk of bias.
[c]Two additional studies were rated high risk of bias.
[d]The additional study rated as high risk of bias found similar results as the medium-risk-of-bias studies. Meta-analysis including all three found a higher risk of headache with naltrexone than with acamprosate: RD –0.087 (–0.159 to –0.015).
[e]Meta-analysis including the two additional studies rated as high or unclear risk of bias found a higher risk of nausea with naltrexone than with acamprosate: RD –0.096 (–0.178 to –0.015).
Abbreviations: AE=adverse effect; CI=confidence interval; RCT=randomized controlled trial; RD=risk difference.
Source. Jonas et al. 2014, Table D–35.

- **Directness:** *Direct*. Studies measured common side effects and dropouts due to adverse events.
- **Consistency:** *Inconsistent*. As indicated by the high values of I^2, there was substantial heterogeneity in the reported adverse events among the trials.
- **Precision:** *Imprecise*. Confidence intervals for studies are wide in many studies and cross the threshold for clinically significant harms of the intervention.
- **Dose-response relationship:** *Unknown*. Studies used a single dose of acamprosate and naltrexone.
- **Confounding factors (including likely direction of effect):** *Absent*. No known confounding factors are present that would be likely to modify adverse events of the intervention.
- **Publication bias:** *Not identified*. No publication bias was noted by the AHRQ review; however, they note that they were unable to assess for publication bias for early clinical trials (prior to the release of https://clinicaltrials.gov).
- **Overall strength of research evidence:** *Low*. Several RCTs have been conducted, some of which have assessed adverse events in a systematic and predefined fashion. Many of the RCTs are funded by governmental agencies. However, findings are imprecise and inconsistent, making it difficult to draw conclusions about differences in side effects between the two medications.

Data Abstraction: Acamprosate Versus Naltrexone

Studies comparing acamprosate and naltrexone are listed in Table B–13.

STATEMENT 10: Disulfiram

APA *suggests* **(2C)** that disulfiram be offered to patients with moderate to severe alcohol use disorder who

- have a goal of achieving abstinence,
- prefer disulfiram or are intolerant to or have not responded to naltrexone and acamprosate,
- are capable of understanding the risks of alcohol consumption while taking disulfiram, and
- have no contraindications to the use of this medication.

Benefits of Disulfiram

Evidence for the benefits of disulfiram comes from randomized controlled double-blind and open-label trials as well as expert opinion. The AHRQ review (Jonas et al. 2014) included four studies conducted at Veterans Health Administration Medical Centers and found no statistically significant difference between disulfiram 250 mg/day and sham comparators (i.e., placebo, disulfiram 1 mg/day, riboflavin). In the two trials included in the AHRQ review that assessed percentage of drinking days, one reported no significant difference among treatment groups. The other trial limited its reporting to a subset of subjects (those who drank during the trial and who also completed all assessments) and found that disulfiram was associated with fewer drinking days ($p=0.05$) than for those who received a comparator (49% with disulfiram 250 mg/day vs. 75.4% with disulfiram 1 mg/day and 86.5% with riboflavin). In the two RCTs included in the AHRQ analysis that had a medium risk of bias (Fuller and Roth 1979, 1986), treatment adherence was associated with abstinence, regardless of whether the subject was assigned to active disulfiram or control treatment. Some shorter RCTs of disulfiram have also been associated with benefits on drinking-related outcomes (Jørgensen et al. 2011).

In a medium-risk-of-bias trial conducted in Japan (Yoshimura et al. 2014), subjects (total $N=109$) were randomly assigned according to a 2×2 design with disulfiram 200 mg/day vs. placebo and

TABLE B–13. Studies related to acamprosate versus naltrexone head-to-head comparison

Author and year; trial name	Study characteristics	Treatment administered, including study arm, dose (mg/day), sample size (N), and co-intervention	Rx duration, weeks (follow-up)	Sample characteristics, including diagnostic inclusions and major exclusions	Outcome measures, main results, and overall percent attrition	Risk of bias
Anton et al. 2006; Donovan et al. 2008; LoCastro et al. 2009; COMBINE	Design: DBRCT Setting: 11 academic outpatient sites Country: United States Funding: govt, meds	ACA 3,000+CBI+MM (151); ACA 3,000+MM (152); NTX100+CBI+MM (155); NTX 100+MM (154); PBO+CBI+MM (156); PBO+MM (153) Other Tx: as randomized; community support group participation (e.g., AA) encouraged	16 (68)	DSM-IV alcohol dependence Mean age: 44 years 23% Nonwhite 31% Female Other Dx: NR	Differences between ACA and NTX were percent drinking days: 1 (95% CI –3.12, 5.12), return to any drinking: 0.03 (95% CI –0.04, 0.09), and return to heavy drinking: 0.03 (95% CI –0.05, 0.1). ACA showed no effect; NTX, CBI, or both had the best outcomes. Complete within-treatment drinking data were provided by 94% of study subjects.	Low
Anton and COMBINE Study Research Group 2003	Design: DBRCT Setting: 11 academic outpatient sites Country: United States Funding: govt, meds	ACA 3,000+CBI+MM (9); ACA 3,000+MM (9); NTX 100+CBI+MM (9); NTX 100+MM (9); PBO+CBI+MM (9); PBO+MM (8) Other Tx: as randomized	16	DSM-IV alcohol dependence Mean age: 38–42 years 17%–22% Nonwhite 22%–33% Female Other Dx: NR	ACA-NTX group adherence was equal to, or better than, adherence with PBO, ACA alone, or NTX alone. Adverse events were comparable in all groups. Attrition: 31%	Medium

TABLE B–13. Studies related to acamprosate versus naltrexone head-to-head comparison (continued)

Author and year; trial name	Study characteristics	Treatment administered, including study arm, dose (mg/day), sample size (N), and co-intervention	Rx duration, weeks (follow-up)	Sample characteristics, including diagnostic inclusions and major exclusions	Outcome measures, main results, and overall percent attrition	Risk of bias
Greenfield et al. 2010; Fucito et al. 2012; COMBINE	Design: secondary data analysis Setting: 11 academic outpatient sites Country: United States Funding: govt, meds	ACA 3,000+CBI+MM (151); ACA 3,000+MM (152); NTX100+CBI+MM (155); NTX 100+MM (154); PBO+CBI+MM (156); PBO+MM (153) Other Tx: as randomized; community support group participation (e.g., AA) encouraged	68	DSM-IV alcohol dependence Mean age: 44 years 23% Nonwhite 31% Female Other Dx: 0%	There was a significant NTX by CBI interaction for women on two primary outcomes (percent days abstinent and time to first heavy drinking day) and also secondary outcome measures (good clinical response, percent heavy drinking days, and craving). Only the NTX by CBI interaction was significant for percent days abstinent. The NTX by CBI interaction was significant for time to first heavy drinking day in men (p=0.048), with each treatment showing slower relapse times; a nonsignificant trend was present in women. NTX or CBI alone was superior to groups receiving neither in the percent of heavy drinking days. Complete within-treatment drinking data were provided by 94% of study subjects.	Low
Kiefer et al. 2003, 2004, 2005	Design: DBRCT Setting: 1 outpatient site Country: Germany Funding: univ, meds	ACA1,998 (40); NTX50 (40); PBO (40); ACA 1,998+NTX 50 (40) Other Tx: group therapy	12	DSM-IV alcohol dependence without any withdrawal symptoms Exclusions: homelessness Mean age: 46 years % Nonwhite NR 26% Female Other Dx: 0%	Time to relapse or time to first drink did not differ between ACA- and NTX-treated groups by survival analysis, although the combination of the drugs was associated with better outcomes than PBO (p<0.01) or than ACA alone (p=0.04). Attrition: 53%	Low

TABLE B–13. Studies related to acamprosate versus naltrexone head-to-head comparison *(continued)*

Author and year; trial name	Study characteristics	Treatment administered, including study arm, dose (mg/day), sample size (N), and co-intervention	Rx duration, weeks (follow-up)	Sample characteristics, including diagnostic inclusions and major exclusions	Outcome measures, main results, and overall percent attrition	Risk of bias
Laaksonen et al. 2008	Design: OLRCT Setting: 6 outpatient sites in 5 cities Country: Finland Funding: govt	ACA 1,998 or 1,333 (81); DIS 100 to 200 (81); NTX 50 (81) Other Tx: manual-based CBT	Up to 52 (119)	ICD-10 alcohol dependence Mean age: 43 years 0% Nonwhite 29% Female Other Dx: NR	During the continuous medication period (1–12 weeks), the DIS group did significantly better than the NTX and ACA groups in time to first heavy drinking day (p=0.001), days to first drinking (p=0.002), abstinence days, and average weekly alcohol intake. During the targeted medication period (13–52 weeks), there were no significant differences between the groups in time to first heavy drinking day and days to first drinking, whereas the DIS group reported significantly more frequent abstinence days than the ACA and NTX groups. During the whole study period (1–52 weeks), the DIS group did significantly better in the time to the first drink compared with the other groups. Attrition: 52%	High
Mann et al. 2013; PREDICT	Design: DBRCT Setting: NR Country: Germany Funding: govt, meds	ACA 1,998 (172); NTX 50 (169); PBO (86) Other Tx: MM	12	Alcohol dependence Mean age: 45 years % Nonwhite NR 23% Female Other Dx: NR	Difference between ACA and NTX for return to heavy drinking: 0.01 (95% CI −0.1, 0.11) Point estimates for heavy drinking relapse-free survival from the Kaplan-Meier curves were 48.3% for ACA, 49.1% for NTX, and 51.8% for PBO. Attrition: 34%	Medium

TABLE B–13. Studies related to acamprosate versus naltrexone head-to-head comparison *(continued)*

Author and year; trial name	Study characteristics	Treatment administered, including study arm, dose (mg/day), sample size (M), and co-intervention	Rx duration, weeks (follow-up)	Sample characteristics, including diagnostic inclusions and major exclusions	Outcome measures, main results, and overall percent attrition	Risk of bias
Morley et al. 2006, 2010	Design: DBRCT Setting: 3 outpatient intensive substance use treatment sites Country: Australia Funding: govt	ACA 1,998 (55); NTX 50 (53); PBO (61) Other Tx: all offered 4–6 sessions of manualized compliance therapy; uptake/attendance NR	12	DSM-IV alcohol dependence or abuse and with alcohol abstinence for 3–21 days Mean age: 45 years % Nonwhite NR 30% Female Other Dx: substantial levels of emotional distress (anxiety, stress, and depression); 3% severe concurrent illness (psychiatric or other)	There was no significant difference between treatments with respect to the number of days to first relapse (Breslow test: $t_2 = 0.4$, $P = 0.81$) or the number of days to first relapse (Breslow test: $t_2 = 2.9$, $P = 0.23$) by survival analysis. Regardless of medication group, significant effects for time were found for drinks per drinking day ($F_{1,159} = 6.8$, $P < 0.01$) and dependence severity ($F_{1,103} = 12.81$, $P < 0.001$) but not for craving ($F_{1,103} = 2.0$, $P = 0.16$). Attrition: 35%	Low
Narayana et al. 2008	Design: prospective cohort Setting: military, outpatient Country: India Funding: NR	ACA 1,332 to 1,998 (28); NTX 50 (26); TOP 100 to 125 (38) Other Tx: various psychotherapies were offered	52	ICD-10 alcohol dependence Mean age: 38 years 100% Nonwhite 0% Female Other Dx: NR	TOP (76.3%) was significantly more effective ($p < 0.01$) in sustaining abstinence, although 57.7% NTX and 60.7% ACA maintained complete abstinence. 7 TOP subjects (18.4%) reported decreased relapses compared with 8 NTX (30.8%) and 9 ACA (32.1%) subjects. Attrition: 18%	High

TABLE B–13. Studies related to acamprosate versus naltrexone head-to-head comparison *(continued)*

Author and year; trial name	Study characteristics	Treatment administered, including study arm, dose (mg/day), sample size (M), and co-intervention	Rx duration, weeks (follow-up)	Sample characteristics, including diagnostic inclusions and major exclusions	Outcome measures, main results, and overall percent attrition	Risk of bias
Rubio et al. 2001	Design: SBRCT Setting: outpatient Country: Spain Funding: govt	ACA 1,665–1,998 (80); NTX 50 (77) Other Tx: supportive group therapy weekly, weekly visits with a psychiatrist for 3 months, then biweekly until end of study	52	DSM-III-R alcohol dependence Exclusions: previous NTX or ACA treatment Mean age: 44 years % Nonwhite NR 0% Female Other Dx: 0%	At the end of 1 year, 41% receiving NTX and 17% receiving ACA had not relapsed (*P*=0.0009), and the accumulated abstinence was greater for NTX compared with ACA (mean number of days: 243 vs. 180). NTX had longer survival until first relapse than ACA (63 days vs. 42 days, *p*=0.02). Relapse to some alcohol use occurred on average 12 days later in the NTX group (SD=16) vs. after 6 days in the ACA group (SD=8). Survival analysis of time to first alcohol consumption showed no significant differences between the two groups (the mean number of days: 44 for the NTX group and 39 for the ACA group; *p*=0.34). Attrition: 17%	High

Note. Unless noted elsewhere, subjects were excluded if they had contraindications for specific medications; were pregnant, breastfeeding, or unreliable in using contraception; were receiving psychotropic medications; or had another substance use disorder (except nicotine dependence), other psychiatric conditions, suicidal or homicidal ideas, or significant physical illness (including renal or hepatic disease). Industry-sponsored studies list the name of the pharmaceutical company.
Abbreviations: AA=Alcoholics Anonymous; ACA=acamprosate; CBI=combined behavioral intervention; CI=confidence interval; COMBINE=Combined Pharmacotherapies and Behavioral Interventions for Alcohol Dependence; DBRCT=double-blind, randomized controlled trial; DIS=disulfiram; Dx=diagnosis; govt=governmental; meds=medications supplied by pharmaceutical company; MM=medical management; NOS=not otherwise specified; NR=not reported; NTX=naltrexone; OLRCT=open-label, randomized controlled trial; PBO=placebo; TOP=topiramate; SBRCT=single-blind, randomized controlled trial; SD=standard deviation; Tx=treatment; univ=university.

receipt of educational material on drinking harms and craving management vs. no such education. At 26 weeks, there were no differences among groups in the percent of individuals who remained abstinent. However, this study may have limited generalizability because individuals were randomly assigned to disulfiram after a 2- to 3-month inpatient stay.

A single study in the AHRQ review (Petrakis et al. 2005) compared disulfiram, naltrexone, placebo, and the combination of disulfiram plus naltrexone for 12 weeks in Veterans Health Administration outpatient settings (Table B–14). Naltrexone was given in a double-blind fashion, but disulfiram was administered as an open-label medication. The trial found no statistically significant difference between disulfiram and naltrexone for number of subjects achieving total abstinence (51 vs. 38, $p=0.11$), percentage of days abstinent (96.6 vs. 95.4, $p=0.55$), or percentage of heavy drinking days (3.2 vs. 4, $p=0.65$).

A meta-analysis (Skinner et al. 2014) differed from the AHRQ analysis in including RCTs that were open-label as well as randomized controlled double-blind trials. Skinner and colleagues (2014) hypothesized that in a double-blind trial, subjects in both disulfiram and placebo groups would avoid drinking because of having been warned of the potential for adverse events regardless of actual treatment assignment. They included 22 studies (2,414 subjects) and found a significant overall effect but no difference between disulfiram and control groups in the double-blind RCTs. When only open-label trials were considered, disulfiram was significantly better than controls on alcohol-related outcomes (Hedges' $g=0.70$; 95% CI=0.46–0.93), for which control conditions included acamprosate, naltrexone, and no disulfiram. Individual comparisons for each of these control conditions were also statistically significant. In studies where medication adherence was assured through supervised administration, the effect of disulfiram was large. As with the double-blind RCTs, however, only a small proportion of women were included in the open-label trials, which limits generalizability.

Grading of the Overall Supporting Body of Research Evidence for Efficacy of Disulfiram

- **Magnitude of effect:** No effect in double-blind studies, moderate effect in open-label studies.
- **Risk of bias:** *High.* Studies are RCTs and a meta-analysis that includes open-label trials. RCTs are of medium to high risk of bias, and open-label studies have not been formally rated but are likely to be of high risk of bias.
- **Applicability:** The included trials all involve individuals with AUD, by either prior diagnostic criteria or other evidence of harmful levels of drinking. The double-blind studies primarily included subjects from the U.S. Veterans Health Administration Medical Centers that are overrepresented among study locations, and the vast majority of subjects are men. The doses of disulfiram used in the studies appear to be representative of outpatient clinical practice.
- **Directness:** *Direct.* Studies measured abstinence and alcohol consumption.
- **Consistency:** *Inconsistent.* There was considerable heterogeneity in the trial findings in both the AHRQ meta-analysis and the meta-analysis by Skinner et al. (2014), which included open-label trials.
- **Precision:** *Imprecise.* Confidence intervals for studies cross the threshold for clinically significant benefit of the intervention.
- **Dose-response relationship:** *No data available to assess.*
- **Confounding factors (including likely direction of effect):** *Present.* As noted above, the subjects' knowledge of treatment assignment may be important in the desire to maintain abstinence to avoid an aversive experience when drinking.
- **Publication bias:** *Possible.* The meta-analysis of Skinner et al. (2014), which included open-label trials, noted funnel plot asymmetry, suggesting a potential for publication bias. Virtually all of the disulfiram trials were conducted prior to the advent of https://clinicaltrials.gov.

TABLE B–14. Disulfiram compared with control

Outcome	Number of studies; number of subjects	Risk of bias; design	Consistency	Directness	Precision	Summary effect size (95% CI)	NNT[d]	Strength of evidence grade
Return to any drinking	2;[a] 492	Medium; RCTs	Consistent[b]	Direct	Imprecise	RD 0.04 (−0.11 to 0.03)	NA	Low
Return to heavy drinking	0; 0	NA	NA	NA	NA	NA	NA	Insufficient
Drinking days	2; 290	Medium; RCTs	Inconsistent	Indirect[c]	Imprecise	1 study reported similar percentages and no significant difference; the other reported that DIS was favored among the subset of subjects who drank and had a complete set of assessment interviews (N=162/605 subjects), p=0.05	NA	Insufficient
Heavy drinking days	0; 0	NA	NA	NA	NA	NA	NA	Insufficient
Drinks per drinking day	0; 0	NA	NA	NA	NA	NA	NA	Insufficient
Accidents	0; 0	NA	NA	NA	NA	NA	NA	Insufficient
Injuries	0; 0	NA	NA	NA	NA	NA	NA	Insufficient
Quality of life or function	0; 0	NA	NA	NA	NA	NA	NA	Insufficient
Mortality	0; 0	NA	NA	NA	NA	NA	NA	Insufficient

[a]One additional study was rated high risk of bias.
[b]Inclusion of the study rated high risk of bias would have made this inconsistent, although it would not have changed the conclusion (the meta-analysis still found no statistically significant difference between groups).
[c]We considered this indirect because the larger study did not report the outcome for the randomized sample; it reported this outcome only for the subset (162/605) who drank and who had a complete set of assessment interviews.
[d]NA entry for NNT indicates that the risk difference (95% CI) was not statistically significant, so we did not calculate a NNT, or that the effect measure was not one that allows direct calculation of NNT (e.g., WMD).
Abbreviations: CI=confidence interval; DIS=disulfiram; NA=not applicable; NNT=number needed to treat; RCT=randomized controlled trial; RD=risk difference; WMD=weighted mean difference.
Source. Jonas et al. 2014, Table D–2.

- **Overall strength of research evidence:** *Low.* A small number of RCTs have been conducted, most of which have medium to high risk of bias; open-label studies also are likely to have a high risk of bias. The available evidence is limited in its generalizability because of the location of the trials and the small proportion of women in the studies. The imprecision and inconsistency of findings are additional limitations.

Harms of Disulfiram

The data on harms from the studies included in the AHRQ report were insufficient to conduct meta-analyses. One study showed a greater rate of drowsiness in patients receiving versus not receiving disulfiram (8% vs. 2%, $p=0.03$). Several patients discontinued disulfiram because of increased levels of hepatic enzymes. A four-arm study (2×2, disulfiram vs. placebo, naltrexone vs. placebo) showed greater rates of specific side effects in patients taking any study medication but no differences between groups. In this study, patients taking disulfiram and placebo experienced 6 of 14 serious adverse events. In the study of Yoshimura and colleagues (2014), 1/53 disulfiram treated subjects had a dermatological problem, 2/53 had liver enzyme elevations, and 1/53 had renal dysfunction, whereas no adverse events were noted in placebo-treated subjects. In the study of Petrakis and colleagues (2005), which compared disulfiram, naltrexone, placebo, and the combination of disulfiram plus naltrexone, fever was more common in the disulfiram group than in the naltrexone group ($p=0.03$), whereas nervousness ($p=0.005$) and restlessness ($p=0.03$) were more common in the naltrexone group than in the disulfiram group.

In the meta-analysis of Skinner et al. (2014), data from randomized, controlled, open-label trials showed considerable heterogeneity but showed a significantly greater number of adverse events with disulfiram as compared with control conditions.

Additional information on potential harms of disulfiram comes from the product labelling (Rising Pharmaceuticals 2016), which notes that disulfiram should not be given to individuals who have recently received metronidazole, paraldehyde, alcohol (within 12 hours), or alcohol-containing preparations. It is also noted to be contraindicated in the presence of severe myocardial disease or coronary occlusion. When alcohol is taken within 14 days of disulfiram ingestion, it can produce the following:

> flushing, throbbing in head and neck, throbbing headache, respiratory difficulty, nausea, copious vomiting, sweating, thirst, chest pain, palpitation, dyspnea, hyperventilation, tachycardia, hypotension, syncope, marked uneasiness, weakness, vertigo, blurred vision, and confusion. In severe reactions, there may be respiratory depression, cardiovascular collapse, arrhythmias, myocardial infarction, acute congestive heart failure, unconsciousness, convulsions, and death.

Disulfiram is noted to be contraindicated in the presence of psychosis or in individuals with hypersensitivity to disulfiram or thiuram derivatives used in pesticides and rubber production. Hepatic toxicity is also reported to have occurred in individuals receiving disulfiram.

Grading of the Overall Supporting Body of Research Evidence for Harms of Disulfiram

- **Magnitude of effect:** *Small.* When instructions for avoiding disulfiram-alcohol reactions are followed, the proportion of individuals who experience adverse events is small.
- **Risk of bias:** *High.* Studies do not prespecify harm outcomes and do not report them consistently.
- **Applicability:** The included trials all involved individuals with AUD by prior diagnostic criteria. The vast majority of study subjects are men, which limits the generalizability of the findings. The doses of disulfiram used in the trials appear to be representative of outpatient clinical practice.

- **Directness:** *Indirect.* Studies generally measured adverse events as a general category or assessed the numbers of individuals who required intervention because of an adverse effect.
- **Consistency:** *Inconsistent.* There was considerable heterogeneity in the findings of the meta-analysis by Skinner et al. (2014), which included open-label trials.
- **Precision:** *Imprecise.* Confidence intervals for studies cross the threshold for clinically significant benefit of the intervention.
- **Dose-response relationship:** *No data are available to assess.*
- **Confounding factors (including likely direction of effect):** *Not identified.*
- **Publication bias:** *Possible.* The meta-analysis of Skinner et al. (2014), which included open-label trials, noted funnel plot asymmetry, suggesting a potential for publication bias. Virtually all of the disulfiram trials were conducted prior to the advent of https://clinicaltrials.gov.
- **Overall strength of research evidence:** *Low.* A small number of double-blind RCTs have been conducted, but measures of adverse events were minimal and not systematically defined. With data from open-label trials, the imprecision and inconsistency of findings are limitations, in addition to the high risk of bias associated with an open-label study design.

Data Abstraction: Disulfiram

Studies related to disulfiram are listed in Table B–15.

STATEMENT 11: Topiramate or Gabapentin

APA *suggests* **(2C)** that topiramate or gabapentin be offered to patients with moderate to severe alcohol use disorder who

- have a goal of reducing alcohol consumption or achieving abstinence,
- prefer topiramate or gabapentin or are intolerant to or have not responded to naltrexone and acamprosate, and
- have no contraindications to the use of these medications.

Benefits of Topiramate

Evidence for topiramate comes from multiple randomized controlled trials, some of which included subjects with co-occurring conditions. The AHRQ review (Jonas et al. 2014) included three studies of topiramate versus placebo and one study of topiramate versus naltrexone versus placebo. The latter study (Baltieri et al. 2008, 2009) was rated as having a high risk of bias and showed no significant differences in the two treatments on drinking outcomes. The two placebo-controlled trials (total $N=521$) that had a low or medium risk of bias were included in the AHRQ meta-analysis (Johnson et al. 2003, 2007). These trials had a duration of 12–14 weeks and were both conducted in the United States. On the basis of this meta-analysis, the AHRQ review concluded that there was a moderate strength of evidence for topiramate efficacy on drinks per drinking days (WMD: –1.10, 95% CI –1.75 to –0.45), percentage of heavy drinking days (WMD: –11.53, 95% CI –18.29 to –4.77), and percentage of drinking days. For the latter outcome, it was not possible to combine the results of the two trials, but each showed a comparable mean difference (WMD: –8.5, 95%, CI –15.9 to –1.1; mean difference –11.6, 95% CI –3.98 to –19.3). Findings from sensitivity analyses were similar when high-risk-of-bias studies were included.

A number of subsequent randomized controlled trials (not included in Table B–16) have also examined effects of topiramate. In a low-risk-of-bias U.S. government–funded trial, topiramate in doses of up to 200 mg/day ($N=67$) was compared with placebo ($N=71$) and was associated with a

TABLE B–15.   Studies related to disulfiram

Author and year; trial name	Study characteristics	Treatment administered, including study arm, dose (mg/day), sample size (N), and co-intervention	Rx duration, weeks (follow-up)	Sample characteristics, including diagnostic inclusions and major exclusions	Outcome measures, main results, and overall percent attrition	Risk of bias
Carroll et al. 1993	Design: OLRCT Setting: outpatient Country: United States Funding: govt	DIS 250 (9); NTX 50 (9) Other Tx: weekly individual psychotherapy 100%	12	DSM-III-R alcohol abuse/dependence and cocaine dependence Mean age: 32 years 39% Nonwhite 72% Female Other Dx: cocaine dependence 100%	Subjects taking DIS reported lower percentage of alcohol use days compared with those taking NTX (4.0% vs. 26.3%, t=3.73, p<0.01). Subjects taking DIS also reported fewer total days using alcohol (2.4 vs. 10.4 days, t=3.00, p<0.01), fewer total drinks (2.3 vs. 27.0, t=−2.00, p=0.06), and more total weeks of abstinence (mean 7.2 vs. 1.1 weeks, t=4.72, p<0.001) compared with those taking NTX. Attrition: 67%	High
De Sousa and De Sousa 2004	Design: OLRCT Setting: outpatient Country: India Funding: NR	DIS 250 (50); NTX 50 (50) Other Tx: supportive group psychotherapy	52	DSM-IV alcohol dependence Exclusions: previous NTX and/or DIS treatment Mean age: 43–47 years % Nonwhite NR 0% Female Other Dx: NR	DIS was associated with greater reduction in relapse, greater survival time until the first relapse, and more days of abstinence than NTX. At study endpoint, relapse was 14% with DIS vs. 56% with NTX. NTX reported lower composite craving scores than DIS. Attrition: 3%	High
De Sousa and De Sousa 2005	Design: OLRCT Setting: outpatient; private psychiatric hospital Country: India Funding: NR	ACA 1,998 (50); DIS 250 (50) Other Tx: weekly supportive group psychotherapy offered	35	DSM-IV alcohol dependence Exclusions: previous DIS or ACA treatment Mean age: 42–43 years 100% Nonwhite 0% Female Other Dx: NR	DIS had a lower relapse rate than ACA (88% vs. 46%, p=0.0001) and a longer mean time to first relapse (123 days vs. 71 days, p=0.0001). ACA had lower craving scores than DIS. Attrition: 7%	High

TABLE B–15. Studies related to disulfiram *(continued)*

Author and year; trial name	Study characteristics	Treatment administered, including study arm, dose (mg/day), sample size (*N*), and co-intervention	Rx duration, weeks (follow-up)	Sample characteristics, including diagnostic inclusions and major exclusions	Outcome measures, main results, and overall percent attrition	Risk of bias
De Sousa et al. 2008	Design: OLRCT Setting: inpatient and outpatient alcohol treatment center Country: India Funding: NR	TOP 150 (50); DIS 250 (50) Other Tx: weekly supporting group psychotherapy offered	39	DSM-IV alcohol dependence Exclusions: previous TOP or DIS treatment Mean age: 43 years 100% Nonwhite 0% Female Other Dx: NR	DIS had greater mean time to first relapse than TOP (133 days vs. 79 days, $p=0.0001$) and a lower relapse rate at study endpoint (10% vs. 44%; $p=0.0001$). TOP had less craving than DIS. Attrition: 8%	High
Fuller and Roth 1979	Design: DBRCT Setting: outpatient; VA Country: United States Funding: VA	DIS 250 (43); DIS 1 (43); RIB 50 (42) Other Tx: counseling (unspecified) 100%	52	Admitted for alcohol-related illness or requesting treatment for alcoholism Mean age: 43 years 61% Nonwhite 0% Female Other Dx: NR	Complete abstinence rates did not differ between regular dose (23%) and no DIS (12%). Median percentages of drinking days among the DIS 500/250 mg, DIS 1 mg, and no DIS groups were 31%, 32%, and 37%, respectively. Attrition: NR	Medium

Author and year; trial name	Study characteristics	Treatment administered, including study arm, dose (mg/day), sample size (N), and co-intervention	Rx duration, weeks (follow-up)	Sample characteristics, including diagnostic inclusions and major exclusions	Outcome measures, main results, and overall percent attrition	Risk of bias
Fuller et al. 1986	Design: DBRCT Setting: outpatient; 9 VA medical centers Country: United States Funding: VA	DIS 250 (202); DIS 1 (204); RIB 50 (199) Other Tx: counseling (loosely defined) % NR	52	Requesting alcohol treatment and meeting National Council on Alcoholism criteria Mean age: 41–42 years 47% Nonwhite 0% Female Other Dx: NR	No significant differences were found among the groups with respect to percentages of those remaining abstinent for the full year: 18.8%, 22.5%, and 16.1% ($p=0.25$) and in the time to first drinking day ($p=0.26$). Of those who reported drinking and provided all scheduled interviews, subjects taking 250 mg of DIS had significantly fewer total drinking days (49 ± 8 days) compared with those taking either 1 mg of DIS (75 ± 12 days) or no DIS (86.5 ± 14 days). Of those who reported drinking and provided six or fewer interviews, the differences among the groups in total drinking days were not statistically significant. Attrition: 5%	Medium

TABLE B–15. Studies related to disulfiram (continued)

Author and year; trial name	Study characteristics	Treatment administered, including study arm, dose (mg/day), sample size (N), and co-intervention	Rx duration, weeks (follow-up)	Sample characteristics, including diagnostic inclusions and major exclusions	Outcome measures, main results, and overall percent attrition	Risk of bias
Laaksonen et al. 2008	Design: OLRCT Setting: 6 outpatient sites in 5 cities Country: Finland Funding: govt	ACA 1,998 or 1,333 (81); DIS 100 to 200 (81); NTX 50 (81) Other Tx: manual-based CBT	Up to 52 (119)	ICD-10 alcohol dependence Mean age: 43 years 0% Nonwhite 29% Female Other Dx: NR	During the continuous medication period (1–12 weeks), the DIS group did significantly better than the NTX and ACA groups in time to first heavy drinking day ($p=0.001$), days to first drinking ($p=0.002$), abstinence days, and average weekly alcohol intake. During the targeted medication period (13–52 weeks), there were no significant differences between the groups in time to first heavy drinking day and days to first drinking, whereas the DIS group reported significantly more frequent abstinence days than the ACA and NTX groups. During the whole study period (1–52 weeks), the DIS group did significantly better in time to the first drink compared with the other groups. Attrition: 52%	High

TABLE B–15. Studies related to disulfiram (*continued*)

Author and year; trial name	Study characteristics	Treatment administered, including study arm, dose (mg/day), sample size (N), and co-intervention	Rx duration, weeks (follow-up)	Sample characteristics, including diagnostic inclusions and major exclusions	Outcome measures, main results, and overall percent attrition	Risk of bias
Ling et al. 1983	Design: DBRCT Setting: outpatient; VA Country: United States Funding: VA	DIS 250 + methadone (41); PBO + methadone (41) Other Tx: methadone 100% as randomized	37	Two of four consecutive >0.05% alcohol readings in subjects on methadone maintenance or at risk of clinic discharge for problem behavior Mean age: 39 years % Nonwhite NR % Female NR Other Dx: heroin use 80%, marijuana use 36%, other drug use 67%, depression 83%, moderate to high depression 50%	Both groups reported fewer episodes of morning drinking, alcoholic blackouts, fights, binge drinking, hospitalizations, and alcohol-related arrests. Attrition: 57% at 12 weeks; 55% lost to follow-up	High
Nava et al. 2006	Design: OLRCT Setting: outpatient Country: Italy Funding: govt	GHB 50 (28); NTX 50 (24); DIS 200 (28) Other Tx: CBT	52	DSM-IV-TR alcohol dependence Exclusions: any withdrawal syndrome, HIV antibodies, homelessness Mean age: 38.5–42.7 years % Nonwhite NR 15% Female Other Dx: 0%	At the end of the study, no statistical difference was found among groups in terms of the number of withdrawn, abstinent, nonabstinent, and relapsed patients. Significant reduction in alcohol intake, craving, and laboratory markers of alcohol abuse was found in all groups. The GHB group showed greater decreases in alcohol craving and in laboratory markers of alcohol abuse compared with the NTX and DIS groups. Attrition: 31%	High

TABLE B–15. Studies related to disulfiram (continued)

Author and year; trial name	Study characteristics	Treatment administered, including study arm, dose (mg/day), sample size (N), and co-intervention	Rx duration, weeks (follow-up)	Sample characteristics, including diagnostic inclusions and major exclusions	Outcome measures, main results, and overall percent attrition	Risk of bias
Petrakis et al. 2005, 2006, 2007; Ralevski et al. 2007; VAMIRECC	Design: DBRCT Setting: outpatient VA Country: United States Funding: govt	DIS 250 (66); NTX 50 (59); PBO (64); NTX 50+DIS 250 (65) Other Tx: psychiatric treatment as usual 100%	12	DSM-IV alcohol dependence and other Axis I disorder Exclusions: psychosis Mean age: 47 years 26% Nonwhite 3% Female Other Dx: Axis I disorder 100%	Difference between DIS and PBO for return to any drinking: –0.12 (95% CI –0.27, 0.04) High rates of abstinence were present in all groups, but there were no differences by group. Fever was more likely in those taking DIS vs. NTX. DIS+NTX had the highest rates of adverse effects as compared with other groups. Attrition: 35%	High
Yoshimura et al. 2014	Design: DBRCT Setting: outpatient Country: Japan Funding: govt	DIS 200+letter (28); DIS 200 no letter (26); PBO+letter (29); PBO no letter (26) Other Tx: proportion of subjects received letter discussing harms of alcohol use and approaches to manage craving	26	ICD-10 alcohol dependence Mean age: 52.1 years % Nonwhite NR 0% Female Other Dx: NP	No difference in the proportion achieving abstinence at 26 weeks Attrition: 25%	Medium

Note. Unless noted elsewhere, subjects were excluded if they had contraindications for specific medications; were pregnant, breastfeeding, or unreliable in using contraception; were receiving psychotropic medications; or had another substance use disorder (except nicotine dependence), other psychiatric conditions, suicidal or homicidal ideas, or significant physical illness (including renal or hepatic disease). Industry-sponsored studies list the name of the pharmaceutical company.

Abbreviations: ACA=acamprosate; CBT=cognitive-behavioral therapy; CI=confidence interval; DBRCT=double blind, randomized controlled trial; DIS=disulfiram; Dx=diagnosis; GHB=gamma-hydroxybutyrate; govt=governmental; NR=not reported; NTX=naltrexone; OLRCT=open label, randomized controlled trial; PBO=placebo; RIB=riboflavin; TOP=topiramate; Tx=treatment; VA=U.S. Department of Veterans Affairs; VAMIRECC=Veterans Affairs Mental Illness Research Education Clinical Centers.

larger ($p=0.001$) and more rapid ($p=0.0001$) reduction in heavy drinking and a larger ($p=0.03$) and more rapid ($p=0.01$) increase in the number of days abstinent (Kranzler et al. 2014a). Topiramate subjects were more likely to have had no heavy drinking days in the last 4 weeks of treatment (35.8% vs. 16.9% with placebo, OR=2.75, 95% CI 1.24–6.10) and to have abstained from alcohol use at the end of treatment (OR=2.57, 95% CI 1.13–5.84). The odds of a heavy drinking day were greater in the placebo group than the topiramate group (OR=5.33, 95% CI 1.68–7.28) by the last week of treatment. These benefits of topiramate appeared to be limited to individuals who were homozygous for the rs2832407 C-allele of *GRIK1* (which encodes the kainate GluK1 receptor subunit). However, at 3- and 6-month follow-up, the beneficial effects of topiramate on percent heavy drinking days and percent days abstinent were no longer significant (Kranzler et al. 2014c). Topiramate (300 mg/day; $N=21$) was also one of the treatment arms in a 14-week medium-risk-of-bias, double-blind, randomized controlled trial of several other anticonvulsant agents that included levetiracetam ($N=21$), zonisamide 400 mg/day ($N=19$), and placebo ($N=24$) (Knapp et al. 2015). For topiramate as compared with placebo, significant treatment effects were seen for weekly percent days drinking ($P<0.0001$), percent days heavy drinking ($P<0.0001$), and drinks consumed per day ($P=0.0007$). A 12-week, medium-risk-of-bias, double-blind, randomized placebo-controlled trial of topiramate (260 mg/day average dose) conducted in Thailand (total $N=106$) was limited by 50% attrition rates but showed no significant difference between the treatments in heavy drinking days, time to first heavy drinking day, or secondary drinking outcomes (Likhitsathian et al. 2013).

Several smaller studies of topiramate have been conducted in individuals with a co-occurring psychiatric disorder. A small (total $N=30$) double-blind, randomized placebo-controlled trial of flexibly dosed topiramate (up to 300 mg/day) was conducted at a Veterans Affairs Medical Center in individuals with co-occurring PTSD (Batki et al. 2014) (Table B–16). This low-risk-of-bias study showed a 51% decrease in drinking days with topiramate as compared with placebo as well as reductions in standard drinks per week but no effect on the percent of heavy drinking days. Another U.S. government–funded, low-risk-of-bias, double-blind, randomized placebo-controlled trial of topiramate (300 mg/day) enrolled individuals with co-occurring cocaine dependence (Kampman et al. 2013). During the 13-week trial, 41/87 (47%) of placebo-treated subjects were lost to follow-up versus 29/83 (35%) with topiramate. However, on primary outcome measures of weekly differences in percent days drinking, percent days heavy drinking, and mean drinks per drinking day, there was no difference between the placebo and topiramate-treated groups. An additional study in individuals with co-occurring bipolar disorder reported the results of 12 randomly assigned participants but had difficulty recruiting subjects because of problems with topiramate tolerability (Sylvia et al. 2016).

Grading of the Overall Supporting Body of Research Evidence for Efficacy of Topiramate

- **Magnitude of effect:** *Moderate.* When present for specific outcomes, the magnitude of the effect is moderate.
- **Risk of bias:** *Medium.* Studies are RCTs of low to high bias based on their described randomization and blinding procedures and descriptions of study dropouts, with the largest trials having low to medium risk of bias.
- **Applicability:** The included trials all involve individuals with AUD, by either prior diagnostic criteria or other evidence of harmful levels of drinking. The studies include subjects from around the world, including North America. The doses of topiramate appear to be representative of outpatient clinical practice.
- **Directness:** *Direct.* Studies measured abstinence and heavy drinking rates as well as measures of alcohol consumption.
- **Consistency:** *Inconsistent.* There was considerable heterogeneity in the study findings, with a proportion of trials showing no effect of topiramate.

TABLE B–16.   Topiramate compared with placebo

Outcome	Number of studies; number of subjects	Risk of bias; design	Consistency	Directness	Precision	Summary effect size (95% CI)	Strength of evidence grade
Return to any drinking	0;[a] 0	NA	NA	NA	NA	NA	Insufficient
Return to heavy drinking	0; 0	NA	NA	NA	NA	NA	Insufficient
Drinking days	2;[b] 521	Low; RCTs	Consistent	Direct	Imprecise	Trial 1: WMD: –8.5 (–15.9 to –1.1)[b] Trial 2: mean difference –11.6 (–3.98 to –19.3)	Moderate[b]
Heavy drinking days	2;[b] 521	Low; RCTs	Consistent	Direct	Imprecise	WMD: –11.53 (–18.29 to –4.77)	Moderate[b]
Drinks per drinking day	2;[b] 521	Low; RCTs	Consistent	Direct	Imprecise	WMD: –1.10 (–1.75 to –0.45)	Moderate[b]
Accidents	0; 0	NA	NA	NA	NA	NA	Insufficient
Injuries	1; 371	Low; RCT	Unknown	Direct	Imprecise	4.4% (TOP) vs. 11.7% (PBO); p=0.01	Insufficient
Quality of life or function	0; 0	NA	NA	NA	NA	NA	Insufficient
Mortality	1; 371	Low; RCT	Unknown	Direct	Imprecise	0 (TOP) vs. 1 (PBO)	Insufficient

[a]One study conducted in Brazil, rated as high risk of bias, reported this outcome. It reported that more patients treated with TOP returned to any drinking than with PBO (24/52 vs. 15/54).

[b]One additional study reporting this outcome was rated as high risk of bias. Our meta-analysis found a lower percentage of drinking days for patients treated with TOP than for those who received PBO both without and with including the trial rated as high risk of bias (WMD –9.7; 95% CI –16.4 to –3.1). Our meta-analysis found a lower percentage of heavy drinking days for patients treated with topiramate than for those who received placebo both without and with including the trial rated as high risk of bias (WMD –11.4; 95% CI –20.4 to –2.4). Our meta-analysis found no statistically significant difference between TOP and PBO when only including the trial rated as low risk of bias but found a statistically significant reduction of 1.2 drinks per drinking day when including the trial rated as high risk of bias (WMD –1.2; 95% CI –2.2 to –0.2). We were unable to include "trial 2" (N=150), rated as medium risk of bias, in our meta-analyses because of differences in the type of data reported, but its findings are shown in the SOE table and were generally consistent with those of the low risk of bias trial ("trial 1," N=371).

Abbreviations: CI=confidence interval; NA=not applicable; PBO=placebo; RCT=randomized controlled trial; SOE=strength of evidence; TOP=topiramate; WMD=weighted mean difference.

Source.   Jonas et al. 2014, Table D–26.

- **Precision:** *Imprecise.* Confidence intervals for studies cross the threshold for clinically significant benefit of the intervention.
- **Dose-response relationship:** *Unclear.* No dose-response relationship studies were done.
- **Confounding factors (including likely direction of effect):** *Unclear.* One study suggests a possible effect of genetic polymorphisms on treatment response, which could confound study interpretation.

- **Publication bias:** *Not identified.* No publication bias was noted by the AHRQ review; however, they note that they were unable to assess for publication bias for early clinical trials (prior to the advent of https://clinicaltrials.gov).
- **Overall strength of research evidence:** *Moderate.* A number of RCTs have been conducted, with low to high risk of bias. Several of the RCTs are funded by governmental agencies. Other studies show inconsistent findings or had high rates of attrition.

Harms of Topiramate

Studies of topiramate in other disorders have reported a number of treatment-related side effects. In the studies of topiramate for AUD that were included in the AHRQ report (Jonas et al. 2014), the most notable side effects of topiramate as compared with placebo were cognitive dysfunction and numbness/tingling/paresthesias (Table B–17). In the study of Likhitsathian et al. (2013), paresthesias were more common in the topiramate group as compared with placebo (45.3% vs. 17%). Kampman et al. (2013) also found a greater frequency of paresthesias in topiramate-treated subjects as compared with placebo-treated subjects (20% vs. 3%). Knapp et al. (2015) also noted paresthesias in 19% of topiramate subjects and erectile dysfunction in 14% of topiramate subjects. In addition, Knapp et al. (2015) found a significant effect of topiramate on the mental slowing subscale of the A-B Neurotoxicity Scales relative to placebo ($P=0.008$). Batki et al. (2014) found no significant differences in side effects between topiramate- and placebo-treated subjects.

Grading of the Overall Supporting Body of Research Evidence for Harms of Topiramate

- **Magnitude of effect:** *Moderate.* When present, the magnitude of effect is moderate for cognitive dysfunction and for numbness/tingling/paresthesias.
- **Risk of bias:** *High.* Studies are RCTs of low to high bias based on their described randomization and blinding procedures and descriptions of study dropouts. However, methods for determining harms are not well specified, and there is potential for selective reporting of results.
- **Applicability:** The included trials all involve individuals with AUD, by either prior diagnostic criteria or other evidence of harmful levels of drinking. The studies include subjects from around the world, including North America. The doses of topiramate appear to be representative of outpatient clinical practice.
- **Directness:** *Direct.* Studies measured common side effects and dropouts due to adverse events.
- **Consistency:** *Consistent.* For adverse events that showed a significant effect (cognitive dysfunction and numbness/tingling/paresthesias), the findings were consistent across trials.
- **Precision:** *Precise.* Confidence intervals for cognitive dysfunction and for numbness/tingling/paresthesias are relatively narrow.
- **Dose-response relationship:** *Unknown.* Dose response information on side effects was not well described.
- **Confounding factors (including likely direction of effect):** Possible and may reduce reported side effects. Given the high rates of attrition in some of the studies and the lack of systematic assessment of side effects, it is possible that attrition occurred because of unrecognized adverse events.
- **Publication bias:** *Not identified.* No publication bias was noted by the AHRQ review; however, they note that they were unable to assess for publication bias for early clinical trials (prior to the advent of https://clinicaltrials.gov).
- **Overall strength of research evidence:** *Moderate.* A number of RCTs have been conducted, but few have assessed adverse events in a systematic and predefined fashion. Many of the RCTs are funded by governmental agencies. Nevertheless, the studies are relatively consistent in reporting increased likelihood of cognitive dysfunction and numbness/tingling/paresthesias with topiramate, which is consistent with reported side effects in clinical trials for other indications.

Outcome	N trials	N subjects	RD	95% CI	I²	Strength of evidence grade
Withdrawal due to adverse events	2	521	0.06	–0.12 to 0.25	93.4%	Low
Withdrawal due to adverse events—SA	3	599	0.06	–0.06 to 0.18	86.9%	
Anorexia	1	371	0.13	0.06 to 0.20	NA	Insufficient
Cognitive dysfunction	2	521	0.08	0.01 to 0.16	38.5%	Moderate
Diarrhea	1	371	0.04	–0.03 to 0.10	NA	Insufficient
Diarrhea—SA	2	477	0.00	–0.07 to 0.08	61.1%	Insufficient
Dizziness	2	521	0.10	–0.01 to 0.22	65.0%	Low
Dizziness—SA	3	627	0.08	0.01 to 0.14	51.5%	Low
Headache	1	371	-0.08	–0.17 to 0.01	NA	Insufficient
Insomnia	1	371	0.03	–0.05 to 0.11	NA	Insufficient
Insomnia—SA	2	477	0.03	–0.03 to 0.10	0.0%	Insufficient
Nausea	1	371	–0.06	–0.13 to 0.01	NA	Insufficient
Nausea—SA	2	477	–0.02	–0.11 to 0.06	62.0%	Insufficient
Numbness/tingling/paresthesias	2	521	0.40	0.32 to 0.47	0.0%	Moderate
Numbness/tingling/paresthesias—SA	3	627	0.29	0.05 to 0.52	93.1%	Moderate
Taste abnormalities	1	371	0.18	0.11 to 0.25	NA	Insufficient

Note. Positive risk differences favor placebo. Sensitivity analyses include studies rated as high risk of bias.

Abbreviations: CI=confidence interval; *N*=number of trials or subjects contributing data; NA=not applicable; RD=risk difference; SA=sensitivity analysis.

Source. Jonas et al. 2014, Table 31; values for strength of evidence are from Table D–37.

Data Abstraction: Topiramate

Studies related to topiramate are listed in Table B–18.

Benefits of Gabapentin

The AHRQ review (Jonas et al. 2014) did not include any studies with a primary focus on gabapentin. In one included study (Anton et al. 2011), gabapentin was added in one treatment arm as an adjunct to naltrexone during the initial 6 weeks of the trial and was associated with improved outcomes at 6 weeks but not at the end of the trial. Several small randomized trials of shorter duration also showed benefit of gabapentin on alcohol-related outcomes (Anton et al. 2009; Furieri and Nakamura-Palacios 2007).

A government-funded low-risk-of-bias, double-blind, randomized controlled dose-ranging trial (Mason et al. 2014) compared gabapentin at 900 mg/day (*N*=54) and 1,800 mg/day (*N*=47) with placebo (*N*=49). The primary study outcomes, which were rate of complete abstinence (chi square=4.19; *P*=.04) and rate of no heavy drinking (chi square=5.39; *P*=.02), increased linearly with

Author and year	Study characteristics	Treatment administered, including study arm, dose (mg/day), sample size (N), and co-intervention	Rx duration, weeks	Sample characteristics, including diagnostic inclusions and major exclusions	Outcome measures, main results, and overall percent attrition	Risk of bias
Baltieri et al. 2008, 2009	Design: DBRCT Setting: outpatient Country: Brazil Funding: govt	TOP to 200–400 (52); NTX 50 (49); PBO (54) Other Tx: psychosocial 100%; AA recommended	12	ICD-10 alcohol dependence Mean age: 44–45 years 29% Nonwhite 0% Female Other Dx: tobacco use 66%	Time to first relapse was greater with TOP than PBO (7.8 weeks vs. 5.0 weeks). NTX was not significantly different from either of the other groups (5.7 weeks). Cumulative abstinence duration was also greater with TOP (8.2 weeks vs. NTX 6.6 weeks vs. PBO 5.6 weeks), as was the mean number of weeks with heavy drinking, but the rate of complete abstinence at study endpoint was comparable in the 3 groups. Smokers relapsed more rapidly than nonsmokers. Attrition: 45%	High
Batki et al. 2014	Design: DBRCT Setting: outpatient Country: United States Funding: govt	TOP to 300 (14); PBO (16) Other Tx: MM	12	DSM-IV alcohol dependence and PTSD Mean age: NR 47% Nonwhite 7% Female Other Dx: PTSD 100%; SUD 33%	TOP was associated with 51% fewer drinking days but showed no effect on heavy drinking days. No difference in adverse events between groups or cognition at end of trial. PTSD severity was reduced in TOP group. Attrition: 10%	Low
DeSousa et al. 2008	Design: OLRCT Setting: inpatient and outpatient alcohol treatment center Country: India Funding: NR	TOP 150 (50); DIS 250 (50) Other Tx: weekly supporting group psychotherapy offered	39	DSM-IV alcohol dependence Exclusions: previous TOP or DIS treatment Mean age: 43 years 100% Nonwhite 0% Female Other Dx: NR	DIS had greater mean time to first relapse than TOP (133 days vs. 79 days, p=0.0001) and a lower relapse rate at study endpoint (10% vs. 44%; p=0.0001). TOP had less craving than DIS. Attrition: 8%	High

TABLE B–18. Studies related to topiramate *(continued)*

Author and year	Study characteristics	Treatment administered, including study arm, dose (mg/day), sample size (N), and co-intervention	Rx duration, weeks	Sample characteristics, including diagnostic inclusions and major exclusions	Outcome measures, main results, and overall percent attrition	Risk of bias
Flórez et al. 2008	Design: OLRCT Setting: outpatient substance use disorders clinic Country: Spain Funding: NR	TOP up to 200 (51); NTX 50 (51) Other Tx: therapy based on relapse prevention model 100%	26	ICD-10 alcohol dependence Mean age: 47 years 0% Nonwhite 15% Female Other Dx: personality disorders 27%	TOP and NTX were both effective but did not differ in efficacy as measured by a composite alcohol use metric. Adverse effects, particularly weight loss, were greater with TOP vs. NTX. Attrition: 10%	High
Flórez et al. 2011	Design: OLRCT Setting: outpatient substance use disorders clinic Country: Spain Funding: NR	TOP 200 (91); NTX 50 (91) Other Tx: BRENDA 100%; at least monthly meeting with psychiatrist 100%	26	ICD-10 alcohol dependence Mean age: 47–48 years % Nonwhite NR 15% Female Other Dx: personality disorders 23%	At 3 and 6 months, patients with TOP reported lower scores than those with NTX on craving and alcohol-related measures; those with TOP also scored less on disability related measures at 6 months. TOP was also associated with fewer drinks per drinking day and fewer heavy drinking days at 3 and 6 months compared with NTX. The percentage of days abstinent and total drinking days were comparable for TOP and NTX. A greater proportion of TOP subjects reported adverse effects at 3 months but not 6 months. Attrition: 10%	High

TABLE B–18.   Studies related to topiramate *(continued)*

Author and year	Study characteristics	Treatment administered, including study arm, dose (mg/day), sample size (N), and co-intervention	Rx duration, weeks	Sample characteristics, including diagnostic inclusions and major exclusions	Outcome measures, main results, and overall percent attrition	Risk of bias
Johnson et al. 2003, 2004a; Ma et al. 2006	Design: DBRCT Setting: 1 outpatient site Country: United States Funding: Ortho-McNeil	TOP 25–300 (75); PBO (75) Other Tx: brief behavioral compliance enhancement therapy	12	DSM-IV alcohol dependence Mean age: 41.5 years 36% Nonwhite 29% Female Other Dx: 0%	Differences between TOP and PBO were drinks per drinking day: –1.2 (95% CI –2.023, –0.3777) and percent heavy drinking days: –14.9 (95% CI –22.556, –7.244). TOP had significant improvements on all drinking outcomes, including 27% fewer heavy drinking days compared with PBO (*p*<0.001) as well as improvements on reported abstinence and not seeking alcohol (OR=2.63; 95% CI 1.52, 4.53; *p*=0.001). Craving was significantly less with TOP vs. PBO. TOP also improved the odds of overall well-being (OR=2.17; 95% CI 1.16, 2.60; *p*=0.01) and overall life satisfaction (OR=2.28; 95% CI 1.21, 4.29; *p*=0.01) and reduced harmful drinking consequences (OR= –0.07; 95% CI –0.12, –0.02; *p*=0.01) relative to PBO. TOP had more frequent adverse events compared with PBO: dizziness (28.0% vs. 10.7%; *p*=0.01), paresthesia (57.3% vs. 18.7%; *p*<0.001), psychomotor slowing (26.7% vs. 12.0%; *p*=0.02), memory or concentration impairment (18.7% vs. 5.3%; *p*=0.01), and weight loss (54.7% vs. 26.7%; *p*=0.001). Attrition: 35%	Medium

Author and year	Study characteristics	Treatment administered, including study arm, dose (mg/day), sample size (N), and co-intervention	Rx duration, weeks	Sample characteristics, including diagnostic inclusions and major exclusions	Outcome measures, main results, and overall percent attrition	Risk of bias
Johnson et al. 2007, 2008	Design: DBRCT Setting: 17 academic outpatient sites Country: United States Funding: Ortho-McNeil	TOP 50–300, mean 171 (183); PBO (188) Other Tx: brief behavioral medication compliance enhancement therapy 100%	14	DSM-IV alcohol dependence Exclusions: >4 unsuccessful inpatient treatment attempts Mean age: 47–48 years 15% Nonwhite 26%–28% Female Other Dx: NR	Differences between TOP and PBO were drinks per drinking day: –0.93 (95% CI –1.986, 0.126), percent drinking days: –8.5 (95% CI –15.88, –1.12), and percent heavy drinking days: –8 (95% CI –15.919, –0.081). Paresthesia, taste abnormalities, loss of appetite, and problems with concentration were more frequent with TOP vs PBO. Attrition: 31%; 6% lost to follow-up	Low
Kampman et al. 2013	Design: DBRCT Setting: outpatient Country: United States Funding: govt	TOP to 300 (83); PBO (87) Other Tx: individual cognitive-behavioral coping skills (Project MATCH)	13	In 30-day period in past 90 days had at least 48/60 drinks (women/men), with 2 or more heavy drinking days; DSM-IV cocaine dependence Mean age: 44 years 83% Nonwhite 21% Female Other Dx: cocaine dependence 100%	No differences were found in weekly percent days drinking, weekly percent days heavy drinking, and mean drinks per drinking day. Paresthesias occurred in 20% of TOP-treated subjects and 3% of PBO subjects. Attrition: 59%	Low

TABLE B–18. Studies related to topiramate (*continued*)

Author and year	Study characteristics	Treatment administered, including study arm, dose (mg/day), sample size (N), and co-intervention	Rx duration, weeks	Sample characteristics, including diagnostic inclusions and major exclusions	Outcome measures, main results, and overall percent attrition	Risk of bias
Knapp et al. 2015	Design: DBRCT Setting: outpatient Country: United States Funding: govt	TOP 300 (21); levetiracetam 2,000 (21); zonisamide 400 (19); PBO (24) Other Tx: brief behavioral compliance enhancement treatment	14	DSM-IV alcohol dependence Mean age: 47 years 9% Nonwhite 43.5% Female Other Dx: NR	Significant treatment effects were seen for weekly percent days drinking ($P<0.0001$), percent days heavy drinking ($P<0.0001$), and drinks consumed per day ($P=0.0007$) for TOP as compared with PBO. Significant effect of TOP was seen on the mental slowing subscale of A-B Neurotoxicity Scales ($p=0.008$). Paresthesias (19%) and erectile dysfunction (14%) were more common with TOP. Attrition: 24%	Medium
Kranzler et al. 2014a	Design: DBRCT Setting: outpatient Country: United States Funding: VA	TOP to 200 (67); PBO (71) Other Tx: MM	12	Average weekly use of standard drinks >23 for men and >17 for women; goal of reducing but not abstaining from alcohol; majority with DSM-IV alcohol dependence Mean age: 51.1 years 12% Nonwhite 38% Female Other Dx: lifetime MDD 19%	TOP was associated with a larger and more rapid decrease in heavy drinking and days with drinking. At the end of treatment, TOP group was more likely to have abstained from alcohol use (OR=2.57; 95% CI 1.13, 5.84) and had no heavy drinking days (35.8% vs. 16.9% with PBO, OR=2.75; 95% CI 1.24, 6.10). TOP subjects reported significantly higher rates of adverse events, specifically numbness/tingling, change in taste, loss of appetite, weight loss, difficulty concentrating, and difficulty with memory. Attrition: 15%	Low
Likhitsathian et al. 2013	Design: DBRCT Setting: outpatient Country: Thailand Funding: govt	TOP up to mean dose 260 (53); PBO (53) Other Tx: MET and MM	12	At least 1 of 4 weeks prior to admission with more than 34 standard drinks per week Mean age: 41.5 years % Nonwhite NR 0% Female Other Dx: NR	Both groups had reduced drinking, but there was no difference in heavy drinking days or time to first heavy drinking day between groups. Paresthesias were more common with TOP (45.3% vs. 17%). Attrition: 50%	Medium

TABLE B–18.   Studies related to topiramate *(continued)*

Author and year	Study characteristics	Treatment administered, including study arm, dose (mg/day), sample size (N), and co-intervention	Rx duration, weeks	Sample characteristics, including diagnostic inclusions and major exclusions	Outcome measures, main results, and overall percent attrition	Risk of bias
Narayana et al. 2008	Design: prospective cohort Setting: military, outpatient Country: India Funding: NR	ACA 1,332–1,998 (28); NTX 50 (26); TOP 100–125 (38) Other Tx: various psychotherapies offered	52	ICD-10 alcohol dependence Mean age: 38 years 100% Nonwhite 0% Female Other Dx: NR	TOP (76.3%) was significantly more effective (*p*<0.01) in sustaining abstinence, although 57.7% NTX and 60.7% ACA maintained complete abstinence. 7 TOP subjects (18.4%) reported decreased relapses compared with 8 NTX (30.8%) and 9 ACA (32.1%) subjects. Attrition: 22%	High
Rubio et al. 2009	Design: DBRCT Setting: outpatient Country: Spain Funding: govt	TOP 250 (31); PBO (32) Other Tx: supportive group therapy offered	12	DSM-IV alcohol dependence Mean age: 42 years % Nonwhite NR 0% Female Other Dx: NR	Differences between TOP and PBO were drinks per drinking day: –2.3 (95% CI –4.715, 0.115), percent drinking days: –14.9 (95% CI –30.07, 0.27), and percent heavy drinking days: –17.6 (95% CI –30.565, –4.635). Attrition: 5%	High

Note.   Unless noted elsewhere, subjects were excluded if they had contraindications for specific medications; were pregnant, breastfeeding, or unreliable in using contraception; were receiving psychotropic medications; or had another substance use disorder (except nicotine dependence), other psychiatric conditions, suicidal or homicidal ideas, or significant physical illness (including renal or hepatic disease). Industry-sponsored studies list the name of the pharmaceutical company.

Abbreviations: AA=Alcoholics Anonymous; ACA=acamprosate; BRENDA=Biopsychosocial evaluation, Report of findings to patient, Empathetic understanding of patient's situation, Needs to be addressed, Direct advice to patient on how to meet those needs, and Assessing reaction/behaviors of patient to advice and adjusting treatment plan as necessary for best care; CI=confidence interval; DBRCT=double blind, randomized controlled trial; DIS=disulfiram; Dx=diagnosis; govt=governmental; MDD=major depressive disorder; MET=motivational enhancement therapy; MM=medical management; NR=not reported; NTX=naltrexone; OLRCT=open-label, randomized controlled trial; OR=odds ratio; PBO=placebo; PTSD=posttraumatic stress disorder; SUD=substance use disorder; TOP=topiramate; Tx=treatment; VA=U.S. Department of Veterans Affairs.

the dose of gabapentin. Sustained 12-week abstinence was 4.1% (95% CI 1.1%–13.7%) with placebo, 11.1% (95% CI 5.2%–22.2%) with 900 mg/day of gabapentin, and 17.0% (95% CI 8.9% –30.1%; NNT=8) with 1,800 mg/day gabapentin with a NNT of 8 for increased rate of abstinence at a dose of 1,800 mg daily. Corresponding rates of no heavy drinking were 22.5% (95% CI 13.6%–37.2%), 29.6% (95% CI 19.1%–42.8%), and 44.7% (95% CI 31.4%–58.8%; NNT=5), respectively, with a NNT of 5 for reduction in heavy drinking days at a dose of 1,800 mg daily. Significant dose-dependent reductions were also noted in the prespecified secondary outcomes: levels of GGT, alcohol craving, sleep, and depression. For subjects who completed the trial, rates of complete abstinence, drinks per week, and number of heavy drinking days per week were sustained at 24-week follow-up. The most frequent adverse events were fatigue (23%), insomnia (18%), and headache (14%), but rates of these side effects did not differ among the three study arms. In addition, there were no differences in the number, severity, or type of reported adverse effects (Mason et al. 2014). Insufficient information was available on side effects of gabapentin to grade the overall supporting body of research evidence for harms.

Grading of the Overall Supporting Body of Research Evidence for Efficacy of Gabapentin

- **Magnitude of effect:** *Moderate.* When present for specific outcomes, the magnitude of the effect is moderate.
- **Risk of bias:** *Low.* One large RCT accounts for the preponderance of findings and has a low risk of bias based on the described randomization and blinding procedures and descriptions of study dropouts.
- **Applicability:** The included trials all involve individuals with AUD, by either prior diagnostic criteria or other evidence of harmful levels of drinking. The studies include subjects from North America. The doses of gabapentin are representative of outpatient clinical practice.
- **Directness:** *Direct.* Studies measured abstinence and heavy drinking rates as well as measures of alcohol consumption.
- **Consistency:** *Not applicable.* Data are predominantly from a single study.
- **Precision:** *Imprecise.* Confidence intervals for some outcomes cross the threshold for clinically significant benefit of the intervention.
- **Dose-response relationship:** *Present.* Linear increases in efficacy are noted with increases in gabapentin dose for multiple outcomes.
- **Confounding factors (including likely direction of effect):** *Not identified.*
- **Publication bias:** *Not identified.*
- **Overall strength of research evidence:** *Low.* Findings are predominantly from a single study with a low risk of bias, a large sample size, and a significant dose-response relationship. Other support for gabapentin is from trials of short duration or combination treatments, rather than gabapentin alone.

Data Abstraction: Gabapentin

Studies related to gabapentin are listed in Table B–19.

Author and year	Study characteristics	Treatment administered, including study arm, dose (mg/day), sample size (N), and co-intervention	Rx duration, weeks	Sample characteristics, including diagnostic inclusions and major exclusions	Outcome measures, main results, and overall percent attrition	Risk of bias
Mason et al. 2014	Design: DBRCT Setting: outpatient Country: United States Funding: govt, meds	Gabapentin 900 (54); gabapentin 1,800 (47); PBO (49) Other Tx: manual guided weekly counseling	12	DSM IV alcohol dependence Mean age: 44.5 years 19% Nonwhite 43% Female Other Dx: 0%	Gabapentin dose showed linear increases with rate of complete abstinence (P=0.04), rate of no heavy drinking (P=0.02), sustained 12-week abstinence (17.0% with NNT=8 for 1,800 mg/day), and rates of no heavy drinking with PBO (44.7% NNT=5 for 1,800 mg/day). Adverse events did not differ among groups, with the predominant side effects of fatigue (23%), insomnia (18%), and headache (14%). Attrition: 43%	Low

Note. Unless noted elsewhere, subjects were excluded if they had contraindications for specific medications; were pregnant, breastfeeding, or unreliable in using contraception; were receiving psychotropic medications; or had another substance use disorder (except nicotine dependence), other psychiatric conditions, suicidal or homicidal ideas, or significant physical illness (including renal or hepatic disease). Abbreviations: DBRCT=double-blind, randomized controlled trial; Dx=diagnosis; govt=governmental; meds=medications supplied by pharmaceutical company; NNT=number needed to treat; NR=not reported; PBO=placebo; Tx=treatment.

Recommendations Against Use of Specific Medications

STATEMENT 12: Antidepressants

APA *recommends* **(1B)** that antidepressant medications not be used for treatment of alcohol use disorder unless there is evidence of a co-occurring disorder for which an antidepressant is an indicated treatment.

Benefits of Antidepressants

Evidence for this recommendation comes from a number of studies of serotonin reuptake inhibitors and tricyclic antidepressants that assessed alcohol-related outcomes in individuals with alcohol dependence and a depressive or anxiety disorder (Jonas et al. 2014). On the basis of a substantial number of trials that directly assess the efficacy of antidepressant medications in treating AUD, the strength of research evidence is rated as moderate.

The AHRQ review (Jonas et al. 2014) included seven trials comparing placebo with sertraline in doses of 50–200 mg/day and treatment durations of 12–26 weeks. Of the seven studies, five were done in the United States, three included only individuals with major depressive disorder and alcohol dependence, and one included individuals with PTSD and alcohol dependence. Meta-analysis did not show a benefit of sertraline on the alcohol-related outcomes, and for the outcome of percent of heavy drinking days the comparison favored placebo (low strength of research evidence; WMD: 1.85 [0.70 to 3.0]). An additional study (total $N=170$) compared placebo with naltrexone alone, sertraline alone, or the combination of naltrexone and sertraline and reported no difference between sertraline and placebo conditions on abstinence rates (Pettinati et al. 2010). The combination of naltrexone plus sertraline showed greater abstinence rates than either treatment alone ($p=0.001$) as well as a longer time to relapse to heavy drinking. A subsequent double-blind RCT of sertraline 200 mg/day ($N=32$) versus placebo ($N=37$) was conducted in individuals with co-occurring PTSD and alcohol dependence (Hien et al. 2015). Treatment in this low-risk-of-bias trial also included 12 sessions of a "Seeking Safety" intervention. At the end of treatment, at 6-month follow-up, and at 12-month follow-up, both sertraline and placebo subjects showed a decreased number of drinks per drinking day, a decrease in heavy drinking days, and an increase in 7-day abstinence rate. PTSD symptoms showed greater improvement with sertraline than placebo, but there was no specific effect of sertraline treatment as compared with placebo on alcohol-related outcomes.

The AHRQ review included two trials (Naranjo et al. 1995; Tiihonen et al. 1996) of 12–13 weeks duration that compared citalopram 40 mg/day with placebo. Both trials were rated as having a high risk of bias, and neither trial showed an effect of citalopram on drinking-related outcomes. A subsequent medium-risk-of-bias 12-week trial of citalopram 40 mg/day ($N=138$) versus placebo ($N=127$) found worse outcomes with citalopram than placebo in terms of the percentage decrease in the frequency of alcohol consumption ($p=0.016$), the percentage decrease in the quantity of alcohol consumed per drinking day ($p=0.025$), the average number of heavy drinking days ($p=0.007$), drinks per drinking day ($p=0.03$), and money spent on alcohol ($p=0.041$) (Charney et al. 2015). When individuals with depression were compared with those without depression, the findings in both subgroups were consistent with findings for the overall sample. In another 12-week study in which all subjects (total $N=138$) received naltrexone (up to 100 mg/day), there was no significant difference on alcohol use or depression-related outcomes between subjects who were randomly assigned to citalopram (up to 60 mg/day) and those assigned to placebo (Adamson et al. 2015).

The AHRQ review (Jonas et al. 2014) included three U.S. trials lasting 12–15 weeks and comparing placebo with fluoxetine in doses from 20 mg to 60 mg per day (Cornelius et al. 1995; Kabel and Petty 1996; Kranzler et al. 1995). In one of the trials, in which all subjects ($N=51$) had major depressive disorder, subjects treated with fluoxetine had fewer drinking days (WMD –11.6; 95% CI –22.7 to –0.5) and fewer heavy drinking days (4.8 versus 16, $p=0.04$) than those who received placebo (Cornelius et al. 1995). When the two medium-risk-of-bias trials were combined (Cornelius et al. 1995; Kranzler et al. 1995), meta-analysis found no difference between fluoxetine and placebo in drinking days (WMD –3.2; 95% CI –18.2 to 11.9) or heavy drinking days (WMD –1.2; 95% CI –4.6 to 2.2).

In a single European trial of fluvoxamine 100–300 mg/day as compared with placebo, there was no difference at 12 weeks of treatment or at 52 weeks of follow-up in the percent of subjects who had returned to drinking or the percent who returned to heavy drinking (Chick et al. 2004). At 12 weeks, fluvoxamine-treated patients had more drinking days in the prior month than placebo-treated patients, but the groups did not differ on this outcome at 52 weeks of follow-up.

One randomized trial compared paroxetine (10–60 mg/day, mean dose 45 mg/day) with placebo in individuals with social anxiety disorder, of whom 79% of 42 subjects also had a co-occurring diagnosis of alcohol dependence (Book et al. 2008; Thomas et al. 2008). After 16 weeks (12 weeks at final paroxetine dose), there was no difference in the mean number of drinks per drinking day or the proportion of drinking days or heavy drinking days for paroxetine-treated patients as compared with placebo-treated patients. In an additional high-risk-of-bias trial (Petrakis et al. 2012), paroxetine with and without naltrexone was compared with desipramine with and without naltrexone in subjects with co-occurring alcohol dependence and PTSD. Individuals who received paroxetine had more heavy drinking days ($p=0.009$) and drinks per drinking day ($p=0.027$) than those who received desipramine. Although all groups showed reductions in PTSD symptoms, combination treatment with naltrexone and an antidepressant was associated with reduced craving as compared with groups treated with antidepressant plus placebo (Petrakis et al. 2012).

Another U.S. study with a medium-risk-of-bias compared desipramine (median dose=200 mg/day) with placebo. In this trial, 39% also had a diagnosis of depression (Mason et al. 1996). Although 12% of desipramine-treated patients returned to heavy drinking as compared with 32% of placebo-treated patients, this difference was not statistically significant. A medium-risk-of-bias-study of imipramine 50–300 mg/day (mean dose=262 mg/day) as compared with placebo in individuals with depression and alcohol dependence found no significant difference between imipramine and placebo groups on percent return to any drinking, percent heavy drinking, or number of drinks per drinking day (McGrath et al. 1996).

Grading of the Supporting Body of Research Evidence for Efficacy of Antidepressants

- **Magnitude of effect:** *None.* When differences were present for specific outcomes, the magnitude of the effect is small and the effect favored placebo.
- **Risk of bias:** *Medium.* Studies are RCTs of medium to high bias based on their described randomization and blinding procedures and descriptions of study dropouts.
- **Applicability:** The included trials all have a substantial proportion of subjects with AUD, by either prior diagnostic criteria or other evidence of harmful levels of drinking. In most of the studies, subjects also had a co-occurring diagnosis of depression or an anxiety disorder. The studies include subjects from around the world, including North America. The doses of antidepressant medications appear to be representative of outpatient clinical practice.
- **Directness:** *Direct.* Studies measured abstinence and heavy drinking rates as well as measures of alcohol consumption. Most studies also included measures related to symptoms of co-occurring disorders.
- **Consistency:** *Consistent.* Although meta-analysis was not conducted across all studies of antidepressant medications, the main findings of the studies were consistent.
- **Precision:** Not able to assess because confidence intervals were not calculated for the majority of the studies.
- **Dose-response relationship:** *Unclear.* Studies typically adjusted medication doses on the basis of clinical response.
- **Confounding factors (including likely direction of effect):** *Not identified.*
- **Publication bias:** *Not identified.*
- **Overall strength of research evidence:** *Moderate.* A number of RCTs have been conducted, most of which had medium to high risk of bias and moderate sample sizes. Many of the RCTs were funded by governmental agencies. Despite the inclusion of different antidepressants of different classes and subjects with different co-occurring conditions, the studies are consistent in showing minimal effect or a slightly detrimental effect of antidepressant medication on alcohol-related outcomes.

Data Abstraction: Antidepressants

Studies related to antidepressants are listed in Table B–20.

TABLE B–20. Studies related to antidepressants (listed alphabetically by medication name)

Author and year; trial name	Study characteristics	Treatment administered, including study arm, dose (mg/day), sample size (N), and co-intervention	Rx duration, weeks (follow-up)	Sample characteristics, including diagnostic inclusions and major exclusions	Outcome measures, main results, and overall percent attrition	Risk of bias
Charney et al. 2015	Design: DBRCT Setting: outpatient Country: Canada Funding: govt	Citalopram 40 (138); PBO (127) Other Tx: weekly individual and group psychotherapy	12	DSM-IV alcohol abuse or dependence Mean age: 45.4 years % Nonwhite NR 30% Female Other Dx: depression only 22%; anxiety only 27%; mixed anxiety and depression 38%; personality disorder 42%	Citalopram was associated with worse outcomes than PBO on frequency of alcohol consumption ($p=0.016$), quantity of alcohol consumed per drinking day ($p=0.025$), average number of heavy drinking days ($p=0.007$), drinks per drinking day ($p=0.03$), and money spent on alcohol ($p=0.041$). Median survival time to first relapse was not significantly different with treatment in depressed or nondepressed subjects. Attrition: 47%	Medium

TABLE B–20. Studies related to antidepressants (listed alphabetically by medication name) *(continued)*

Author and year; trial name	Study characteristics	Treatment administered, including study arm, dose (mg/day), sample size (N), and co-intervention	Rx duration, weeks (follow-up)	Sample characteristics, including diagnostic inclusions and major exclusions	Outcome measures, main results, and overall percent attrition	Risk of bias
Naranjo et al. 1995	Design: DBRCT Setting: outpatient research center Country: Canada Funding: govt; Lundbeck A/S	Citalopram 40 (53); PBO (46) Other Tx: brief psychosocial intervention 100%	12 (20)	Mild to moderate alcohol dependence with at least 28 drinks per week Mean age: 45 years % Nonwhite NR 44% Female Other Dx: NR	Both treatment groups showed a significant decrease in alcohol intake ($p<0.001$) (35.1% citalopram vs. 38.8% PBO). Citalopram had a significant initial effect; reduced alcohol intake during the first week of the treatment period by 47.9% from baseline compared with 26.1% ($p<0.01$) decrease in the PBO group. During weeks 2–12, the effects of citalopram and PBO were similar; reductions in alcohol intake were 33.4% and 40.5%, respectively. Percentage of abstinent days in the citalopram group increased from baseline to 27.3%±3.6 ($p<0.001$). The PBO group increased their abstinent days from 7.1%±2.3 at baseline to 23.5%±3.1 ($p<0.001$); drinks per drinking day decreased from baseline for citalopram (from 7.6±0.6 to 5.4±0.4, $p<0.001$) and PBO (from 6.4±0.4 to 4.7±0.4, $p<0.001$). Attrition: 37%	High

Author and year; trial name	Study characteristics	Treatment administered, including study arm, dose (mg/day), sample size (N), and co-intervention	Rx duration, weeks (follow-up)	Sample characteristics, including diagnostic inclusions and major exclusions	Outcome measures, main results, and overall percent attrition	Risk of bias
Tiihonen et al. 1996	Design: DBRCT Setting: outpatient; community-based alcohol rehabilitation center Country: Finland Funding: Lundbeck	Citalopram 40 (31); PBO (31) Other Tx: supportive psychotherapy intervention 100%	13 (17)	DSM-III-R alcohol dependence Mean age: 45–47 years % Nonwhite NR 0% Female Other Dx: 0%	The citalopram group reported better outcomes than PBO in dropout rates, GGT changes, and the reports of patients and relatives: significant differences in dropout rates (32% vs. 58%, $p<0.05$) and in relatives' reports (26% vs. 7%, $p<0.05$). Attrition: 45%	High
Mason et al. 1996	Design: DBRCT Setting: psychiatry outpatient departments at 2 urban medical centers Country: United States Funding: govt	DMI median 200 (37); PBO (34) Other Tx: AA and other psychosocial treatments encouraged	26	DSM-III-R alcohol dependence Mean age: 40 years 38% Nonwhite 17% Female Other Dx: depression 39%	Kaplan-Meier survival curves showed a significant difference between PBO and DMI in time to relapse ($P=0.03$). There were more relapses on PBO than on DMI among depressed patients (40% vs. 8.3%) and among nondepressed patients (26.6% vs. 14.3%), but the differences were not statistically significant. Patients who relapsed had more severe alcohol dependence than those who did not (mean±SD: 24.46±8.8 and 18.7±6.9, respectively) Attrition: 52%	High

TABLE B–20. Studies related to antidepressants (listed alphabetically by medication name) *(continued)*

Author and year; trial name	Study characteristics	Treatment administered, including study arm, dose (mg/day), sample size (N), and co-intervention	Rx duration, weeks (follow-up)	Sample characteristics, including diagnostic inclusions and major exclusions	Outcome measures, main results, and overall percent attrition	Risk of bias
Petrakis et al. 2012	Design: DBRCT Setting: outpatient; multiple psychiatric centers, primarily VA Country: United States Funding: VA	DMI 200+PBO (24); paroxetine 40+PBO (20); DMI 200+NTX 50 (22); paroxetine 40+NTX 50 (22) Other Tx: clinical management; compliance enhancement therapy 100%	12	DSM-IV alcohol dependence and PTSD Exclusions: psychosis Mean age: 47 years 25% Nonwhite 9% Female Other Dx: PTSD 100%	Compared with paroxetine, DMI significantly reduced the percentage of heavy drinking days ($F_{1,84}=7.22$, $p=0.009$) and drinks per drinking days ($F_{1,84}=5.04$, $p=0.027$). There was a significant interaction for time by DMI/paroxetine treatment on drinks per week ($ATS_{6,82}=2.46$, $p=0.018$): DMI subjects had a greater reduction in their drinking over time compared with paroxetine subjects. NTX, compared with PBO, significantly decreased craving ($F_{1582.0}=6.39$, $p=0.012$; NTX=19.88 [SD=12.89] and PBO=21.1 [SD=12.89] at baseline vs. NTX=6.7 [SD=14.07] and PBO=8.3 [SD=13.38] at endpoint). GGT declined more in the DMI-treated participants ($F_{1229.5}=5.08$, $p=0.02$; DMI baseline=55.2, paroxetine baseline=86.4; DMI week 4=48.7, paroxetine week 4=46.1; DMI week 8=41.7, paroxetine week 8=47.1; DMI week 12=37.5, paroxetine week 12=57.1). Attrition: 44.3%	High

TABLE B–20. Studies related to antidepressants (listed alphabetically by medication name) *(continued)*

Author and year; trial name	Study characteristics	Treatment administered, including study arm, dose (mg/day), sample size (N), and co-intervention	Rx duration, weeks (follow-up)	Sample characteristics, including diagnostic inclusions and major exclusions	Outcome measures, main results, and overall percent attrition	Risk of bias
Cornelius et al. 1995, 1997	Design: DBRCT Setting: inpatient psychiatric institute Country: United States Funding: govt	Fluoxetine 20–40 (25); PBO (26) Other Tx: usual care: psychotherapy 100%	12	DSM-III-R alcohol dependence and major depression Mean age: 35 years 53% Nonwhite 49% Female Other Dx: MDD 100%	Differences between fluoxetine and PBO were drinks per drinking day: –3 (95% CI –5.4, –0.6), percent drinking days: –11.6 (95% CI –22.71, –0.49), and return to any drinking: –0.13 (95% CI –0.35, 0.1). Fluoxetine produced more improvement in depressive symptoms on the Ham-D but not on the BDI. Attrition: 10%	Medium
Kabel and Petty 1996	Design: DBRCT Setting: inpatient substance abuse treatment Country: United States Funding: govt	Fluoxetine 20–60 (15); PBO (13) Other Tx: NR	15	Alcohol dependence Mean age: 47 years 46% Nonwhite 0% Female Other Dx: cocaine use 14%; an average of 4 DSM-III-R personality disorders	Difference between fluoxetine and PBO for return to any drinking: 0.16 (95% CI –0.2, 0.51) Abstinence was maintained at 12 weeks in 53% of fluoxetine subjects and 69% of PBO subjects (*p*=NSD). Craving was significantly reduced with fluoxetine vs. PBO. Attrition: 42%	High

TABLE B–20. Studies related to antidepressants (listed alphabetically by medication name) *(continued)*

Author and year; trial name	Study characteristics	Treatment administered, including study arm, dose (mg/day), sample size (*N*), and co-intervention	Rx duration, weeks (follow-up)	Sample characteristics, including diagnostic inclusions and major exclusions	Outcome measures, main results, and overall percent attrition	Risk of bias
Kranzler et al. 1995	Design: DBRCT Setting: outpatient Country: United States Funding: govt	Fluoxetine 20–60, mean 47 (51); PBO (50) Other Tx: group psychotherapy 79%; individual psychotherapy 21%	12 (38)	DSM-III-R alcohol dependence Mean age: 40 years 5% Nonwhite 20% Female Other Dx: major depression 14%	Difference between fluoxetine and PBO for drinks per drinking day: 0.5 (95% CI –1.61, 2.61), percent drinking days: 3.8 (95% CI –2.08, 9.68). Survival analysis showed no difference between groups on proportion remaining abstinent. There were no significant differences in adverse effects except more reports of reduced sexual interest with fluoxetine vs. PBO. Attrition: 16%	Medium
Chick et al. 2004	Design: DBRCT Setting: 10 outpatient sites Country: United Kingdom, Ireland, Austria, Switzerland Funding: Solvay-Duphar	Fluvoxamine 100–300 (261); PBO (260) Other Tx: psychosocial treatment	52	DSM-III-R alcohol dependence Exclusions: not wishing to aim for total abstinence Mean age: 42 (19–72) years % Nonwhite NR 35% Female Other Dx: NR	There was no difference in abstinence at week 52 (fluvoxamine: *n*=75, 55% vs. PBO: *n*=117, 63%; *p*=0.24 by LOCF analysis). At week 12, the percentage of days not drinking since the last assessment was 69% for fluvoxamine and 77% for PBO (*p*=0.009). The mean dependence severity was more favorable for the PBO group (*p*=0.029). Attrition: 64% noncompleters; 21% lost to follow-up	Medium

TABLE B–20. Studies related to antidepressants (listed alphabetically by medication name) *(continued)*

Author and year; trial name	Study characteristics	Treatment administered, including study arm, dose (mg/day), sample size (N), and co-intervention	Rx duration, weeks (follow-up)	Sample characteristics, including diagnostic inclusions and major exclusions	Outcome measures, main results, and overall percent attrition	Risk of bias
McGrath et al. 1996	Design: DBRCT Setting: university-based depression research clinic Country: United States Funding: govt	IMI 50–300; mean 262 (36); PBO (33) Other Tx: weekly relapse prevention psychotherapy	12	DSM-III-R alcohol dependence or abuse and with major depression, dysthymia, or depressive disorder NOS Exclusions: history of mania Mean age: IMI 37 years, PBO 11 years[a] 17%–22% Nonwhite 49%–53% Female Other Dx: MDD 71%–72%, bipolar 11%–12%, atypical depression 70%–72%, other substance abuse 16%	CGI response to IMI (52%; 95% CI, 33%–70%) was significantly better than response to PBO (21%; 95% CI, 9%–38%). Patients receiving IMI were significantly less depressed than patients taking PBO by the Ham-D. IMI and PBO did not differ in rates of alcohol abstinence in either the last week (44% vs. 22%) or the last 4 weeks (31% vs. 21%) and did not differ in percent of days drinking, percent days of heavy drinking, or standard drinks per drinking day. Attrition: 23%	Medium
Book et al. 2008; Thomas et al. 2008	Design: DBRCT Setting: outpatient Country: United States Funding: govt, meds	Paroxetine titration over 4 weeks 10–60; average 45 (20); PBO (22) Other Tx: MM 100%; optional one individual therapy session 67%	16	DSM-IV alcohol use disorder (abuse: 21% and dependence: 79%) and social anxiety disorder, generalized type Mean age: 28–30 years 0%–18% Nonwhite 45%–50% Female Other Dx: social anxiety disorder 100%, MDD ~10%	Drinking outcomes did not change with paroxetine or PBO. Liebowitz Social Anxiety Scale scores were improved with paroxetine vs. PBO by week 7 through week 16. Attrition: 37%	Medium

Author and year; trial name	Study characteristics	Treatment administered, including study arm, dose (mg/day), sample size (*N*), and co-intervention	Rx duration, weeks (follow-up)	Sample characteristics, including diagnostic inclusions and major exclusions	Outcome measures, main results, and overall percent attrition	Risk of bias
Brady et al. 2005	Design: DBRCT Setting: outpatient Country: United States Funding: meds	SERT 150 (49); PBO (45) Other Tx: CBT 100%	12	DSM-IV alcohol dependence and current PTSD in response to civilian trauma Mean age: 37 years % Nonwhite NR 43%–49% Female Other Dx: PTSD 100%, depressive disorder 51%, anxiety disorder 38%	Differences between SERT and PBO were percent heavy drinking days: 1.8 (95% CI 0.65, 2.95) and drinks per drinking day: 0.5 (95% CI –2.42, 3.42). No side-effect differences were reported between groups. Attrition: 34%	Medium
Coskunol et al. 2002	Design: DBRCT Setting: inpatient (mean 1 month) followed by 6 months outpatient; substance abuse treatment unit Country: Turkey Funding: Pfizer	SERT 100 (30); PBO (29) Other Tx: thiamine 500 mg/day 100%; pyridoxine 500 mg/day 100%; AA during inpatient 100%	26	DSM-III-R alcohol dependence Mean age: 44 years % Nonwhite NR 0% Female Other Dx: 0%	Difference between SERT and PBO for return to heavy drinking: –0.19 (95% CI –0.44, 0.06). Relapse rates at 6 months were 50% SERT and 69% PBO. Attrition: 5%	Medium
Gual et al. 2003	Design: DBRCT Setting: 1 outpatient site Country: Spain Funding: NR	SERT 50–150 (44); PBO (39) Other Tx: NR	24	DSM-IV and ICD-10 criteria for alcohol dependence and for major depression or dysthymia or both Mean age: 47 years % Nonwhite NR 47% Female Other Dx: depression/dysthymia 100%	Differences between SERT and PBO were percent drinking days: 0.6 (95% CI –46.17, 47.37) and return to heavy drinking: 0.09 (95% CI –0.1, 0.28). Rates of adverse effects did not differ between the groups. Attrition: 45%	Medium

TABLE B–20. Studies related to antidepressants (listed alphabetically by medication name) *(continued)*

Author and year; trial name	Study characteristics	Treatment administered, including study arm, dose (mg/day), sample size (N), and co-intervention	Rx duration, weeks (follow-up)	Sample characteristics, including diagnostic inclusions and major exclusions	Outcome measures, main results, and overall percent attrition	Risk of bias
Hien et al. 2015	Design: DBRCT Setting: outpatient Country: United States Funding: govt	SERT 200 (32); PBO (37) Other Tx: "Seeking Safety" 12 sessions	12 (12)	DSM-IV-TR alcohol dependence or alcohol abuse with 2 heavy drinking days in past 90 days; additional inclusion criteria based on consumption patterns Co-occurring DSM-IV-TR PTSD Mean age: 42.2 years 59% Nonwhite 81% Female Other Dx: PTSD or subthreshold PTSD 100%; other SUD 55%	Decreased number of drinks per drinking day, a decrease in heavy drinking days, and an increase in 7-day abstinence rate in both groups; no effect of SERT Seeking safety plus SERT led to greater reduction in PTSD symptoms than seeking safety plus PBO (79% vs. 48%). Attrition: 42%	Low
Kranzler et al. 2011, 2012b	Design: DBRCT Setting: outpatient; university health center Country: United States Funding: govt, meds	SERT 50–200 (63); PBO (71) Other Tx: coping skills training 100%	12 (26)	DSM-IV alcohol dependence Mean age: 48 years 8% Nonwhite 19% Female Other Dx: cannabis use disorder 17%; cocaine use disorder 19%; past MDD 21%	Differences between SERT and PBO were percent heavy drinking days: 6.6 (95% CI –4.63, 17.83) and percent drinking days: 3.8 (95% CI –7.95, 15.55). Attrition: 38%	Medium

TABLE B–20. Studies related to antidepressants (listed alphabetically by medication name) *(continued)*

Author and year; trial name	Study characteristics	Treatment administered, including study arm, dose (mg/day), sample size (N), and co-intervention	Rx duration, weeks (follow-up)	Sample characteristics, including diagnostic inclusions and major exclusions	Outcome measures, main results, and overall percent attrition	Risk of bias
Moak et al. 2003	Design: DBRCT Setting: 1 outpatient site Country: United States Funding: govt, meds	SERT 50–200 (38); PBO (44) Other Tx: CBT	12	Mild to moderate alcohol dependence or alcohol abuse and DSM-III-R major depressive episode or dysthymic disorder Exclusions: bipolar affective or psychotic disorder; treatment-resistant depression Mean age: 41 years 1% Nonwhite 39% Female Other Dx: depression/dysthymia 100%	Differences between SERT and PBO were percent drinking days: 0 (95% CI –11.39, 11.39) and drinks per drinking day: –1.2 (95% CI –2.56, 0.16). Kaplan-Meier survival analysis showed no difference in time to first heavy drinking day. Attrition: 41%	Medium

TABLE B–20. Studies related to antidepressants (listed alphabetically by medication name) *(continued)*

Author and year; trial name	Study characteristics	Treatment administered, including study arm, dose (mg/day), sample size (N), and co-intervention	Rx duration, weeks (follow-up)	Sample characteristics, including diagnostic inclusions and major exclusions	Outcome measures, main results, and overall percent attrition	Risk of bias
O'Malley et al. 2008	Design: DBRCT Setting: Alaskan outpatient site Country: United States Funding: govt, meds	NTX 50 (34); PBO (34); NTX 50+SERT 100 (33) Other Tx: MM 100%	16	DSM-IV alcohol dependence Mean age: 40 years 70% Nonwhite 34% Female Other Dx: NR	There was a statistically significant advantage of NTX over PBO but no additional benefit from the addition of SERT to NTX on total abstinence (NTX vs. PBO, $p=0.04$; NTX vs. NTX+SERT, $p=0.56$) or the percentage who reported a drinking-related problem during treatment (NTX vs. PBO, $p=0.04$; NTX vs. NTX+SERT, $p=0.85$). Time to first heavy drinking day was longer but not significantly greater for NTX compared with PBO (NTX vs. PBO, $p=0.14$; NTX vs. NTX+SERT, $p=0.84$). Treatment efficacy was not dependent on the presence of an Asn40 allele. Attrition: 33%	Medium

TABLE B–20. Studies related to antidepressants (listed alphabetically by medication name) *(continued)*

Author and year; trial name	Study characteristics	Treatment administered, including study arm, dose (mg/day), sample size (N), and co-intervention	Rx duration, weeks (follow-up)	Sample characteristics, including diagnostic inclusions and major exclusions	Outcome measures, main results, and overall percent attrition	Risk of bias
Pettinati et al. 2001	Design: DBRCT Setting: outpatient Country: United States Funding: govt, meds	SERT 200 (50); PBO (50) Other Tx: 12-step facilitation	14	DSM-III-R alcohol dependence Mean age: 44 years 80% Nonwhite 48% Female Other Dx: depression 47%	Difference between SERT and PBO for percent drinking days: –1.27 (95% CI –11.59, 9.05). Sexual disturbance, headache, and fatigue were more common with SERT vs. PBO. Survival analysis showed time to relapse was longer with SERT vs. PBO and was more prominent in those without a history of MDD. Attrition: 42%	Medium
Pettinati et al. 2010	Design: DBRCT Setting: outpatient Country: United States Funding: govt, meds	SERT 200 (40); NTX 100 (49); PBO (39); SERT 200+NTX 100 (42) Other Tx: CBT 100%	14	DSM-IV alcohol dependence and major depression Mean age: 43 years 35% Nonwhite 38% Female Other Dx: depression 100%	SERT vs. PBO total abstinence: 27.5% abstinent vs. 23.1%. Time (days) to relapse to heavy drinking: median 23 vs. 26; mean 39.9 vs. 41.7. SERT+NTX was associated with a higher rate of abstinence and longer time to heavy drinking relapse than PBO or either drug alone. Rates of adverse effects were not significantly different among groups. Attrition: 43%	Medium

Note. Unless noted elsewhere, subjects were excluded if they had contraindications for specific medications; were pregnant, breastfeeding, or unreliable in using contraception; were receiving psychotropic medications; or had another substance use disorder (except nicotine dependence), other psychiatric conditions, suicidal or homicidal ideas, or significant physical illness (including renal or hepatic disease). Industry-sponsored studies list the name of the pharmaceutical company.

[a]The study reported 11 years, but it was clearly a reporting error; likely 31 or 41 years.

Abbreviations: AA=Alcoholics Anonymous; ATS=ANOVA-type statistic; BDI=Beck Depression Inventory; CBT=cognitive-behavioral therapy; CGI=Clinical Global Impression Scale; DBRCT=double-blind, randomized controlled trial; DMI=desipramine; Dx=diagnosis; GGT= gamma-glutamyl transferase; govt=governmental; Ham-D=Hamilton Rating Scale for Depression; IMI=imipramine; LOCF=last observation carried forward; MDD=major depressive disorder; meds=medications supplied by pharmaceutical company; MM=medical management; NOS=not otherwise specified; NR=not reported; NSD=no significant difference; NTX=naltrexone; PBO=placebo; PTSD=posttraumatic stress disorder; SD=standard deviation; SERT=sertraline; Tx=treatment; VA=U.S. Department of Veterans Affairs

STATEMENT 13: Benzodiazepines

APA *recommends* **(1C)** that in individuals with alcohol use disorder, benzodiazepines not be used unless treating acute alcohol withdrawal or unless a co-occurring disorder exists for which a benzodiazepine is an indicated treatment.

Evidence for this recommendation is indirect and is based primarily on expert opinion. Consequently, the strength of research evidence is rated as low. The systematic review of the literature did not yield any references that dealt directly with the use of a benzodiazepine to treat AUD, except in the context of alcohol withdrawal or alcohol detoxification. A Cochrane review of pharmacotherapy for co-occurring AUD and anxiety disorders also did not find any randomized trials of benzodiazepines for anxiety disorders in this population, although studies of naltrexone, acamprosate, and disulfiram were excluded from the review (Ipser et al. 2015). One small open-label study (Bogenschutz et al. 2016) assessed use of lorazepam in combination with disulfiram and manual-based MM in individuals with DSM-IV alcohol dependence and symptoms of anxiety. Subjects had reductions in anxiety, depression, and craving and had no signs of misuse or dose escalations for lorazepam, but two-thirds of the 41 subjects were no longer adherent to treatment at 16 weeks.

STATEMENT 14: Pharmacotherapy in Pregnant or Breastfeeding Women

APA *recommends* **(1C)** that for pregnant or breastfeeding women with alcohol use disorder, pharmacological treatments not be used unless treating acute alcohol withdrawal with benzodiazepines or unless a co-occurring disorder exists that warrants pharmacological treatment.

Evidence for this recommendation is indirect and is based on data from case reports, registries, case control studies of birth outcomes, and, in some instances, animal studies of teratogenicity and neurodevelopmental effects of medication exposure during pregnancy. Consequently, the strength of research evidence is rated as low. Additional evidence that was considered in making this recommendation was the relatively small effect sizes of these medications for treatment of AUD as discussed with Statements 9, 10, and 11.

Data in pregnant animals suggest a moderate risk for use of naltrexone, high risk for use of acamprosate, and possible risks for use of gabapentin and topiramate (Briggs and Freeman 2015). For disulfiram, Briggs and colleagues (Briggs and Freeman 2015) noted that there are no animal data available. Data for the use of these medications in pregnant women is limited (Briggs and Freeman 2015); however, an increased risk of malformation does appear to be associated with use of topiramate (Alsaad et al. 2015; Briggs and Freeman 2015; Tennis et al. 2015; Weston et al. 2016) but not gabapentin (Weston et al. 2016). No clustering of birth defects has been seen when disulfiram is taken by pregnant women, but samples have been small (Briggs and Freeman 2015).

Little data are available on the use of these medications in breastfeeding women, but there may be potential for toxicity with disulfiram and naltrexone (Briggs and Freeman 2015; Sachs and Committee on Drugs 2013) as well as topiramate (Briggs and Freeman 2015), whereas acamprosate and gabapentin are noted to be "probably compatible" (Briggs and Freeman 2015) with breastfeeding.

STATEMENT 15: Acamprosate in Severe Renal Impairment

APA *recommends* **(1C)** that acamprosate not be used by patients who have severe renal impairment.

Evidence for this statement comes from a pharmacokinetic study (Sennesael 1992), which shows increases in terminal elimination half-life and peak plasma concentration with decreases in renal clearance of drug from plasma after a single dose of 666 mg of acamprosate. Individuals with moderate (CrCl of 1.8–3.6 L/h/1.73 m^2) or severe (CrCl of 0.3–1.74 L/h/1.73 m^2) renal impairment had a mean terminal elimination half-life of 33.4 hours and 46.6 hours, respectively, as compared with 18.2 hours for healthy volunteers (with CrCl of >4.5 L/h/1.73 m^2). Peak plasma concentrations were 198 mcg/L for healthy volunteers, as compared with 398 mcg/L and 813 mcg/L for individuals with moderate or severe renal impairment, respectively. On the basis of the significant curvilinear relationship between renal impairment and pharmacokinetic properties, the overall strength of research evidence was viewed as low.

STATEMENT 16: Acamprosate in Mild to Moderate Renal Impairment

APA *recommends* (1C) that for individuals with mild to moderate renal impairment, acamprosate not be used as a first-line treatment and, if used, the dose of acamprosate be reduced compared with recommended doses in individuals with normal renal function.

Evidence for this statement also comes from a pharmacokinetic study (Sennesael 1992), as described in Statement 15 above. Evidence for reducing the dose of acamprosate, if it is used, comes from basic principles of pharmacokinetics.

STATEMENT 17: Naltrexone in Acute Hepatitis or Hepatic Failure

APA *recommends* (1C) that naltrexone not be used by patients who have acute hepatitis or hepatic failure.

Evidence for this recommendation is indirect. Direct data are not available for the conditions specified in this recommendation (i.e., acute hepatitis, hepatic failure) because individuals with these conditions were excluded from clinical trials. Consequently, the strength of research evidence is rated as low. In early studies of other conditions (e.g., obesity, dementia), some patients had severalfold elevations in hepatic transaminase levels with naltrexone treatment (Knopman and Hartman 1986; Malcolm et al. 1985; Mitchell et al. 1987; Pfohl et al. 1986; Verebey and Mulé 1986). The FDA initially included a black box warning on the package labeling discussing potential hepatotoxicity and recommending that naltrexone not be used in individuals with acute hepatitis or hepatic failure. However, subsequent studies suggested that elevations of hepatic enzymes in individuals treated with naltrexone occurred at about the same frequency as in individuals treated with placebo (Brewer and Wong 2004; Lucey et al. 2008; Vagenas et al. 2014; Yen et al. 2006). In addition, a small study suggested that hepatic enzymes did not change and that reducing the dose of naltrexone was not needed in individuals with mild to moderate hepatic impairment (Turncliff et al. 2005). Consequently, the FDA removed the black box warning (Stoddard and Zummo 2015), although the potential for adverse hepatic effects continues to be noted in the package labeling for naltrexone.

STATEMENT 18: Naltrexone With Concomitant Opioid Use

APA *recommends* (1C) that naltrexone not be used as a treatment for alcohol use disorder by individuals who use opioids or who have an anticipated need for opioids.

Evidence for this recommendation is indirect, and consequently, the strength of research evidence is rated as low. Multiple studies have used opioid antagonists to hasten opioid discontinuation in individuals with opioid use disorder (Gowing et al. 2009, 2010). Although opioid antagonist administration was reliable in producing opioid withdrawal, the extent of any benefit was unclear, and potential for complications was noted (Gowing et al. 2009, 2010). These findings suggest that naltrexone not be given to individuals who are currently using opioids unless there is a clinically appropriate period of opioid abstinence before naltrexone initiation. Expert opinion is consistent with this recommendation. Clinical experience also suggests a need for adjustment to typical regimens for pain management in individuals who are receiving naltrexone (R. Chou et al. 2016; Vickers and Jolly 2006) because of the effects of naltrexone in blocking opioid receptors.

Treatment of Alcohol Use Disorder and Co-occurring Opioid Use Disorder

STATEMENT 19: Naltrexone for Co-occurring Opioid Use Disorder

APA *recommends* **(1C)** that in patients with alcohol use disorder and co-occurring opioid use disorder, naltrexone be prescribed to individuals who

- wish to abstain from opioid use and either abstain from or reduce alcohol use and
- are able to abstain from opioid use for a clinically appropriate time prior to naltrexone initiation.

Evidence for this statement is primarily indirect from research findings of naltrexone efficacy in AUD (see Statement 9) and separate studies of naltrexone in individuals with opioid use disorder. Consequently, the strength of research evidence is rated as low. Efficacy has been reported in several studies of long-acting injectable or implanted naltrexone (Krupitsky et al. 2011, 2012, 2013; Larney et al. 2014; Sullivan et al. 2015; Syed and Keating 2013; Timko et al. 2016), with minimal responses to oral naltrexone (Minozzi et al. 2011), likely related to high percentages of attrition.

One double-blind, placebo-controlled trial (Mannelli et al. 2011) randomly assigned individuals with opioid dependence who were undergoing a methadone taper to very low dose naltrexone (0.125 or 0.250 mg/day). Of the subjects, 79 of 174 also had problem drinking, and this group had reduced withdrawal symptoms, less treatment discontinuation, and less resumption of alcohol use after treatment as compared with those who received placebo. However, the relevance of this study to the guideline statement is limited by the use of low-dose naltrexone and the short duration of the trial in the context of methadone tapering.

In a nonblinded trial, persons infected with HIV with AUD and/or opioid use disorder were randomly assigned to treatment as usual or to extended-release naltrexone (Korthuis et al. 2017). Of 35 subjects with AUD, 8 also had opioid use disorder. Only two-thirds of those assigned to extended-release naltrexone initiated treatment, but of those who did initiate treatment, the medication was well tolerated, and rates of treatment retention were greater than in subjects who received treatment as usual. Given the fact that the study had a small sample and was limited to individuals infected with HIV, the relevance to other individuals with co-occurring AUD and opioid use disorder is unclear.

Appendix C: Additional Study Characteristics Relevant to Risk of Bias Determinations

TABLE C–1. Recruitment, randomization, and attrition

Author and year	Treatment	Recruitment method	Was randomization adequate?	Was allocation concealment adequate?	Were groups similar at baseline?	Was there high overall or differential attrition?
Batki et al. 2014	TOP vs. PBO	VA hospital	Yes	Yes	Yes	No
Charney et al. 2015	Citalopram vs. PBO	Academic center, addiction center, and patients	Not well described	Not described	Yes, but citalopram group needed more benzodiazepine treatment before the trial	Yes, high attrition
Chen et al. 2014; Morgenstern et al. 2012	NTX vs. PBO	Online and print advertisements	Yes	Yes	Yes	No
Foa and Williams 2010; Foa et al. 2013; McLean et al. 2014; Zandberg et al. 2016	NTX vs. PBO	Advertisements, anxiety treatment program, and VA hospital	Yes	Not described	More nonwhite subjects in exposure condition	Yes, high attrition
Fridberg et al. 2014; King et al. 2012	NTX vs. PBO	Internet, print, and radio advertisements	Unclear; computer randomized but exact method not specified	Unclear	Unclear	Unclear
Hien et al. 2015	Sertraline vs. PBO	Newspaper and radio advertisements, flyers, and outpatient mental health center referrals	Yes	Yes	Yes	No
Higuchi and Japanese Acamprosate Study Group 2015	Acamprosate vs. PBO	Hospitalized patients referred to study after discharge	Not well described	Yes, independent	Yes	Yes, high attrition but long study duration
Kampman et al. 2013	TOP vs. PBO	Advertisements and professional referrals	Yes	Yes	Yes	Yes, differential attrition that was greater with PBO

TABLE C–1. Recruitment, randomization, and attrition *(continued)*

Author and year	Treatment	Recruitment method	Was randomization adequate?	Was allocation concealment adequate?	Were groups similar at baseline?	Was there high overall or differential attrition?
Knapp et al. 2015	TOP vs. levetiracetam vs. zonisamide vs. PBO	Radio or newspaper advertisements	Yes	Yes	Yes	No
Kranzler et al. 2014a	TOP vs. PBO	Advertisements	Yes	Yes	Yes, except PBO group slightly older (mean age 52.8 years vs. 49.3 years)	No
Likhitsathian et al. 2013	TOP vs. PBO	Inpatient residential alcohol treatment program	Yes	Yes	Yes	Yes; high attrition
Mason et al. 2014	Gabapentin vs. PBO	Print and Internet advertisements	Yes	Yes	Yes	No
Oslin et al. 2015	NTX vs. PBO	Advertisements, physician referrals, and self-referrals	Yes, block randomization created prior to study	Yes	Yes	No
Yoshimura et al. 2014	DIS vs. PBO	Recruited during 2- to 3-month inpatient stay	Not described	Psychosocial treatment status known to patient	Yes	No

Note. Abbreviations: DIS=disulfiram; NTX=naltrexone; PBO=placebo; TOP=topiramate; VA=U.S. Department of Veterans Affairs.

TABLE C–2. **Intervention fidelity, adherence, and masking**

Author and year	Was intervention fidelity adequate?	Was adherence to the intervention adequate?	Were outcome assessors masked?	Were care providers masked?	Were patients masked?
Batki et al. 2014	Yes	No; only 63% adherent to total prescribed dose	Yes	Yes	Yes
Charney et al. 2015	Yes	Not described	Yes	Yes	Yes
Chen et al. 2014; Morgenstern et al. 2012	Yes	Yes	Yes (for NTX)	Yes (for NTX)	Yes (for NTX)
Foa and Williams 2010; Foa et al. 2013; McLean et al. 2014; Zandberg et al. 2016	Yes	Yes	Yes	Yes for NTX condition	Yes for NTX condition
Fridberg et al. 2014; King et al. 2012	Yes	Yes	Yes	Yes	Yes
Hien et al. 2015	Yes	Yes	Yes	Yes	Yes
Higuchi and Japanese Acamprosate Study Group 2015	Yes	Yes	Yes	Yes	Yes
Kampman et al. 2013	Yes	Yes	Yes	Yes	Yes
Knapp et al. 2015	No	Yes	NR	NR	NR
Kranzler et al. 2014a	No	Yes	Yes	Yes	Yes
Likhitsathian et al. 2013	Yes	Yes	Yes	Yes	Yes
Mason et al. 2014	Yes	Yes	Yes	Yes	Yes
Oslin et al. 2015	Yes	Yes; but less with Asp40/NTX than Asn40/NTX group	Yes	Yes	Yes
Yoshimura et al. 2014	Yes	Yes	Yes	Yes	No

Note. Abbreviations: NR=not reported; NTX=naltrexone.

TABLE C–3. **Outcome characteristics, statistical methods, and risk of bias**

Author and year	Were outcome measures equal, valid, and reliable?	Did the study have cross-overs or contamination raising concern for bias?	Did the study use acceptable statistical methods?	Was an appropriate method used to handle missing data?	Risk of bias
Batki et al. 2014	Yes	No	Yes	Yes	Low
Charney et al. 2015	Yes	No	Yes	Yes	Moderate
Chen et al. 2014; Morgenstern et al. 2012	Yes	No	Yes	Not needed because <1% of data was missing	Moderate
Foa and Williams 2010; Foa et al. 2013; McLean et al. 2014; Zandberg et al. 2016	Yes	No	Yes	Yes	Moderate
Fridberg et al. 2014; King et al. 2012	Yes	No	Yes	Yes	Moderate
Hien et al. 2015	Yes	No	Yes	Yes	Low
Higuchi and Japanese Acamprosate Study Group 2015	Yes	No	Unclear	Unclear	Low
Kampman et al. 2013	Yes	No	Yes	Yes	Low
Knapp et al. 2015	Yes	No	Yes	Yes	Moderate
Kranzler et al. 2014a	Yes	No	Yes	Yes	Low
Likhitsathian et al. 2013	Yes	No	Yes	Yes	Moderate
Mason et al. 2014	Yes	No	Yes	Yes	Low
Oslin et al. 2015	Yes	No	ITT	Yes	Low
Yoshimura et al. 2014	Yes	No	Yes	Not stated	Moderate

Note. Abbreviations: ITT=intention to treat.

TABLE C–4. Study harms

Author and year	Were harms prespecified and defined?	Were ascertainment techniques for harms adequately described?	Were ascertainment techniques for harms equal, valid, and reliable?	Was the duration of follow-up adequate for harms assessment?
Batki et al. 2014	Yes	Yes	Yes	Yes
Charney et al. 2015	Not well described	Not well described	Unclear	Yes
Chen et al. 2014; Morgenstern et al. 2012	No	No	Unclear	Yes
Foa and Williams 2010; Foa et al. 2013; McLean et al. 2014; Zandberg et al. 2016	No	No	Not specified	Yes
Fridberg et al. 2014; King et al. 2012	No	No	No	Yes
Hien et al. 2015	Not applicable	Not applicable	Not applicable	Not applicable
Higuchi and Japanese Acamprosate Study Group 2015	No	Not well described	Not well described	Yes
Kampman et al. 2013	Yes	Yes	Yes	Yes
Knapp et al. 2015	Yes	Yes	Yes	Yes
Kranzler et al. 2014a	No	No	Unclear	Yes
Likhitsathian et al. 2013	Yes	Yes	Yes	Yes
Mason et al. 2014	Yes	Yes	Yes	Yes
Oslin et al. 2015	Unclear	No	Unclear	Unclear
Yoshimura et al. 2014	No	Yes	Yes	Yes